Good House[

Family Guide to Prescription Medicines

Pamela Mason BSc, MSc PhD, MRPharmS
with
Dr Marion Newman MBBS, BSc, MRCGP

TED SMART

First published in 1999

1 3 5 7 9 10 8 6 4 2

Text © Ebury Press Limited 1999

First published in the United Kingdom in 1999 by Ebury Press
Random House, 20 Vauxhall Bridge Road, London SW1V 2SA.

A TED SMART Publication 1999

Random House Australia (Pty) Limited
20 Alfred Street, Milsons Point, Sydney, New South Wales 2061, Australia

Random House New Zealand Limited
18 Poland Road, Glenfield, Auckland 10, New Zealand

Random House South Africa (Pty) Limited
Endulini, 5a Jubilee Road, Parktown 2193, South Africa

Random House UK Ltd Reg. No. 954009

A catalogue record for this book is available from the British Library.

Consultant Pharmacists: Dr Judith Hall and Dr Ian Morton
Designer: Paul Saunders
Editors: Catherine Bradley and Slaney Begney
Proofreader: Peter Gibbs

Printed and bound by Mackays of Chatham plc, in Chatham, Kent

Contents

Introduction   1

1. Understanding and Using Prescription Medicines   5

2. Prescription Medicines Directory   22

   The Brain and the Nervous System   24
   The Cardiovascular System   77
   The Gastrointestinal System   111
   The Respiratory System   132
   Bones, Joints and Muscles   144
   The Endocrine System   162
   The Reproductive System   177
   The Urinary System   196
   The Skin   200
   The Eye   223
   The Ear, Nose and Throat   234
   Infection   245
   Allergy   284
   Cancer   290
   Anaemias and other Nutritional Deficiencies   310

3. Vaccinations   319

   Index   339

ACKNOWLEDGMENTS

This book would not have been possible without the help and hard work of a number of people. I would like to thank in particular my co-author, Dr Marion Newman, our two consultants, Dr Judith Hall and Dr Ian Morton, and our editor, Catherine Bradley.

INTRODUCTION

A LARGER NUMBER of people than ever before are taking prescription medicines. Recent figures are as high as 43 per cent of adults in their own homes, increasing to 71 per cent between 65 and 74 years of age, and 82 per cent of the over-75s. Total NHS spending on prescription medicines is now about £5,200m and accounts for about 10 per cent of total NHS spending. In the community, prescribed medicines account for about 50 per cent of total healthcare costs.

During the last 50 years, medicine has undergone an enormous revolution and the growth in the number of prescription products on the market has been dramatic. Before the Second World War, doctors had very few medicines with which they could treat their patients effectively. Aspirin, a few other painkillers, a few sedatives, sulphonamides, cough and stomach mixtures were about all that was available. Today, it is a very different story. More than 1,000 different drugs are available on NHS prescription, whilst the number of branded prescription products now exceeds 2,000. Antibiotics, which were just starting to appear at the end of the 1940s, have saved millions of lives by curing infection. Many heart conditions can also be controlled with medicines now, adding years to people's lives.

The growth and development of prescription medicines has indeed revolutionised our lives, and the pharmaceutical industry is one of the UK's most successful industries. In 1996, the average number of prescription items dispensed was eight per person per year, with children on average receiving five and the elderly an astonishing average of 22 items. However, it is important to realise that the increased life expectancy that we have experienced in the UK is due as much – if not more – to clean water supplies, better diet and vaccination. Medicines certainly help, but many other factors significantly influence our health.

DRUGS AND MEDICINES

There is often confusion about the difference between drugs and medicines. In fact the term drug is used by pharmacists, doctors and nurses in exactly the same way as the term medicine. Health professionals mean precisely the same thing by either of these two words. Strictly speaking, a drug is a chemical substance and what we call the active ingredient in a medicine. A medicine consists of a drug together with other substances such as starch and sugar. These other substances are known as inactive ingredients.

However, you may think of drugs primarily as substances of addiction – heroin and cannabis, for example. These substances certainly are drugs, but so in medical terms is paracetamol. Additionally, some people think of medicines as liquids only. In fact, a tablet or capsule is just as much of a medicine as a cough linctus. Indeed the term medicine is starting to be used much more frequently to describe all those items you obtain on a prescription or buy over the counter.

In a legal sense, the word medicine has a very precise meaning. It is a substance that affects the body and is used to maintain or improve health, and it has been licensed to do so. Medicines are not just for treating illnesses. Vaccines, anaesthetics, contraceptives and some diagnostic tests come under this definition.

WHERE DO MEDICINES COME FROM?

For many centuries of medical history, most drugs came from plants. Both morphine and codeine, for example, were originally derived from the opium poppy. Herbalism, the study of plants with a medicinal value, was practised by the Chinese more than 5,000 years ago, and herbal remedies are being increasingly used today.

Nowadays, most prescription medicines are made in the laboratory. However, plants are increasingly being researched as sources of new drugs. Although most antibiotics, for example, were originally produced by fermentation with moulds and yeasts, many are now partly synthetic. Some drugs are still discovered quite by chance, for example paracetamol was discovered during the manufacture of dyes. Other drugs are discovered after years of directed scientific research, and the development of one drug may lead to the discovery of others with similar uses. The discovery of the sedative diazepam led to the discovery of several other similar drugs, such as nitrazepam and temazepam.

When a new drug has been discovered, it can take many years – not to mention a great deal of money – to get it on to the market. The drug is thoroughly tested to see how good it is at treating the disease it is supposed to treat, and the risk of side effects is carefully studied. Both of these aspects of the drug will be improved where possible. The drug will be tested initially on animals and later in clinical trials on human beings. Provided there is good evidence that the new drug is safe, effective and of adequate quality, an application to market it will be made in the UK to the body known as the Committee on Safety of Medicines (CSM). If approval is given, the new drug will be licensed by the licensing authority, which is known as the Medicines Control Agency (MCA) and is a branch of the Department of Health. At the time of licensing, a drug will typically have been tested on 1,000 to 3,000 patients under strictly controlled conditions. This means that most of its side effects will be known. However, the efficacy and side effects will be monitored throughout the life of the drug, and, if serious side effects come to light as the drug is used, it will sometimes be withdrawn from the market.

Since 1998, the MCA has been licensing only those medicines intended solely for the UK market. If a pharmaceutical company wants to have its product licensed throughout the European Union (EU) – as, increasingly, many do – they must apply to the European Medicines Evaluation Agency, which is based in London. A licence granted through this route is then valid in every member state of the EU.

The EU has for some years been moving towards the harmonisation of pharmaceuticals. Proposals on labelling, patient information leaflets, advertising and distribution have been considered, and some aspects have been implemented. However, if you are travelling round EU countries you will still find some differences, for example in what is and what is not available on prescription. In some Mediterranean countries antibiotics can be bought without a prescription, which is not the case in the UK. If you are travelling anywhere, particularly in more remote areas of the world, it is always best to take sufficient supplies of any medicines – especially those prescribed by your doctor – with you.

DRUG NAMES

Drugs are named in several ways and according to several different systems.

At the start of a drug's life in the laboratory, it is given what we call a chemical name. This can be quite long and complicated. The chemical name for the drug called atenolol, for example, is 4-(2-hydroxy-3-isopropylaminopropoxy)phenylacetamide.

Later in its development, a drug is given a generic name. Atenolol is an example. This is the official medical name, and the name which doctors often use when writing prescriptions.

Then, there is the brand name or proprietary name. This is chosen by the manufacturer alone and intended to be easily remembered, pronounced and written. Tenormin is one brand name for atenolol. There are often many different brand names for one generic drug, all produced by different manufacturers. In addition, some medicines can be both prescribed by doctors and bought over the counter and have a different brand name for each circumstance. For example, Brufen is a brand name for ibuprofen on prescription, and Nurofen is a brand name for ibuprofen bought over the counter. Confusingly, both generic and trade names may be different in some other countries, such as the US.

HOW DRUGS ARE CLASSIFIED

Drugs can be grouped together or classified in several different ways depending on who is doing the classifying! The ways in which they can be classified include:

- chemical structure
- legal category
- use or effect on the body
- body system

Chemical structure

Scientists, including pharmacologists and chemists who work in laboratories, are interested in chemistry and chemical structure. They therefore tend to classify drugs according to chemical structure. You may have heard of a group of drugs called tricyclic antidepressants. All the drugs in this group have a similar chemical structure. Amitriptyline and imipramine are examples.

Legal category

All drugs are categorised legally to control how they can be supplied to the public. Prescription-only medicines (POMs), as their name implies, can only be supplied on a doctor's prescription. Most – but not all – of the drugs described in this book are prescription-only medicines. Pharmacy medicines (Ps) are obtained in a pharmacy under the supervision of a pharmacist. General sale list medicines (GSL) can be bought in both pharmacies and other outlets, such as general stores, supermarkets or garage forecourts. However, some P medicines and some GSL medicines are also available on prescription.

Use or effect on the body

Pharmacists and doctors, both of whom are concerned with the use of a drug (its *indications*), tend to classify drugs according to their use or effects in the body. Thus drugs used to treat high blood pressure are all grouped together and known as antihypertensives, whilst drugs used to treat constipation are known as laxatives. Most drugs fit into one group, but there is some overlap. For example, atenolol is used both as an antihypertensive and as a drug to treat angina.

Body system

A broader method of classifying drugs is to group drugs together that treat disease of one body system. Drugs such as antihypertensives are really treating a disorder of the cardiovascular system. Many other drugs, apart from antihypertensives, are used to treat disease in the cardiovascular system. Glyceryl trinitrate, for example, is a drug used to treat angina – another cardiovascular system disease. Thus, anti-hypertensives and drugs used in angina would be grouped together as examples of types of drugs used in the treatment of disease in the cardiovascular system. Laxatives and indigestion remedies would be grouped together as examples of drugs used in the treatment of disease in the gastrointestinal system.

HOW TO USE THIS BOOK

This book consists of three main chapters. The first tells you how drugs work and how to use them. The second covers most of the drugs available on prescription in the UK. However, we have not included drugs used *exclusively* in hospital, such as general anaesthetics, drugs to treat acute heart attack and various diagnostic testing medicines. This book is largely about medicines you can obtain on prescription from your GP. The third chapter covers vaccines and immunisation.

Finally, as you use this book, remember that medical science is one of the greatest benefits of modern living. If you respect prescribed medicines and use them wisely, they can be of enormous value to your general health and quality of life.

CHAPTER 1

UNDERSTANDING AND USING PRESCRIPTION MEDICINES

MEDICINES HAVE a wide range of effects on the body, and the way they produce these effects is often very complex. Our understanding of the action of medicines has grown dramatically in the last 20 years – almost as fast as the growth in the number of medicines themselves. New medicines, acting in novel ways, are now regularly introduced. However, medical science still has some way to go in fully understanding the action of every medicine on the market.

Medicines are used in several different ways, sometimes to cure but more often to alleviate symptoms or prevent a disease from getting worse. Indeed, relatively few medicines actually cure disease. Antibacterials – medicines that kill or eliminate infectious micro-organisms – are the most dramatic examples of medicines that do cure disease, and they do this very effectively. Other medicines, such as painkillers and cold and flu remedies, help you feel better by relieving your symptoms while the condition gets better on its own. Some medicines are very useful in controlling, or managing, disease. If you suffer from a chronic condition, such as high blood pressure, heart failure, asthma or rheumatoid arthritis, medicines can be used to control that condition and in many cases to prolong life, but they do not actually cure the condition. A few medicines, notably vaccines, prevent disease, whilst others, such as aspirin and cholesterol-lowering medicines, are used to prevent possible heart attacks and strokes.

HOW MEDICINES WORK

Most medicines are needed to work *inside* the body, at the heart, the kidney, the brain, and so on. There are a variety of ways in which a drug can get to the appropriate place. For medicines that work inside the body, almost the first thing they need to do is to enter the blood. Our blood travels, or circulates, round the body to every single part of the body, delivering the medicine to the organ that needs it. Medicines that travel through the bloodstream and work inside the body are said to have a systemic action.

Once a medicine gets into the bloodstream, it doesn't simply travel to the site of action (ie the place where we want it to go), but to other parts of the body too.

This can be a good thing, because it means a medicine can have more than one use. The same antibiotic, for example, can be used to treat an infection in the respiratory tract or an infection in the bladder. However, medicines that work systemically can also create problems by reaching parts of the body where we don't want them to be. This is why we may get side effects.

Consider antihistamines, for example – medicines used to treat hayfever, amongst other conditions. The main side effect of many of them is drowsiness, because antihistamines reach the nervous system – where we don't want them to work – as well as the site of action in the respiratory system.

However, the site of action is not always inside the body. A medicine may also be applied directly to a location on or near the surface of the body. If you have a skin problem such as acne, you can put a cream or lotion straight on to the site of action, that is the skin. If you have an eye infection, you can put eye drops directly into the eye. Medicines that can be applied directly to the site of action are called locally acting medicines.

The effect of a locally acting medicine is ideally limited to the site of the disorder and there is less chance of it reaching another part of the body where we don't want it to work. However, just to complicate matters, medicines that are *intended* to act locally may also, *unintentionally*, act systemically. Thus inhaled steroids, although applied to the lungs for a local effect, can also be absorbed into the bloodstream where they can act systemically.

In addition, do not always assume that a medicine applied to the skin is always intended to have a local effect. HRT patches and glyceryl trinitrate patches, for example, are applied to the skin, but they are intended to act systemically (ie *inside* the body). Medicines are absorbed from these patches into the blood.

Whatever way a medicine enters the body, the end result should be the same. The medicine needs to travel as efficiently as possible to its intended site of action and produce the desired effect. This can be quite complicated to arrange. In the case of heart disease, for example, a doctor needs to get the medicine to the heart. If an injection is given, or the medicine is taken by mouth, that medicine will travel in the bloodstream everywhere round the body. How can doctors know that it will work on the appropriate organ or organs?

The answer to this fascinating, complex question lies in some tiny structures called receptors – special places in the cell membrane. They have a specific shape – rather like a lock – which can only be opened by the appropriate key. The 'keys' that open receptors may be natural body chemicals, such as neurotransmitters, that work by attaching themselves to receptors. Or they may be opened by a medicine containing a chemical of exactly the right 'shape'. There are lots of different receptors in cells, all with different shapes, each designed to take different chemicals and achieve different effects.

Noradrenaline is one of the body's own chemical 'keys', a neurotransmitter that works by attaching itself to and unlocking a receptor. One effect of noradrenaline is to increase the heart rate, and it achieves this by having the right shape to key into receptors in the heart. Many medicines also produce their effects by attaching themselves to specific receptors, for which they have to be exactly the right shape. They may seek to mimic the action of the natural body chemical and are called agonists. Others, known as antagonists, block the action of the natural body chemical, latching on to the receptor and preventing the natural body chemical from getting to it. Thus a medicine that *mimics* noradrenaline will increase the heart rate, and a medicine that *blocks* noradrenaline will reduce the heart rate. An example of the latter are medicines known as beta-blockers. Used extensively in cardiovascular medicine for conditions such as angina and high blood pressure, beta-blockers work by keying into receptors to block the action of the natural body chemical noradrenaline.

Many receptors, particularly those where medicines are known to work, have been given names. The medicine codeine, for example, which like many of our older medicines was extracted from the opium poppy, works at receptors called opioid receptors. Beta-blockers, as you might imagine, key into receptors known as beta receptors.

The action of medicines at receptors is not quite so simple as the analogy of a front door key with the specific shape to open your front door. Your door key, after all, will open nobody else's door – or should not do. However, with medicines there tends to be a lot of overlap in the receptors to which they respond. Some medicines will consequently fit into more than one receptor.

A medicine that fits very well into a receptor is said to possess a high affinity for that receptor. However, a particular medicine may have affinity for several receptors. This may be a problem, as a medicine with an affinity for several receptors can have several effects, including unwanted side effects.

Fortunately, some medicines do fit into only one receptor type. We say that these medicines have a high specificity for that receptor, and it is, as you might imagine, a desirable characteristic for a medicine to possess. If it fits only one receptor, a medicine will only have one major effect and few side effects. Unfortunately, few medicines are like this.

However, attaching themselves to receptors is not the only way in which medicines work. They can also be used to interfere with the action of hormones in the body. Diabetes, for example, is often treated by giving injections of the hormone insulin, which corrects the lack of the natural hormone in the body. Other medicines adopt a more lateral approach to a condition – some medicines given in diabetes, for instance, work not by replacing insulin but by increasing its production. These medicines, known as oral hypoglycaemics, help to reduce blood sugar by boosting the production of insulin.

Sometimes there is a need to reduce the production of a hormone in the body. In some forms of thyroid disease, for example, the thyroid gland produces too much hormone. This can be reduced by the use of medicines such as carbimazole.

Other medicines work by influencing the production or action of enzymes. Enzymes, like neurotransmitters, are natural body chemicals, and they are responsible for a whole host of chemical reactions that take place in our bodies. One of the uses of medicines known as angiotensin-converting enzyme (ACE) inhibitors, for example, involves the inhibition of an enzyme with this name. This enzyme has a role in raising blood pressure, and restricting its action in this way helps to lower blood pressure.

Yet another way in which medicines act is to alter the actual movement of chemicals in and out of body cells. Calcium channel blockers, for example, are medicines that alter the transport of calcium in and out of cells. These medicines are used to treat various heart conditions, such as angina. Similarly, the antidepressants known as specific serotonin re-uptake inhibitors (SSRIs), as their name suggests, work by inhibiting the uptake of the brain neurotransmitter serotonin into the nerves.

Finally, some medicines work by killing micro-organisms or preventing them from multiplying. All antibiotics, antifungals and antivirals work in this way. Because these medicines eliminate the root cause of a disease, they do actually cure, rather than alleviating symptoms or controlling the condition.

ENTERING THE BODY

Medicines can be delivered to their site of action in several ways. Known as routes of administration, these are:

• oral (by mouth)
• parenteral (by injection)
• rectal (by the rectum)
• inhalation (by the lungs)
• transdermal (through the skin)
• topical (directly to skin, eye, ear, nose, mouth, lungs, rectum, vagina)

Oral

In the UK most medicines are taken by mouth. The medicine passes down the food pipe (oesophagus) and into the stomach. From the stomach the medicine progresses into the intestine, from where it is absorbed into the blood. The advantages of the oral route are that it is cheap, convenient and safe. However, it is unsuitable for people who are vomiting or unconscious and also for certain medicines that are destroyed by stomach acids (eg insulin).

Several different types of medicines are given by the oral route. These include both solid and liquid formulations.

Tablets are the most common form of oral medicine. A tablet is a solid medicine that contains one – or occasionally more than one – active ingredient together with several inactive ingredients, such as diluents, flavours, colours, disintegrants and binders. Most tablets are designed to disintegrate in the stomach and to release the medicine for absorption in the intestine.

Tablets come in many different shapes, sizes and colours. Some are plain and uncoated; certain types are made to dissolve in water, while others are chewable. Some tablets are coated, however, which helps to protect the tablet from destruction in the stomach – it can then get into the intestine from where it is absorbed into the blood. Other tablets are known as modified-release tablets. These release the medicine slowly over a longer period of time than a plain tablet, and this allows you to take the tablet once or twice a day instead of, say, three or four times a day. Then there are sublingual tablets, which are placed under the tongue, from where the medicine is absorbed straight into the blood. This type of tablet, of which glyceryl trinitrate (for angina) is the best-known example, produces a rapid action because the medicine does not need to pass through the gut first. Buccal tablets are somewhat similar in that they are placed between the teeth and the cheek from where the medicine is absorbed into the blood.

Other solid formulations given by the oral route include capsules, granules and powders.

There are several different types of liquids for oral doses of medicines. These include elixirs, linctuses, suspensions, emulsions and oral drops. Liquids are often easier to take than solids, simply because they slip down the throat without difficulty. They are certainly easier to administer to young children. They also tend to act faster than tablets – because they do not have to disintegrate in the stomach before absorption of the medicine. However, oral liquids are usually dispensed in large bottles – sometimes glass, sometimes plastic – and they are not always convenient to carry.

Parenteral (by injection)

An injection is a means of introducing a medicine directly into one of the body's tissues. Injections can be given into a vein (intravenous), into a muscle (intramuscular), under the skin (subcutaneous), into a joint (intra-articular), into a space around the spinal cord (epidural) and into a variety of other body tissues.

The medicine contained in an injection does not have to be absorbed from the gastrointestinal tract first in order to get into the blood. Various types of equipment are available for giving injections, the most basic being a needle and syringe. The parenteral route is an advantage for medicines that are destroyed by the gastric juices of the stomach (eg insulin). Injections are a useful route for people who cannot swallow, either because of surgery or disease of the stomach and digestive tract. An injection is also useful in circumstances where people need a medicine to act very rapidly.

Some injections are available in the form of what is known as depot injections, which can be given infrequently, for example once a week or once a month. The medicine is deposited in a pool under the skin at the site of the injection, and the medicine is slowly released from that pool into the blood. This can be useful for people who find it difficult to comply with a course of treatment and who will be asked to go to a surgery or clinic for an injection, thus making sure that they take the medicine. Some drugs used for schizophrenia and some contraceptives are given in this way.

Rectal

Medicines can be given rectally in the form of suppositories, rectal solutions or enemas. The advantage of this route of administration is that it avoids the stomach, so is useful for medicines that upset the stomach or are destroyed by the stomach. This method is also useful if a person is too ill to take a medicine by mouth, or is vomiting. However, it may be inconvenient and medicine absorption from the rectum tends to be a bit erratic.

Transdermal

Transdermal means 'across the skin'. Some medicines can get through the skin in amounts that can have an effect inside the body – they can enter the bloodstream and so have a systemic effect.

The transdermal route is useful for medicines that work for only a short time following oral administration. Because the skin is quite a good barrier, medicines are absorbed very slowly from skin patches. Some patches are designed to last for a week. This means that a skin patch needs to be applied very much less frequently than a medicine that needs to be taken by mouth. Some hormone replacement therapy (HRT) is used in this way, as are some travel sickness drugs.

Topical

When a medicine is used topically, it should only work where it is applied. In other words, it is intended have a local and not a systemic effect, which helps to reduce the risk of side effects. However, some of the medicine usually does pass into the blood, so do not assume that a topically applied medicine will produce no systemic side effects. The risk is lower, but it can still happen.

Medicines can be applied topically (ie to produce a local effect) to several different body tissues. These are:

- the skin (eg creams, ointments, sprays, powders, liniments, pastes)
- the eyes (eg eye drops and eye ointments)
- the ears (eg ear drops)
- the nose (eg nasal drops and nasal sprays)
- the mouth (eg mouthwashes, sprays, pastilles, lozenges)
- the lungs (eg inhalers). General anaesthetics are also given via the lungs, but are obviously intended to produce a systemic effect.
- the rectum (eg suppositories, enemas, creams and ointments)
- the vagina (eg pessaries and vaginal tablets)

HOW DO MEDICINES LEAVE THE BODY?

Medicines leave the body through two main routes – the liver and the kidneys. Enzymes in the liver process medicines, converting them from active to inactive substances – substances that can no longer work in the ways that medicines do.

The inactive substance then passes in the blood to the kidneys. The kidneys make urine through which many unwanted substances, including medicines, leave the body. Although the urine is the main route out of the body for medicines, they can also leave the body in the sweat, the faeces and even in the breath.

HAZARDS OF DRUGS AND MEDICINES

Everything we do in life involves risks. Statistically, cycling, driving or even crossing the road carries surprisingly high risks. There is, of course, no such thing as an absolutely safe medicine. Almost all medicines can cause unwanted effects and in deciding whether to prescribe a medicine or not, a doctor has to consider the 'risk-benefit ratio'. In other words, he or she assesses the risks to the patient of taking that medicine compared with the expected benefits of the medicine.

In calculating the risks of prescribing a medicine, doctors must weigh up a number of factors. These include:

- the risk of adverse effects of the prescribed medicine
- whether the patient has a disease where the use of a particular medicine is dangerous (eg some medicines should not be taken by diabetics)
- interactions of the prescribed medicine with other medication that the patient may be taking
- the age of the patient
- whether the patient is, or may become, pregnant, or is currently breastfeeding
- the risks of the disease itself – whether it is justified to use a potentially toxic drug for a disease that is life-threatening when less toxic drugs are available

SIDE EFFECTS

Side effects, sometimes called adverse effects, especially when serious, are unwanted or unintended effects of a medicine. These can occur even if the medicine is being used appropriately.

Most medicines are capable of producing some side effects, but not all the possible side effects of any one medicine will be experienced by every individual, or to the same severity in every individual. Some people may well experience none at all. So when you look up medicines in this book and see quite a long list of side effects, do not be unnecessarily alarmed. You may not experience any of them, and even if you do, they may be quite mild.

In addition, not all side effects are very significant. In fact, very few side effects are that serious, because the medicine would not get on to the market in the first place if the risks of serious side effects were substantial. Nevertheless, they can be unpleasant and they certainly exist: as many as 10 per cent of hospital admissions are thought to be associated with side effects of prescribed medicines.

Remember that virtually no medicine is a 'magic bullet' that pinpoints its target entirely in isolation. Undoubtedly, it would be good if we could design a medicine to treat asthma, for example, and do nothing else. However, once a medicine gets into the bloodstream, it inevitably travels everywhere – not just to the lungs where it is needed.

Some side effects may just be inconvenient, and they may fade or become less noticeable with time. Serious side effects are fairly rare, but they do occur, and they may lead to a medicine being withdrawn from the market. Although a medicine is thoroughly tested before reaching the market, not all its side effects may be detected until literally thousands of people have taken it.

Serious reactions to medicines may lead to illness or disease itself. Digoxin, for example, used to treat heart failure, actually causes abnormal heartbeats as a side effect. Oral contraceptives can cause blood clots in a vein. Other medicines can cause major problems if taken in the wrong circumstances. The most notorious recent example is thalidomide, a medicine with great benefits, but which can cause disability to the unborn baby if taken during pregnancy. Nowadays, however, techniques for testing for adverse side effects on the unborn child are much more sophisticated.

Some medicines can even cause death if used unwisely. Paracetamol, a painkiller used successfully by millions of people, has caused death because too much has been taken – often as part of an impulsive gesture without suicidal intentions. Be aware too that paracetamol is found in a wide range of over-the-counter products – cold and flu remedies as well as analgesics. Always read the list of ingredients on the label carefully, and be careful not to take more than one remedy at once that contains paracetamol.

DRUG INTERACTIONS

When two different medicines are taken together, or when a medicine is taken in combination with certain foods or alcohol, this may produce effects different from when the medicine is taken on its own. This is known as a drug interaction.

Many drug interactions are potentially harmful and once you start taking one medicine – whether it is prescribed or you have bought it over the counter – always talk to your doctor or pharmacist before taking another. When you go to your doctor, always tell him or her what medicines you are taking, including ones that the doctor should already know about (because they should be on your medical records). In a pharmacy, it is also important to tell the pharmacist what other medicines you are taking. Remember to include all prescribed and over-the-counter medicines, including vitamin supplements, herbal remedies and other complementary therapies. This will help you to avoid the effects of potentially harmful drug interactions.

Be aware, however, that not all drug interactions are harmful. Sometimes two medicines that are known to interact are given together deliberately. Moreover, doctors may prescribe two interacting drugs to one patient, simply because both medicines are likely to benefit the patient. Thus aspirin interacts with warfarin to increase the tendency to bleed. However, several patients are prescribed both of these medicines and so long as the doses and the effects of the treatment are carefully watched and monitored, the combination is quite safe – and indeed is beneficial to many patients.

Medicines interact in several different ways. Thus a medicine may alter the speed at which another medicine enters (is absorbed by) the body. One medicine may alter the amount of another medicine that travels round in the blood, sometimes competing with the second medicine for a site on a receptor. Some medicines compete to leave the body and one medicine can have an influence on the speed with which another medicine is excreted in the urine. In other circumstances, the effects may simply be additive (eg alcohol and sedatives).

WHO IS MOST AT RISK FROM TAKING MEDICINES?

Different people respond in different ways to medicine treatment. With one medicine, one person may suffer from side effects and another person experience none at all. We don't always know why these differences exist, but certainly some groups of people are more at risk of adverse effects from medicines. Sometimes the reason for differences is known to be genetic; some diseases run in families and may predispose some family members to certain drug adverse effects, as is seen in porphyria (a disease where there is abnormality in the blood pigments). Whole racial groups may be at risk from some drugs for genetic reasons, for example glucose 6-phosphate dehydrogenase deficiency (G6PD deficiency). Other at-risk groups include babies and children, the elderly, pregnant and breastfeeding women, patients with liver or kidney disease and those taking several different medicines.

Babies and children

Babies and children need lower doses of medicines than adults. This is quite simply because babies and children weigh less than adults. In addition, a baby's organs are not so well developed as they are in an adult. This is particularly important as far as the liver and kidneys are concerned. Both the liver and kidneys are involved in getting rid of medicines from the body. In babies and children, because the liver and kidneys are not well developed, medicines do not leave the body so easily as they do in adults. Thus medicine doses must be reduced.

Medicine doses in babies and children are, however, not quite so low as you might expect. Just because a six-month-old baby is about a tenth of the weight of an adult male, this does not mean that the baby is given one tenth of the adult dose of a medicine. This is partly because the composition of a baby's body is different from that of an adult. For example, water makes up 70 per cent of a baby's body but only 55 per cent of an adult body. This means that some medicines are not as concentrated in a baby's body as they are in an adult's. Another factor is that a baby's metabolism is faster than that of an adult. For both these reasons, higher doses relative to the baby's weight may be needed.

Older people

Older people are at particular risk from taking medicines. Firstly, older people's bodies do not always work as efficiently as those of younger adults. For example, the liver and kidneys may not be able to get rid of medicines so easily. Some parts of the body may become more sensitive to the action of medicines.

Secondly, elderly people are often prescribed a large number of medicines. This, of course, increases the likelihood of drug interactions. Thirdly, elderly people do not always take their medicines properly. Sometimes younger people do not either, of course, but the risk of this generally seems to be higher in older people. This is often because older people take so many medicines that it can be difficult for them to remember when to take which medicine. The incidence of confusion and dementia increases with extreme age. Added to which, some medicines can cause confusion and sedation as side effects.

Pregnancy

Great care is needed to protect the unborn child from harm during pregnancy. If a pregnant woman is taking medicines, they can leave her blood and cross the placenta into the baby's blood. Many medicines are known to harm the baby, others are thought to be safe, and for some medicines, there is no firm evidence. However, no medicine has been proved beyond doubt to be safe in pregnancy and doctors have to weigh up the risks and the benefits.

For some pregnant women, for example those with chronic conditions such as asthma or epilepsy, it is more risky not to take their medicines. They have to take medicines for life, whether they are pregnant or not.

Medicines can have different effects on the baby, depending on which part of pregnancy the medicine is taken in. In the first trimester (first three months), some medicines may cause malformations in the baby. This is important because you may take medicines at a time when you do not realise you are pregnant.

So if you know that you might become pregnant, or if you are actively planning to do so, think very carefully about any medicines you take and discuss them with your doctor. In the second and third trimesters, some medicines lead to poor growth in the baby and can have adverse effects on labour. If your doctor thinks you need a particular medicine, you can discuss the likely risks and benefits.

Breastfeeding

Just as medicines pass from the mother to the baby during pregnancy, so medicines can pass from the mother to the baby in the milk during breastfeeding. During a feed, a baby may therefore receive a small dose of any medicine the mother is taking. Often this is not a problem because the dose of medicine received by the baby is too small to do any harm.

However, some medicines can cause adverse effects. Sedatives and alcohol, for example, may make the baby drowsy. Other medicines can reduce the amount of milk produced by the mother and yet others can reduce the ability of the baby to suck at the breast.

So, again, always tell your doctor or pharmacist if you are breastfeeding, so that they can advise you on appropriate medicine should one be necessary.

Liver disease

Many medicines are converted in the liver to inactive substances before being removed from the body. If the liver is not working properly it cannot do this. And this is exactly what can happen in patients with liver disease, for example those with a severe alcohol problem. They cannot get rid of medicines so easily. Medicines therefore tend to circulate round the body for prolonged periods, which can increase the risk of adverse effects. Use of medicines should be kept to a minimum in patients with liver disease. If they cannot be avoided altogether, the dose may often need to be reduced.

Kidney disease

Medicines leave the body in the urine. If your kidneys are not working properly, medicines cannot leave your body very easily. This is a particular problem for patients with kidney disease, and the dose may need to be substantially reduced.

Patients taking several medicines

Patients taking more than one medicine are at particular risk from adverse effects. Some diseases, of course, need to be treated with more than one medicine. Patients with asthma, for example, may need two or three different inhalers.

Taking several medicines is not always a good idea, however. For example, you may be taking a medicine containing codeine for pain and this could cause constipation. It is better to change the codeine for another medicine that does not cause constipation than to start taking a laxative – unless the codeine is absolutely necessary.

HOW TO USE MEDICINES

One of the most important aspects of your treatment is knowing how to use your medicines properly. If you do not use them properly, they will not work as effectively as intended. Listen to any instructions your doctor or pharmacist gives you and read all labels and package inserts very carefully before taking your medicine.

If there is anything you are not clear about, check with your doctor or pharmacist. For example, instructions such as three times a day can be confusing. Does it mean that you should take the medicine every eight hours throughout the whole 24-hour period or does it mean three times a day during the time you are awake? In fact, it does usually mean the latter, but do check with your doctor or pharmacist just in case. And what about a dose to be taken in the morning if you do shift work? Again, check with your doctor, but it may be better to take the medicine before you go to work in the evening. Likewise with a medicine to be taken in the evening. The best time to take such a medicine may be just before you go to bed – whenever that may be. Again, check with your doctor or pharmacist.

Another thing to check if you are taking a number of different medicines is: can they be taken together? Or should they be taken at different times of day? And should you take any of your medicines with food? Some medicines can upset the stomach and this can be prevented if you take your medicine with food. On the other hand, some medicines do not work so well if they are taken with food. Food delays their absorption from the gut and it is important that you take some medicines on an empty stomach.

What about alcohol? Can you have a drink with your medicines or not? If your medicine has a sedative action, drinking alcohol will make you feel even more drowsy, and it would be extremely dangerous to drive under these circumstances. Indeed, it is always a wise precaution when starting on any new medicine to see how it affects you before you try to drive. Many medicines do cause drowsiness and dizziness as a minor side effect, and it can be dangerous to drive or operate machinery. Alcohol can cause an unpleasant reaction with some medicines (eg the antibiotic metronidazole) and your doctor or pharmacist should tell you if this is the case.

What happens if you miss a dose? Or take too much? Quite often this doesn't matter. If you miss a dose take it as soon as you remember. But depending on the medicine – and instructions specific to each medicine are given in chapter 2 – missing one dose does not mean that you should take the missed dose and the next dose together. And if you miss a dose of a medicine that should be taken in the morning, say a water tablet (diuretic), it may cause you a number of trips to the toilet in the middle of the night if you take the missed dose in the evening. So, again, check with your doctor or pharmacist what you should do if you miss a dose.

Medicines are used in different ways. Some, such as painkillers, are intended to be used when you need them whereas others, such as antibiotics, must be taken regularly. You can stop taking some medicines when you feel better; with others you will need to complete the prescribed course (eg antibiotics), and yet others may need to be taken for life. If you have a condition such as asthma, epilepsy, high blood pressure, a heart condition or diabetes, never stop taking your medicines without discussing it with your doctor first. This is because it could make your underlying condition worse.

How to take oral medicines

• Always take tablets, capsules and powders standing up or sitting upright. If you take them when you are lying down they can get stuck in your oesophagus (food pipe) where they can cause damage. Moreover, the medicine will not get to its intended site of action.
• Unless they are intended to be dissolved in water or dissolved in your mouth, always swallow tablets, capsules and powders with a glass of water.
• If you are taking a liquid medicine, always shake the bottle well. This ensures that the active ingredient is well distributed through the liquid and you take the correct dose. Always measure the dose very carefully, using the spoon or oral syringe supplied.
• If your medicine leaves a nasty taste in the mouth, drink a glass of water and this will often mask the taste.

How to use inhalers

• Sit upright or stand and remove the cap of the inhaler.
• Shake the inhaler well and hold it upright with your thumb at the base below the mouthpiece and your forefinger on top of the canister.
• Raise your chin slightly and breathe out.
• Put the mouthpiece to your mouth and close your lips firmly round the mouthpiece without biting it.
• Breathe in slowly and, at the same time, press down on the inhaler button to release the medication.

- Keep breathing in and hold your breath for as long as is comfortable – up to 10 seconds if possible.
- If you require a second puff, wait for 1 minute before repeating the steps above. This will help the second puff to penetrate the lungs more efficiently.

A device known as a spacer is useful, particularly if you have trouble using your inhaler. They are particularly recommended for children. Ask your doctor or pharmacist.

NB Inhaled dry powder capsules require a different technique. To use a dry powder inhaler it is important to close the mouth tightly round the mouthpiece and inhale rapidly.

How to use suppositories

- Wash your hands thoroughly with soap and water.
- Remove the suppository from its wrapping (if there is one) and if you wish put on a disposable glove (available from your pharmacist).
- Lie on your side with your lower leg straight and your upper leg bent forwards towards your stomach.
- Lift your upper buttock to expose the rectum.
- Insert the suppository, pointed end first, until it passes the muscular sphincter of the rectum. This is about one inch inside. If you do not insert the suppository beyond this sphincter it may pop out.
- Hold the buttocks together for a few seconds and remain lying down for about 10 minutes to avoid the suppository coming out.
- Wash your hands thoroughly.

How to use eye drops

- Wash your hands thoroughly with soap and water.
- Stand in front of a mirror so that you can see what you are doing.
- Tilt your head back and pull down the lower eye lid with your index finger to form a pocket.
- Hold the tip of the bottle as close to the eye as possible without touching it.
- Squeeze the dropper gently so that the correct number of drops falls into the pocket you have made with your finger.
- Close your eye for 2 to 3 minutes. Wipe any excess fluid from your face with a tissue.
- Replace the cap on the dropper bottle straight away. Avoid touching the dropper tip at all times. It must be kept clean.
- Wash your hands thoroughly.
- Once you have opened eye drops, always throw them away after 28 days.

NB Having someone else to do this for you is sometimes easier.

How to use eye ointments

• Wash your hands thoroughly with soap and water.
• Stand in front of a mirror so that you can see what you are doing.
• Tilt your head forwards and pull down the lower eye lid with your index finger to form a pocket.
• Hold the tip of the tube as close to the eye as possible without touching it.
• Squeeze a ribbon of eye ointment into the pocket you made with your finger.
• Blink your eye gently and close your eye for 1 to 2 minutes. Wipe any excess fluid from your face with a tissue.
• Replace the cap on the ointment straight away. Avoid touching the tip of the tube at all times. It must be kept clean.
• Wash your hands thoroughly.

NB Having someone else to do this for you is sometimes easier.

How to use ear drops

• Wash your hands thoroughly with soap and water.
• Warm the drops to body temperature by holding the container in your hands for a few minutes.
• Draw the medication into the dropper.
• Tilt the affected ear upwards and lie on your side.
• Hold the tip of the dropper as close to the ear as possible without touching it.
• Place the prescribed number of drops in your ear. Then pull gently on your ear to let the drops run in.
• Keep your ear tilted for a few minutes or plug your ear with cotton wool.
• Replace the cap or dropper on the bottle straight away. Avoid touching the dropper at all times. It must be kept clean.
• Wash your hands thoroughly.

NB Having someone else to do this for you is sometimes easier.

How to use nose drops

• Blow your nose gently and wash your hands thoroughly.
• Tilt your head back as far as possible. You may want to lie down on the bed and hang your head over the edge.
• Place the prescribed number of drops in your nose.
• Bend head forward and move it left and right. Remain in this position for a few minutes.
• Replace the cap or dropper on the bottle right away. Avoid touching the dropper at all times. It must be kept clean.
• Wash your hands thoroughly.

NB Having someone else to do this for you is sometimes easier.

STORING MEDICINES

Most medicines should be stored in a cool dry place away from direct sunlight and out of the reach of children. A locked cabinet is ideal for medicines but this should not be in the bathroom because of the damp. Room temperature is fine for most medicines, but some (eg insulin, antibiotic liquids, some creams and some eye drops) should be stored in the refrigerator. Your pharmacist will give you instructions about this.

Always keep your medicines in their original containers and do not remove or change the labels. This will avoid the possibility of you taking the wrong medicine. Always screw caps back on firmly.

Always dispose of old medicines or medicines that you are no longer using. Most medicines have 'Use-By' dates which should be adhered to, even if the pack has not been opened. Medicines that have become discoloured or changed in consistency or that taste or smell different than when you first obtained them should be discarded. Tablets or capsules more than two years old should also be thrown away. You can do this by returning them to your pharmacist or flushing them down the toilet. Never put medicines in the dustbin.

POISONING

Despite public education programmes and the advent of child-proof containers, accidental poisoning with drugs results in the deaths of 10 to 15 children a year, and many trips to the casualty department. While accidental poisoning in adults does occur, deliberate self-poisoning (often with prescription drugs and alcohol) is much more common and accounts for many hospital admissions every year.

Prevention is much better than cure. Always use lockable drug cabinets and child-proof containers, and return medicines that you no longer need to your doctor or pharmacist. Put medicine containers safely away after each dose has been taken, and, when you are visiting other people's homes, check that there are no tablets on view where inquisitive toddlers can get hold of them. Accidental overdosage in the elderly, who are often on lots of drugs for multiple problems, can be reduced by the provision of a special box with labelled compartments that are filled by the carer or district nurse with the drugs for the day or week. Doctors, too, should play their part by the careful prescribing of drugs to people who are at risk.

What drugs may be implicated in overdosage?

Alcohol – is not a prescription drug, but it is widely available and often taken with other medicines. Although people drink to have a good time, alcohol is basically a sedative, and drinking large quantities will result in sleepiness, unconsciousness and even death, either because people inhale vomit or because they stop breathing. Alcohol taken with other sedative drugs, such as tranquillisers, antidepressants and some painkillers, is more likely to cause unconsciousness and death.

Tranquillisers and antidepressants – these drugs are safe when taken as prescribed but in overdosage may result in unconsciousness. They are more dangerous if taken with alcohol and some may cause fits or irregularity of the heartbeat.

Painkillers – aspirin, which is widely used and available over the counter, is toxic in overdosage, causing stomach pain, vomiting, ringing in the ears, breathlessness and confusion. Overdosage with paracetamol is deceptive because there may be few symptoms initially, but treatment is required to prevent liver damage, which may be fatal. Codeine-based painkillers (which resemble narcotics) may cause unconsciousness with shallow breathing.

Narcotics – drugs such as heroin or morphine (to which drugs such as codeine are related) are used on prescription to treat severe pain, but are widely misused. Addicts are particularly at risk of accidental overdosage because the drugs they obtain are of variable strength, and if they have been drug free for a while they may not tolerate their former dose. Overdosage causes confusion, unconsciousness with shallow breath, or death. Although not strictly relevant to this book, it is worth noting that most of the other 'street drugs' tend to cause irritability, restlessness and wild behaviour, and sometimes hallucinations.

Iron – is a safe drug if used appropriately, but overdose results in irritation of the stomach lining with bleeding, vomiting and diarrhoea. Without treatment, after a delay of a day or two, damage to the internal organs results in collapse, internal bleeding, convulsions and death.

Initial response to an overdose

If you have reason to suspect that someone has taken an overdose, it is important to get advice and help straight away. If the person appears well, speak to your GP or local casualty department, who can get detailed advice from a network of poison information centres based in major city hospitals in the UK. They will find it helpful if you can give an estimate of the number of tablets taken, based on the label on the bottle and any remaining tablets that you find. They may be able to reassure you about the risk and advise you on monitoring at home, or they may tell you to take the patient to hospital. If the patient has taken a deliberate overdose because of depression, then you should try to persuade him or her to go to hospital.

Do **not** make the person vomit, but do collect the empty medicine containers or used syringes to take with you to the hospital.

If the person is unconscious, drowsy or confused, then he or she should go to hospital to be monitored. Check his or her breathing, and then put the person in the 'recovery position', which is essentially lying semi-prone so that any vomit will drain out of the mouth. Dial 999 for an ambulance. Be prepared to give the ambulance controller the exact address and a clear description of the person, saying that he or she has taken an overdose. Let them know if the person is conscious or not.

Stay with the person all the time. If he or she is not breathing, is breathing shallowly or is choking, clear the airway by removing any obvious obstructions, such as broken dentures or vomit. Then lift the tongue away from the back of the throat by gently tilting the head back and using two fingers under the chin to lift it up. Breathe for the person by pinching his or her nostrils together with one hand while continuing to lift the chin with the other. Cover the person's mouth with your mouth, making sure that you get a good seal, and blow in slowly and strongly. It requires some effort and takes about two seconds, but you will be able to see his or her chest rise and then fall. (Allow about four seconds for that.) Give him or her two breaths. If the person starts breathing, put him or her in the recovery position and stay with them. If he or she does not start breathing, then continue with 'mouth to mouth' and check his or her pulse. If you feel a pulse 'mouth to mouth' is enough, but if the pulse is absent you will need to start CPR (cardio-pulmonary resuscitation) as well if you have been taught how to do it. Continue until the ambulance arrives.

Hospital treatment is beyond the scope of this book, but includes activated charcoal to minimise further absorption of the drugs, supportive care, specific antidotes in some cases and often a psychiatric assessment.

CHAPTER 2

PRESCRIPTION MEDICINES DIRECTORY

THIS CHAPTER COVERS most of the drugs available on prescription in the UK. However, we have not included drugs used exclusively in hospital – general anaesthetics, drugs to treat acute heart attack and various diagnostic testing medicines. This book is largely about medicines you can obtain on prescription from your GP.

We have classified the drugs according to the body system in which they have their main action. You will therefore find medicines for stomach ulcers in the gastrointestinal section, medicines for heart failure in the cardiovascular section and so on. However, if you want to find a drug quickly, look it up in the index and this will guide you to the appropriate page number.

In each section of chapter 2, you will find a brief description of the body system – how it works in a healthy person and what can go wrong with it. Then there is a list of common conditions that can affect that body system together with the main types of medicines used to treat them.

The bulk of each of the sections is, however, given to a list of all the prescription medicines that treat diseases and conditions affecting that body system. Moreover, we have grouped the medicines according to type. So, you will find all the laxatives together and all the medicines for asthma together.

Under each medicine type (eg laxatives) you will find a description of what the group of medicines is used for, an explanation of the way in which the group of medicines works to treat the disease or condition, and a list of headings as follows:

How to use: You should always take a prescribed medicine according to the instructions of your doctor, but we have provided some brief details as to what you should do, for example, if you miss a dose, together with any other special instructions. We have not given details of dosage because this can vary, and a dose that is appropriate for you is not necessarily appropriate for someone else. Your doctor will have prescribed the appropriate dose for your individual circumstances.

Precautions: This is basically a list of things you should discuss with your doctor or things you should ensure that your doctor knows about your health. Always tell your doctor if you are pregnant or planning to conceive because some medicines can have adverse effects on the unborn child throughout the term of pregnancy, but particularly in the very early stages. Similarly, always tell your doctor if you are breastfeeding. The list of precautions also covers conditions such as liver disease, heart problems and breathing problems. If you have one or more of the conditions mentioned, it may not be appropriate for you to take that particular medicine, although your doctor will weigh up the risks for you in the light of the expected benefits you will gain from taking the medicine. So do not assume that the precautions listed are definite contraindications to your taking the drug. Although information regarding any conditions you have should be on your medical records, it is a wise policy to discuss your overall health with your doctor before s/he prescribes a medicine for you.

Side effects: Several medicines are associated with a long list of side effects. However, this does not mean that you will experience all – or indeed any – of them. We have included what we consider to be the most likely side effects you could experience, and made special mention of any side effects that you should talk to your doctor about.

Warnings: These are warnings related mainly to alcohol consumption and driving. Alcohol can increase the side effects of certain medicines and in these cases it is not a good idea to mix the two. Although a glass of wine or a pint of beer has no ill effects with many medicines, alcohol can be quite dangerous with others and it can produce some unpleasant effects.

Drug interactions: Many medicines interact with other medicines, and it is important that you always talk to your doctor or pharmacist before starting to take any new medicines – whether prescribed or over the counter. Drug interactions can lead to nasty side effects and sometimes reduce the beneficial effects of the medicines you are taking. Under this heading we have identified important interactions only. Be aware, too, that some interactions are used deliberately by doctors to produce a beneficial effect, so just because two drugs interact, it does not necessarily mean that they should never be taken together.

Following the information about the drug group, you will find an A–Z listing of all the drugs within that group – by generic name. The generic name is used because this is the name that most doctors now use when prescribing. However, when there is a branded product available, we have identified that name too. If there is any additional information specific to the drug that we did not include in the general details about the drug group, it is included along with the drug itself.

The Brain
and the Nervous System

RESEMBLING A HUGE control centre and communications network, the nervous system has the job of co-ordinating all your body's activities. It achieves this by carrying messages rapidly from one part of the body to another and instructing that part of the body to act as necessary.

How it works

The nervous system consists of two main parts – the central nervous system, which is composed of the brain and spinal cord, and the peripheral nervous system, which is a network of nerves connecting the brain and spinal cord to the rest of the body. The most basic unit in the nervous system is the nerve cell – also known as a neurone – and there are more than 10 billion neurones in the brain alone. Every nerve cell has one or more nerve fibres, and these nerve fibres are bundled together and wrapped in tissue to form the nerves.

The central nervous system acts something like a telephone exchange, receiving messages via the nerves from all parts of the body, processing those messages and then passing them on to other parts of the body. The messages are in the form of both electrical and chemical changes that take place within the nerves. Electrical impulses and chemical changes carry messages along the nerves, while chemicals carry messages across the junctions between two nerves. These chemicals are known as neurotransmitters, and many drugs work by stimulating or inhibiting their action.

Your brain is an extremely complex organ, and although it is often compared to a computer, this really does it an injustice. Not only does it receive and process information and decide what to do with it, but the brain also controls consciousness, intelligence, reasoning, memory, personality and sense of identity.

Acting as a monitoring device, the brain also ensures that your body is functioning properly and makes any necessary adjustments. For example, if you go for a walk, your body needs extra oxygen, and to meet this need, the brain sends messages to your lungs which lead to an increase in the speed and depth of breathing. And to speed up the delivery of oxygen round your body, the brain also sends messages to the heart to increase your heart rate.

Unlike your decision to go for a walk – which is normally a voluntary action – these effects on the heart and lungs are completely involuntary and happen automatically. Breathing, emptying the bladder, digestion of food, sweating, production of hormones and alteration of the heart rate are all largely involuntary actions.

They involve not only the brain, but also that part of the peripheral nervous system known as the autonomic nervous system.

What can go wrong

The brain and nervous system can be affected by a variety of disorders – from mental handicap, such as Down's syndrome, and brain damage caused by serious head injury or infection (for example meningitis) to brain tumours.

Mental illnesses, such as anxiety, depression, phobias, mania and schizophrenia, are also disorders that affect the nervous system. These illnesses lead to emotional and behavioural difficulties which vary from feelings of inadequacy and hopelessness in depression to sweating and tremor in anxiety. People with schizophrenia and mania lose touch with reality and suffer delusions and hallucinations. Sleeping problems can be a feature of all types of mental illness, and indeed many other illnesses too.

Epilepsy, a condition in which temporary loss of consciousness occurs, is caused by abnormal, irregular discharge of electricity from nerves inside the brain. Conditions such as dementia, Alzheimer's and Parkinson's disease are thought to be caused by degeneration of brain cells and imbalance in the chemical neurotransmitters.

Multiple sclerosis is caused by damage to the myelin sheath that surrounds the nerves. As a result, the nerves lose their ability to send messages round the body and this leads to the characteristic symptoms of multiple sclerosis which include unsteadiness in walking, uncoordinated movements and blurred vision.

Pain is a symptom of many diseases – it is not a disease in itself, but rather an indication that something is wrong – and the nervous system plays an important role in pain. If a part of the body is damaged or diseased, a message is sent via the nerves to the brain and this message is translated into pain.

Common conditions and drugs used to treat them

Anxiety – benzodiazepines (eg diazepam, chlordiazepoxide, lorazepam); buspirone; beta-blockers (eg propranolol); meprobamate

Insomnia – sedatives/hypnotics including benzodiazepines (eg temazepam, nitrazepam); zolpidem and zopiclone; chloral; chlormethiazole; barbiturates

Depression – tricyclics (eg amitriptyline, imipramine); selective serotonin reuptake inhibitors (SSRIs); monoamine oxidase inhibitors (MAOIs) and noradrenaline re-uptake inhibitors (NARIs)

Schizophrenia and mania – antipsychotics (eg chlorpromazine, haloperidol; antimanic (lithium)

Epilepsy – anticonvulsants (eg phenytoin, carbamazepine, valproate)

Parkinson's disease – antimuscarinics (eg orphenadrine, procyclidine); dopamine-receptor stimulating drugs (eg levodopa, bromocriptine, selegeline)

Alzheimer's disease – acetylcholinesterase inhibitors (eg donepezil)

Pain – analgesics (eg aspirin, paracetomol, morphine)

Migraine – treatment: analgesics, ergotamine, drugs for nausea; $5HT_1$ agonists (eg sumatriptan); prevention: beta-blockers (eg propranolol); pizotifen; tricylic anti-depressants (eg amitriptyline)

Nausea and vomiting – anti-emetics: phenothiazines (eg chlorpromazine); metoclopramide, domperidone, antihistamines.

BENZODIAZEPINES

Benzodiazepines are used in the treatment of anxiety and (as hypnotics) for sleeping problems (see pages 27–29). Although there is some overlap in the benzodiazepines used for these two conditions, different ones do tend to be used in the treatment of anxiety and insomnia. Some of these medicines are also used in the treatment of epilepsy (see page 48), as skeletal muscle relaxants and as sedatives before surgery or uncomfortable diagnostic procedures.

Benzodiazepines are sedatives and work by dampening down excessive brain activity, thus reducing symptoms of anxiety. They do this by increasing the effect of the chemical neurotransmitter called gamma-aminobutyric acid (GABA). GABA reduces the activity of brain cells and benzodiazepines increase its effect.

Benzodiazepines can be classified according to their duration of action in the body. Short-acting ones are removed rapidly from the body and this reduces the risk of a hangover effect. However, short acting benzodiazepines carry a greater risk of withdrawal symptoms than longer acting ones. Longer acting benzodiazepines are more likely to cause hangover effects and to accumulate in the body, but withdrawal is less of a problem than with the shorter acting drugs.

How to use: Take the medicine exactly as prescribed by the doctor. If you miss a dose, take it as soon as you remember. However, if it is almost time for your next dose, skip the missed dose. Do not take double the dose. If you take one dose daily at bedtime, and miss this dose, do not take it the next morning. If you have been taking one of these drugs for longer than two weeks, never stop taking it abruptly because this may cause rebound anxiety and agitation. Your doctor will advise you how to reduce the dose gradually.

Precautions: Tell your doctor if you are pregnant, planning to become pregnant or breastfeeding, or if you have lung disease or breathing difficulties, liver or kidney problems, a history of drug or alcohol abuse, or if you suffer from muscle weakness (especially if you have the condition known as myasthenia gravis).

Side effects: Drowsiness, lightheadedness, confusion, forgetfulness, and hangover effects. Headache, dizziness, blurred vision, rashes, low blood pressure, dry mouth or mouth watering, difficulty in passing urine, changes in libido and digestive disorders may occur, but these tend to be quite rare.

Side effects are often worse in older people than in those who are young or middle aged. Older people are therefore often prescribed a smaller dose.

One of the main problems with benzodiazepines is that you can become physically and psychologically dependent on them. Your doctor is therefore likely to prescribe only very short courses (2–4 weeks) of these drugs in the lowest dose that works for you.

Warnings: Do not drink alcohol while you are taking benzodiazepines because this will increase the sedative effect of the medicine. Do not drive or take part in any activity that requires you to be alert until you know how you react to the medicine.

Interactions: Other sedative medicines (eg drugs used for anxiety and insomnia, antidepressants and antihistamines) increase the effects of benzodiazepines. Several over-the-counter medicines (eg remedies for coughs, colds, hayfever and travel sickness) contain sedatives, so always tell your pharmacist if you are taking a benzodiazepine drug.

Alprazolam

General information: A long acting benzodiazepine. It is used in the short term treatment of anxiety.

Available preparations: Tablets
Brand names: Xanax

Bromazepam

General information: A short acting benzodiazepine. It is used in the short term treatment of anxiety.

Available preparations: Tablets
Brand names: Lexotan

Chlordiazepoxide

General information: A long acting benzodiazepine. It is used in the short term treatment of anxiety and to help acute alcohol withdrawal.

Available preparations: Tablets, capsules
Brand names: Librium

Clorazepate

General information: A long acting benzodiazepine. It is used in the short term treatment of anxiety.

Available preparations: Capsules
Brand names: Tranxene

Diazepam

General information: A long acting benzodiazepine. It is used in the short term treatment of anxiety and insomnia (see page 29), epilepsy (see page 47), as a muscle relaxant (see page 156), to help withdrawal problems in people with acute alcohol poisoning, and as a sedative before surgery or uncomfortable diagnostic procedures.

Available preparations: Tablets, liquid, injection, suppositories, rectal solution
Brand names: Valium

Flunitrazepam

General information: A long acting benzodiazepine. It is used for the short term treatment of insomnia.

How to use: Take the prescribed dose at bedtime.
Available preparations: Tablets
Brand names: Rohypnol

Flurazepam

General information: A long acting benzodiazepine. It is used for the short term treatment of insomnia.

How to use: Take the prescribed dose at bedtime.
Available preparations: Capsules
Brand names: Dalmane

Loprazolam

General information: A short acting benzodiazepine. It is used for the short term treatment of insomnia.

How to use: Take the prescribed dose at bedtime.
Available preparations: Tablets
Brand names: None

Lorazepam

General information: A short acting benzodiazepine. It is used in the short term treatment of anxiety.

Available preparations: Tablets, injection
Brand names: Ativan

Lormetazepam

General information: A short acting benzodiazepine. It is used for the short term treatment of insomnia.

How to use: Take the prescribed dose at bedtime.
Available preparations: Tablets
Brand names: None

Nitrazepam

General information: A long acting benzodiazepine. It is used for the short term treatment of insomnia.

How to use: Take the prescribed dose at bedtime.
Available preparations: Tablets, liquid
Brand names: None

Oxazepam

General information: A short acting benzodiazepine. It is used in the short term treatment of anxiety.

Available preparations: Tablets
Brand names: None

Temazepam

General information: A short acting benzodiazepine. It is used for the short term treatment of insomnia.

How to use: Take the prescribed dose at bedtime.
Available preparations: Tablets, capsules, liquid
Brand names: None

OTHER MEDICINES FOR ANXIETY AND INSOMNIA

Other medicines prescribed for anxiety and sleeping problems are listed in the section below. In addition, beta-blockers (eg propranolol, oxprenolol – see page 82) are used occasionally to treat the physical symptoms of anxiety and panic attacks. They block the action of the neurotransmitter called noradrenaline (excessive noradrenaline is responsible for producing many of the physical symptoms of anxiety, such as rapid heart beat and sweating). Beta-blockers have no direct effect on the psychological symptoms of anxiety.

Some antihistamines (eg diphenhydramine and promethazine) can be bought over the counter for occasional insomnia, but these products should not be used for more than a few days. Promethazine is occasionally prescribed by doctors for children with insomnia.

Barbiturates were at one time quite popular for the treatment of sleeping problems. They are much more dangerous in overdose than the benzodiazepines and are very rarely prescribed these days. Available drugs include amylobarbitone (Amytal) and butobarbitone (Soneryl). It is very easy to become dependent on these drugs, and they can cause excessive sedation.

Buspirone

General information: Used in the short term treatment of anxiety.

How to use: As benzodiazepines (see page 26).
Precautions: As for benzodiazepines. In addition, tell your doctor if you have epilepsy.
Side effects: Nausea, dizziness, headache, nervousness, excitement. Palpitations, rapid heart beat, chest pain, drowsiness, confusion, dry mouth, tiredness and sweating can occur, but these side effects tend to be quite rare.
Warnings and interactions: As benzodiazepines (see page 27).
Available preparations: Tablets
Brand names: Buspar

Chloral

General information: Chloral is a sedative used for the short term treatment of insomnia. This medicine used to be popular for use in children, but is now rarely used.

How to use: Take the prescribed dose at bedtime with plenty of water.
Precautions: As benzodiazepines (see page 26). In addition, tell your doctor if you suffer from heart disease.
Side effects: As benzodiazepines (see page 26). In addition, there is a risk of nausea and vomiting, bloating, wind and delirium.
Warnings and interactions: As benzodiazepines (see page 27).
Available preparations: Tablets, liquid
Brand names: Welldorm

Chlormethiazole

General information: Chlormethiazole is a sedative. It is used for the short term treatment of severe insomnia, restlessness and agitation in older people, and for problems with alcohol withdrawal.

How to use: For insomnia, take the prescribed dose at bedtime. For other conditions take as prescribed.
Precautions: As benzodiazepines (see page 26). In addition, tell your doctor if you have heart disease.
Side effects: As benzodiazepines (see page 26). Other side effects may include nasal congestion and irritation, eye irritation, rash and anaphylaxis (severe allergic reaction).
Warnings and interactions: As benzodiazepines (see page 27).
Available preparations: Capsules, liquid, injection
Brand names: Heminevrin

Meprobamate

General information: Used in the short term treatment of anxiety. However, it is less effective than benzodiazepines and more likely to cause side effects, so is now rarely used.

How to use: As benzodiazepines (see page 26).
Precautions: As for benzodiazepines. In addition, tell your doctor if you have porphyria.
Side effects: As benzodiazepines (see page 26), but the side effects can be more frequent and more severe.
Warnings and interactions: As benzodiazepines (see page 27).
Available preparations: Tablets
Brand names: contained in Equagesic (with analgesics)

Triclofos

General information: Triclofos is a sedative similar to chloral used for the short term treatment of insomnia, but is rarely prescribed.

How to use: Take the prescribed dose at bedtime.
Precautions, side effects, warnings, interactions: As chloral (see page 30).
Available preparations: Liquid
Brand names: None

Zolpidem

General information: Zolpidem is a short acting sedative used for the short term treatment of insomnia.

How to use: Take the prescribed dose at bedtime.
Precautions, side effects, warnings, interactions: As benzodiazepines (see page 26).
Available preparations: Tablets
Brand names: Stilnoct

Zopiclone

General information: Zopiclone is a short acting sedative used for the short term treatment of insomnia.

How to use: Take the prescribed dose at bedtime.
Precautions, side effects, warnings, interactions: As benzodiazepines (see page 26). Additional possible side effects include a bitter or metallic taste, nausea and vomiting, rashes, hallucinations, nightmares and behavioural disturbances (eg aggression).
Available preparations: Tablets
Brand names: Zimovane

ANTIDEPRESSANTS

Drugs used to treat depression include the tricyclics (eg amitriptyline, imipramine), selective serotonin re-uptake inhibitors (SSRIs), monoamine oxidase inhibitors (MAOIs) and the recently introduced noradrenaline re-uptake inhibitors (NARIs). Other drugs used occasionally in depression include flupenthixol (see page 42) and tryptophan. In depression there may be a reduction in the levels of certain chemical neurotransmitters in the brain. All antidepressants work by increasing the levels of these chemicals, although they do this in slightly different ways.

Tricyclics and related drugs

Tricyclics and drugs similar to them are used to relieve depression, including the depression associated with anxiety. They elevate mood and restore interest in life and everyday activities. They work by blocking the re-uptake of the neurotransmitters noradrenaline and serotonin into the nerve endings. They increase the levels of these chemicals in the brain and nervous system and so prolong their action. Some (eg maprotiline, viloxazine) act mainly on noradrenaline, with little influence on serotonin. Tricyclics are also used to treat bedwetting in children (see page 198).

Some tricyclics have a sedative action and are often prescribed for people who have depression and high levels of anxiety and agitation; they may also be useful for some of those with sleep problems. These include amitriptyline, clomipramine, dothiepin, doxepin, maprotiline, mianserin, trazodone and trimipramine. Other tricyclics (eg amoxapine, imipramine, lofepramine, nortriptyline, protriptyline and viloxazine) are less sedating and often prescribed for people with depression who are also lethargic.

How to use: Take the medicine exactly as prescribed by the doctor. It may take several weeks for these medicines to work and produce full benefit. So do not stop taking the medicine in the first few weeks, even if you feel no better. If you miss a dose, take it as soon as you remember. However, if it is almost time for your next dose, skip the missed dose. Do not take double the dose. If you take one dose daily at bedtime, and miss this dose, do not take it the next morning. Do not stop taking the medicine – even if you feel better – without checking with your doctor. Your doctor will advise you how to reduce the dose gradually.

Precautions: Tell your doctor if you are pregnant, planning to become pregnant or breastfeeding, or if you have any heart problems, liver or kidney problems, epilepsy, diabetes, thyroid problems, glaucoma, difficulties in passing urine or constipation.

Side effects: Dry mouth, constipation, blurred vision, increased appetite, weight gain, unpleasant taste, sweating, weakness, palpitations, dizziness, lightheadedness, drowsiness, insomnia, nervousness, reduced libido, problems in passing urine, loss of balance, shaking or trembling, unsteadiness in walking, trouble in swallowing or talking. Rare side effects include breast swelling (in men and women), ringing in the ears, seizures, skin rashes (often caused by sensitivity to sunlight) and itching.

Warnings: Do not drink alcohol while you are taking tricyclics because this will increase the sedative effect of the medicine and will interfere with the antidepressant effect. Do not drive or take part in any activity that requires you to be alert until you know how you react to the medicine. Avoid exposure to the sun or sunlamps until you know how you react to the medicine. The effects of tricyclics can last for up to a week after you have finished taking them so continue to follow all the warnings and precautions during this time. If you have been taking a monoamine oxidase inhibitor (see page 38), you must leave a gap of a least 14 days before starting a tricyclic. An MAOI should not be started within two weeks of stopping a tricyclic.

Interactions: Other sedative medicines (eg drugs used for anxiety, insomnia, antidepressants and antihistamines) increase the effects of tricyclics. Several over-the-counter medicines (eg remedies for coughs, colds, hayfever and travel sickness) contain sedatives, so always tell your pharmacist if you are taking a tricyclic antidepressant. Tricyclics may also influence the effects of drugs used for high blood pressure, and the effects of tricyclics may be influenced by drugs used for epilepsy.

Amoxapine

General information: Amoxapine is used for depression.

Available preparations: Tablets
Brand names: Asendis

Amitriptyline

General information: Amitriptyline is used for depression, particularly when a sedative effect is required. It is also used for nocturnal enuresis (bedwetting) in children.

Available preparations: Tablets, capsules, liquid
Brand names: Lentizol, Tryptizol
Combination preparations: Triptafen and Triptafen M (both contain amitriptyline and perphenazine, an antipsychotic).

Clomipramine

General information: Clomipramine is used for depression and phobias and obsessional conditions.

Available preparations: Tablets, capsules, liquid, injection
Brand names: Anafranil, Anafranil SR

Dothiepin

General information: Dothiepin is used for depression, particularly when a sedative effect is required.

Available preparations: Tablets, capsules
Brand names: Prothiaden

Doxepin

General information: Doxepin is used for depression, particularly when a sedative effect is required.

Available preparations: Capsules
Brand names: Sinequan

Imipramine

General information: Imipramine is used for depression and nocturnal enuresis (bedwetting) in children.

Available preparations: Tablets, liquid
Brand names: Tofranil

Lofepramine

General information: Lofepramine is used for depression.

Available preparations: Tablets, liquid
Brand names: Gamanil

Maprotiline

General information: Maprotiline is used for depression, particularly when a sedative effect is required.

Side effects: As tricyclics (see page 32), but dry mouth, blurred vision, sweating, difficulty in passing urine and effects on the heart may occur less frequently. However, rashes are quite common.
Available preparations: Tablets
Brand names: Ludiomil

Mianserin

General information: Mianserin is used for depression, particularly when a sedative effect is required.

Side effects: As tricyclics (see page 32), but dry mouth, blurred vision, sweating, difficulty in passing urine and effects on the heart may occur less frequently. However, jaundice, blood disorders and arthritic pain may occur.
Warnings: As tricyclics (see page 32). In addition, if you develop fever, sore throat, sore mouth or any signs of infection, tell your doctor immediately. Mianserin can cause blood disorders and you should have a full blood count every 4 weeks during the first 3 months of treatment and at regular intervals after that.
Precautions and interactions: As tricyclics (see pages 32–33).
Available preparations: Tablets
Brand names: None

Mirtazapine

General information: Mirtazapine is used for depression.

Side effects: As tricyclics (see page 32). Increased appetite and weight gain, jaundice, fluid retention, rash and blood disorders may occur.
Warnings: As tricyclics (see page 32). In addition, if you develop fever, sore throat, sore mouth or any signs of infection, tell your doctor immediately.
Precautions and interactions: As tricyclics (see pages 32–33).
Available preparations: Tablets
Brand names: Zispin

Nortriptyline

General information: Nortriptyline is used for depression and nocturnal enuresis (bedwetting) in children.

Available preparations: Tablets
Brand names: Allegron
Combination preparations: Motipress, Motival (both contain nortriptyline and fluphenazine, an antipsychotic).

Protriptyline

General information: Protriptyline is used for depression, particularly in those who are apathetic and lethargic.
Available preparations: Tablets
Brand names: Concordin

Trazodone

General information: Trazodone is used for depression, particularly when a sedative effect is required.

Side effects: As tricyclics (see page 32), but dry mouth, blurred vision, sweating, difficulty in passing urine and effects on the heart may occur less frequently.
Precautions, warnings, interactions: As tricyclics (see pages 32–33).
Available preparation: Tablets, sustained-release tablets, capsules, liquid
Brand names: Molipaxin

Viloxazine

General information: Viloxazine is used for depression.

Side effects: As tricyclics (see page 32), but drowsiness, dry mouth, blurred vision, sweating, difficulty in passing urine and effects on the heart may occur less frequently. Nausea and headache may occur.
Precautions, warnings, interactions: As tricyclics (see pages 32–33).
Available preparations: Tablets
Brand name: Vivalan

SELECTIVE SEROTONIN RE-UPTAKE INHIBITORS (SSRIs) and related antidepressants

SSRIs (of which Prozac is the best-known example) and related drugs are used to relieve depression, including the depression that sometimes occurs with anxiety. Some are also used to treat obsessive-compulsive disorders, panic attacks and bulimia nervosa. SSRIs are no more effective than tricyclics, but they are better tolerated, are less sedative and some side effects (eg blurred vision, constipation, difficulty in passing urine and effects on the heart) occur less frequently. They are also less toxic in overdose and often have a shorter onset of action. SSRIs and drugs which are similar to them elevate mood and restore interest in life and everyday activities. They work by blocking the re-uptake of the neurotransmitter serotonin into the nerve endings. By doing this, they increase the levels of serotonin in the brain and nervous system and so prolong its action.

How to use: Take the medicine exactly as prescribed by the doctor. It make take up to 4 weeks for these medicines to work and produce full benefit. So, do not stop taking the medicine in the first few weeks even if you feel no better. If you miss a dose, take it as soon as you remember. However, if it is almost time for your next dose, skip the missed dose. Do not take double the dose. Do not stop taking the medicine – even if you feel better – without checking with your doctor. Your doctor will advise you how to reduce the dose gradually.

Precautions: Tell your doctor if you are pregnant, planning to become pregnant or breastfeeding, or if you have any heart problems, liver or kidney problems, epilepsy or diabetes.

Side effects: Gastrointestinal effects (eg nausea, vomiting, diarrhoea, constipation or stomach cramps) are quite common. Anxiety, insomnia, nervousness, decreased appetite and weight loss, reduced sexual drive, dizziness, lightheadedness and tiredness may occur. Stop taking the medicine and check with your doctor immediately if you develop a rash or any other allergic reaction. Check with your doctor immediately if you develop palpitations, unsteadiness or shakiness, chills or fever, signs of low blood sugar (such as dizziness, tiredness, shakiness) or fits.

Warnings: Alcohol may increase the sedative effect of SSRIs. Do not drive or take part in any activity that requires you to be alert until you know how you react to the medicine. If you have been taking a monamine oxidase inhibitor (see page 38), you must leave a gap of at least 14 days before starting an SSRI. An MAOI should not be started within two weeks (five weeks with fluoxetine) of stopping an SSRI.

Interactions: Other sedative medicines (eg drugs used for anxiety, insomnia, antidepressants and antihistamines) increase the effects of SSRIs. Several over-the-counter medicines (eg remedies for coughs, colds, hayfever and travel sickness) contain sedatives, so always tell your pharmacist if you are taking an SSRI. SSRIs may also influence the effects of anticoagulants (eg warfarin), lithium, drugs used for epilepsy, theophylline and some drugs used for migraine (eg sumatriptan).

Citalopram

General information: Citalopram is used for depression and panic disorder.

Available preparations: Tablets
Brand names: Cipramil

Fluoxetine

General information: Fluoxetine is used for depression, bulimia nervosa and obsessive-compulsive disorder.

Available preparations: Capsules, liquid
Brand names: Prozac

Fluvoxamine

General information: Fluvoxamine is used for depression and obsessive-compulsive disorder.

Available preparations: Tablets
Brand names: Faverin

Nefazodone

General information: Nefazodone is used for depression.

Precautions, side effects, warnings, interactions: As SSRIs, but also possibility of dry mouth, visual disturbances, burning or tingling hands and feet. Increased risk of heart problems if cisapride is taken at the same time.
Available preparations: Tablets
Brand names: Dutonin

Paroxetine

General information: Paroxetine is used for depression, panic disorder, social anxiety, social phobias and obsessive-compulsive disorder.

Available preparations: Tablets, liquid
Brand names: Seroxat

Sertraline

General information: Sertraline is used for depression.

Available preparations: Tablets
Brand names: Lustral

Venlafaxine

General information: Venlafaxine is used for depression.

Side effects: Nausea, vomiting, constipation, stomach cramps, headache, insomnia,

drowsiness, dizziness, sweating, nervousness, abnormal dreams, reduced sexual ability, visual disturbances, tingling hands and feet, chills, weight changes, palpitations.
Precautions and warnings: As SSRIs (see page 36).
Interactions: Other sedative medicines (eg drugs used for anxiety, insomnia, antidepressants and antihistamines) increase the effects of SSRIs. Several over-the-counter medicines (eg remedies for coughs, colds, hayfever and travel sickness) contain sedatives, so always tell your pharmacist if you are taking venlafaxine.
Available preparations: Tablets, capsules
Brand names: Efexor, Efexor XL

MONOAMINE OXIDASE INHIBITORS (MAOIs)

MAOIs are used to relieve severe depression, but they are used much less frequently than either tricyclics or SSRIs. This is mainly because of the dangers of interactions with other drugs and also with certain foods producing dangerous side effects. Like tricyclics and SSRIs, MAOIs work by increasing the levels of chemical neurotransmitters in the brain. They achieve this by interfering with enzymes that terminate the action of these neurotransmitters.

How to use: Take the medicine exactly as prescribed by the doctor. It make take up to 4 weeks for these medicines to work and produce full benefit, so do not stop taking the medicine if in the first few weeks you feel no better. If you miss a dose, take it as soon as you remember. However, if it is almost time for your next dose, skip the missed dose. Do not take double the dose. Do not stop taking the medicine – even if you feel better – without checking with your doctor.

Precautions: Tell your doctor if you are pregnant, planning to become pregnant or breastfeeding, or if you have any heart problems or have had a stroke, liver problems, epilepsy, diabetes or phaeocromocytoma.

Side effects: Dizziness, dry mouth, drowsiness, insomnia, headache, blurred vision, constipation and other gastrointestinal disturbances, difficulty in passing urine, nervousness, sweating, rash, tingling of hands and feet.

Warnings: Never drink any red wine, particularly Chianti, when taking MAOIs. You must also avoid certain foods (eg cheese, pickled herrings, yeast and yeast extracts, including Bovril, Oxo and Marmite, broad bean pods and foods which are stale or 'going off'). Consuming such foods and drinks while you are taking an MAOI is dangerous because it can lead to an excessive rise in blood pressure. Your pharmacist should give you a card which tells you in detail the foods and drinks which you need to avoid.

Any alcohol may increase the sedative effect of MAOIs. Do not drive or take part in any activity that requires you to be alert until you know how you react to the medicine. If you have been taking any other antidepressant, you must leave a gap before starting the MAOI (check with your doctor). Conversely, you must also leave a gap between stopping an MAOI and starting another antidepressant (again, check with your doctor). The effects of MAOIs can last for up to 2 weeks after you have finished taking them so continue to follow all the warnings and precautions during this time.

Interactions: MAOIs interact with a wide variety of other medicines. Other sedative medicines (eg drugs used for anxiety, insomnia, antidepressants and antihistamines) increase the effects of MAOIs. Several over-the-counter medicines (eg remedies for coughs, colds, hayfever and travel sickness) contain sedatives and other ingredients (eg ephedrine, pseudoephedrine, phenylpropanolamine) which increase the effects of MAOIs. Do not take any other medicine without checking with your doctor or pharmacist.

Isocarboxazid

General information: Isocarboxazid is used for depression.

Available preparations: Tablets
Brand names: None

Moclobemide

General information: Moclobemide is used for depression and social phobia.

Precautions, side effects, warnings, interactions: As MAOIs (see above). However, the risk of interactions with foods and other drugs is thought to be less than that with other MAOIs. Nevertheless, you should still follow the same precautions and warnings. In addition, tell your doctor if you have a thyroid problem. Check with your pharmacist or doctor before taking any analgesics or cimetidine.
Available preparations: Tablets
Brand names: Manerix

Phenelzine

General information: Phenelzine is used for depression.

Available preparations: Tablets
Brand names: Nardil

Tranylcypromine

General information: Tranylcypromine is used for depression.

Available preparations: Tablets
Brand names: Parnate, Parstelin (also contains trifluoperazine, an antipsychotic)

NORADRENALINE RE-UPTAKE INHIBITORS (NARIs)

There is only one drug (ie reboxetine) in this category. It is used for depression. NARIs and drugs which are similar to them elevate mood and restore interest in life and everyday activities. NARIs increase the level of the neurotransmitter noradrenaline in the brain by preventing its re-uptake into nerves.

How to use: Take the medicine exactly as prescribed by the doctor. It make take several weeks for these medicines to work and produce full benefit, so do not stop taking the medicine if in the first few weeks you feel no better. If you miss a dose, take it as soon as you remember. However, if it is almost time for your next dose, skip the missed dose. Do not take double the dose. Do not stop taking the medicine – even if you feel better – without checking with your doctor.

Precautions: Tell your doctor if you are pregnant, planning to become pregnant or breastfeeding, or if you have liver or kidney problems, epilepsy, problems in passing urine or glaucoma.

Side effects: These may include insomnia, sweating, dizziness, tingling of hands and feet, difficulty in passing urine, impotence, dry mouth, constipation, rapid heart beat.

Warnings: Alcohol may increase the sedative effect of NARIs. Do not drive or take part in any activity that requires you to be alert until you know how you react to the medicine. If you have been taking a monamine oxidase inhibitor (see page 38), you must leave a gap of at least 14 days before starting a NARI. Conversely, an MAOI should not be started within one week of stopping a NARI.

Interactions: Other sedative medicines (eg drugs used for anxiety, insomnia, antidepressants and antihistamines) increase the effects of NARIs. Several over-the-counter medicines (eg remedies for coughs, colds, hayfever and travel sickness) contain sedatives. NARIs may also influence the effects of some antibiotics and antifungal medicines. Check with your doctor or pharmacist before taking other medicines, including those available over the counter.

Reboxetine

General information: Reboxetine is used for depression.

Available preparations: Tablets
Brand names: Edronax

ANTIPSYCHOTICS

Antipsychotics, also known as neuroleptics or tranquillisers, are used mainly in the treatment of schizophrenia to control symptoms and prevent relapses. However, they do not cure the disease. They are also used to control symptoms of mania, such as euphoria and delusions of grandeur, and in low doses to sedate people with dementia who are acutely confused and agitated. Antipsychotics work mainly by blocking the effects of the neurotransmitter dopamine. In conditions such as schizophrenia, the activity of dopamine is thought to be excessive, so blocking the action of dopamine may help to control the symptoms. Antipsychotics also affect other neurotransmitters including acetylcholine, histamine, noradrenaline and serotonin.

How to use: Take the medicine exactly as prescribed by the doctor. If you miss a dose, take it as soon as you remember. However, if it is almost time for your next dose, skip the missed dose. Do not take double the dose. Do not stop taking the medicine without checking with your doctor because symptoms may recur. Withdrawal problems can occur if these medicines are stopped abruptly. Your doctor will advise you about gradually reducing the dose.

NB Antipsychotics can be given orally, by rectum or by injection. However, they can also be given in the form of a depot injection. This type of injection releases the drug slowly over several weeks and is particularly useful for people who might forget to take their medicine or might take an overdose.

Precautions: Tell your doctor if you are pregnant, planning to become pregnant or are breastfeeding, or if you have heart or breathing problems, Parkinson's disease, epilepsy, phaeocromocytoma, liver or kidney problems, thyroid disease, glaucoma or prostate problems.

Side effects: Side effects with these drugs are quite common and include drowsiness, dizziness or fainting, blurred vision, constipation, loss of balance, shuffling walk or stiff arms and legs, spasms of neck, face and back, trembling of hands, trouble chewing, talking and swallowing, uncontrolled movements, weakness of arms and legs. Rarer side effects include rash and other allergic reactions, difficulties in passing urine, worsening of glaucoma, sexual problems, infrequent periods, low blood pressure (which can lead to falls and accidents), convulsions, fast or irregular heartbeat, aching muscles and joints, nausea, vomiting, diarrhoea and blood changes. Blood changes are often revealed by symptoms such as sore throat, fever, unusual bruising or bleeding.

If you experience particular problems with spasms, stiffness, trembling and shaking, swallowing, restlessness and abnormal movements in any part of your body, your doctor may prescribe another drug to suppress these symptoms (eg benzhexol or orphenadrine – see pages 52-53).

Warnings: Do not drink alcohol while you are taking antipsychotics because this will increase the sedative effect of the medicine. Do not drive or take part in any activity that requires you to be alert until you know how you react to the medicine. Do not stay in the sun or very hot places, because your risk of heat stroke is increased if you are taking antipsychotics (check with your doctor or pharmacist).

Interactions: Antipsychotics interact with many other medicines, including drugs used for heart conditions and epilepsy and some antibiotics. Other sedative medicines (eg drugs used for anxiety, insomnia, antidepressants and antihistamines) increase the effects of antipsychotics. Several over-the-counter medicines (eg remedies for coughs, colds, hayfever and travel sickness) contain sedatives, so always tell your pharmacist if you are taking an antipsychotic drug.

Amisulpride

General information: Amisulpride is used for schizophrenia.

Available preparations: Tablets
Brand names: Solian

Benperidol

General information: Benperidol is used for the control of deviant anti-social sexual behaviour.

Available preparations: Tablets
Brand names: Anquil

Chlorpromazine

General information: Chlorpromazine is used for schizophrenia and other similar conditions, severe anxiety, mania, and also nausea and vomiting in terminal illness.

Available preparations: Tablets, liquid, suppositories, injection
Brand names: Largactil

Clozapine

General information: Clozapine is used in schizophrenia, but only in cases where other antipsychotics have not worked. This drug is started in hospital and you will be registered with and given full instructions by the Clozaril Patient Monitoring Service while taking this medicine.

Available preparations: Tablets
Brand names: Clozaril

Droperidol

General information: Droperidol is used for rapid calming of manic and severely agitated people.

Available preparations: Tablets, liquid, injection
Brand names: Droleptan

Flupenthixol

General information: Flupenthixol is used for schizophrenia and other similar conditions, particularly in those who are withdrawn or apathetic. It is also used for depression.

Available preparations: Tablets, depot injection
Brand names: Depixol

Fluphenazine

General information: Fluphenazine is used for schizophrenia and other similar conditions, mania, severe anxiety, agitation and severe behavioural disorders, but it should not be used for depression.

Available preparations: Tablets, depot injection
Brand names: Modecate, Moditen

Haloperidol

General information: Haloperidol is used for schizophrenia and other similar conditions, mania, severe anxiety, agitation, severe behavioural disorders and severe hiccup.

Available preparations: Tablets, capsules, liquid, injection, depot injection
Brand names: Dozic, Haldol, Serenace

Loxapine

General information: Loxapine is used for severe psychotic states.

Available preparations: Capsules
Brand names: Loxapac

Methotrimeprazine

General information: Methotrimeprazine is used for schizophrenia and other similar conditions and also for pain, restlessness, distress or vomiting in terminal illness.

Available preparations: Tablets, injection
Brand names: Nozinan

Olanzapine

General information: Olanzapine is used for schizophrenia.

Available preparations: Tablets
Brand names: Zyprexa

Oxypertine

General information: Oxypertine is used for schizophrenia and other similar conditions, mania, severe anxiety, agitation and severe behavioural disorders.

Available preparations: Tablets, capsules
Brand names: None

Pericyazine

General information: Pericyazine is used for schizophrenia and other similar conditions, mania, severe anxiety, agitation and severe behavioural disorders. It is also used in children for severe mental and behavioural disorders.

Available preparations: Tablets, liquid
Brand names: Neulactil

Perphenazine

General information: Perphenazine is used for schizophrenia and other similar conditions, mania, severe anxiety, agitation and severe behavioural disorders. It is also used as an anti-emetic (see page 70) for nausea and vomiting.

Available preparations: Tablets
Brand names: Fentazin

Pimozide

General information: Pimozide is used for schizophrenia and other similar conditions. This drug can cause severe irregularities in heart beat and you should therefore be asked to attend regular appointments for ECG monitoring.

Available preparations: Tablets
Brand names: Orap

Pipothiazine

General information: Pipothiazine is used for schizophrenia and other similar conditions.

Available preparations: Depot injection
Brand names: Piportil

Prochlorperazine

General information: Prochlorperazine is used for schizophrenia and other similar conditions, severe anxiety and also for nausea, vomiting and vertigo, or dizziness (see page 70).

Available preparations: Tablets, effervescent tablets, liquid, suppositories, injection
Brand names: Buccastem, Stemetil

Promazine

General information: Promazine is used for severe agitation and restlessness.

Available preparations: Tablets, liquid, injection
Brand names: None

Quetiapine

General information: Quetiapine is used for schizophrenia.

Available preparations: Tablets
Brand names: Seroquel

Risperidone

General information: Risperidone is used for schizophrenia and other similar conditions.

Available preparations: Tablets, liquid
Brand names: Risperdal

Sulpiride

General information: Sulpiride is used for schizophrenia.

Available preparations: Tablets
Brand names: Dolmatil, Sulparex, Sulpitil

Thioridazine

General information: Thioridazine is used for schizophrenia and other similar conditions, mania, severe anxiety, agitation and severe behavioural disorders.

Available preparations: Tablets, liquid
Brand names: Melleril

Trifluoperazine

General information: Trifluoperazine is used for schizophrenia and other similar conditions, and severe anxiety.

Available preparations: Tablets, capsules, liquid
Brand names: Stelazine

Zotepine

General information: Zotepine is used for the treatment of schizophrenia.

Available preparations: Tablets
Brand names: Zoleptil

Zuclopenthixol

General information: Zuclopenthixol is used for schizophrenia and other similar conditions, mania and agitation.

Available preparations: Tablets, injection, depot injection
Brand names: Clopixol, Clopixol Accuphase

ANTIMANIC DRUGS – LITHIUM

Manic depression – exaggerated mood swings with peaks of elation and troughs of depression – is normally treated with lithium. However, because lithium may take several weeks to work, an antipsychotic medicine (see page 40) or a benzodiazepine (see page 26) may be given at first to give immediate relief of symptoms. Carbamazepine (see page 47) may be used in people who do not respond to lithium. It is useful for the prevention and treatment of mania, prevention of manic depression and prevention of depression. It has an important advantage over lithium in that it is not sedative and it does reduce the frequency of attacks.

Lithium

General information: Lithium is used in mania, manic depression, severe depression and in the treatment of aggressive and self-mutilating behaviour.

How to use: Take the medicine exactly as prescribed by the doctor. It may take several weeks for this medicine to work and produce full benefit. If you miss a dose, take it as soon as you remember. However, if it is almost time for your next dose, skip the missed dose. Do not take double the dose. Do not stop taking the medicine without checking with your doctor – even if you feel better – because symptoms may recur.

Precautions: Tell your doctor if you are pregnant, planning to become pregnant or breastfeeding, or if you have or have had heart problems, liver or kidney problems, thyroid disease or myasthenia gravis.

Side effects: Mild thirst, frequent urination, drowsiness, tremor, mild nausea, fluid retention and weight gain may occur. Check with your doctor immediately if you experience loss of appetite, diarrhoea, vomiting, unsteadiness, difficulty in walking, giddiness, drowsiness and lethargy or unusual muscle weakness.

Warnings: Do not drink alcohol while you are taking lithium because this will increase the sedative effect of the medicine. Do not drive or take part in any activity that requires you to be alert until you know how you react to the medicine. Drink plenty of fluid (8–12 cups or glasses each day), particularly in hot weather. Lithium levels in the blood are affected by the amount of salt you have in your diet, so you should be careful not to increase or decrease your salt intake. You will be asked to attend for regular blood and other tests while you are taking lithium. Do not miss these appointments. Your pharmacist will give you a card which explains exactly what you have to do and what to expect while taking this medicine.

Interactions: Lithium interacts with a wide range of other medicines; diuretics in particular may affect the lithium dose. Do not take any medicine – including those available over the counter – without checking with your doctor or pharmacist.

Available preparations: Tablets, liquid

Brand names: Camcolit, Li-Liquid, Liskonum, Litarex, Priadel

ANTICONVULSANTS

Anticonvulsants are used in the treatment of epilepsy. An epileptic fit (convulsion) occurs when the normal electrical activity in the brain becomes disrupted. There are several drugs used for epilepsy and the choice of drug is governed to some extent by the type of epilepsy, although there is a great deal of overlap in the drugs used. The condition called status epilepticus is an emergency, which is treated with various drugs (eg diazepam and clonazepam). Anticonvulsants inhibit the excessive electrical activity in the brain which is a feature of epilepsy.

How to use: Take the medicine exactly as prescribed by the doctor. If you miss a dose, take it as soon as you remember. Do not stop taking the medicine without checking with your doctor because symptoms may recur. Fits may become more frequent if you take your medicine irregularly.

Precautions: See also individual drugs. However, if you plan to become pregnant discuss with your doctor. Anticonvulsants can cause malformations in the baby and you need to understand the risks and benefits of taking these drugs during pregnancy. In addition you should take a supplement of folic acid from the time you plan to become pregnant until the 12th week of pregnancy. Your doctor will prescribe this supplement for you – it is stronger than those available over the counter.

Side effects: See individual drugs.

Warnings: See also individual drugs. Do not drink alcohol while you are taking anticonvulsants because this will increase the sedative effect of the medicine. Do not drive or take part in any activity that requires you to be alert until you know how you react to the medicine. You will be asked to attend for various tests, including blood tests, while taking these medicines. Do not miss your appointments.

Interactions: Anticonvulsants interact with a wide variety of medicines. Do not take any other medicine, including those available over the counter, without checking with your doctor or pharmacist. Women taking the contraceptive pill should be aware that anticonvulsants can decrease the effectiveness of the pill, and to prevent pregnancy it is necessary to use an additional method of birth control.

Carbamazepine

General information: Carbamazepine is used for certain types of epilepsy. It is also used for trigeminal neuralgia (facial nerve pain), and occasionally for manic depressive illness (see page 46).

How to use: As anticonvulsants (see above).
Precautions: Tell your doctor if you think you could be pregnant, plan to become pregnant or are breastfeeding, or if you have or have had heart problems, liver or kidney problems or glaucoma.
Side effects: Side effects are relatively uncommon with this drug, but the following may occur: nausea and vomiting, constipation, diarrhoea, loss of appetite, dizziness, drowsiness, headache, confusion, agitation and irritability, blurred or double vision.

Warnings: As anticonvulsants (see page 47). In addition, check with your doctor immediately if you experience sore throat, fever, mouth sores, any unusual bleeding or bruising, rash, yellowing of the skin or eyes or dark urine.
Interactions: As anticonvulsants (see page 47).
Available preparations: Tablets, liquid, suppositories
Brand names: Tegretol, Timonil

Clobazam

General information: Clobazam belongs to the benzodiazepine group of drugs which are commonly used in anxiety and insomnia. However, clobazam is also used in epilepsy.

How to use: As anticonvulsants (see page 47).
Precautions: Tell your doctor if you think you could be pregnant, plan to become pregnant or are breastfeeding, or if you have lung, liver or kidney problems.
Side effects: Side effects are common and include drowsiness, dizziness, confusion and lightheadedness.
Warnings: As anticonvulsants (see page 47).
Interactions: As anticonvulsants (see page 47).
Available preparations: Tablets
Brand names: Frisium

Clonazepam

General information: Clonazepam belongs to the benzodiazepine group of drugs which are commonly used in anxiety and insomnia. However, clonazepam is also used in epilepsy.

Precautions: Tell your doctor if you think you could be pregnant, plan to become pregnant or are breastfeeding, or if you have lung, liver or kidney problems.
Side effects: Side effects are common and include drowsiness, dizziness, increased salivation, clumsiness, aggression and irritability.
Warnings: As anticonvulsants (see page 47). In addition, check with your doctor if you develop a rash.
Interactions: As anticonvulsants (see page 47).
Available preparations: Tablets, injection
Brand names: Rivotril

Ethosuximide

General information: Ethosuximide is used to treat a type of epilepsy called absence seizure (petit mal).

How to use: As anticonvulsants (see page 47).
Precautions: Tell your doctor if you think you could be pregnant, plan to become pregnant or are breastfeeding, or if you have or have had liver or kidney problems or porphyria.

Side effects: Side effects are relatively uncommon with this drug, but the following may occur: drowsiness, dizziness, upset stomach, vomiting, constipation, diarrhoea, headache, depression, irritability, insomnia, confusion, swelling of the gums or tongue.

Warnings: As anticonvulsants (see page 47). In addition, check with your doctor immediately if you experience sore throat, fever, mouth sores, any unusual bleeding or bruising, rash, yellowing of the skin or eyes or dark urine.

Interactions: As anticonvulsants (see page 47).

Available preparations: Capsules, syrup

Brand names: Emeside, Zarontin

Gabapentin

General information: Gabapentin is used for certain types of epilepsy.

How to use: As anticonvulsants (see page 47).

Precautions: Tell your doctor if you think you could be pregnant, plan to become pregnant or are breastfeeding, or if you have kidney problems.

Side effects: Side effects are relatively uncommon with this drug, but the following may occur: drowsiness, dizziness, trembling, clumsiness, headache, blurred or double vision, irregular eye movements, nausea and vomiting and runny nose.

Warnings: As anticonvulsants (see page 47).

Interactions: As anticonvulsants (see page 47).

Available preparations: Capsules

Brand names: Neurontin

Lamotrigine

General information: Lamotrigine is used for certain types of epilepsy.

How to use: As anticonvulsants (see page 47).

Precautions: Tell your doctor if you think you could be pregnant, plan to become pregnant or are breastfeeding, or if you have liver or kidney problems.

Side effects: Rashes are common (tell your doctor immediately – see below). The following may also occur: drowsiness, blurred or double vision, conjunctivitis, dizziness, insomnia, headache, irritability, confusion, nausea.

Warnings: As anticonvulsants (see page 47). In addition, check with your doctor immediately if you develop a rash or influenza-like symptoms.

Interactions: As anticonvulsants (see page 47).

Available preparations: Tablets, soluble tablets

Brand names: Lamictal

Phenobarbitone (and methylphenobarbitone)

General information: Phenobarbitone is used for certain types of epilepsy.

How to use: As anticonvulsants (see page 47).

Precautions: Tell your doctor if you think you could be pregnant, plan to become pregnant or are breastfeeding, or you have heart or breathing problems or liver or kidney problems.

Side effects: Side effects are common and include drowsiness, lethargy, depression, confusion, clumsiness, unsteadiness, excitement and restlessness.

Warnings: As anticonvulsants (see page 47). Check with your doctor immediately if you develop a rash.

Interactions: As anticonvulsants (see page 47).

Available preparations: Tablets, liquid, injection

Brand names: None

Primidone

General information: Primidone is used for certain types of epilepsy. It is converted to the active drug phenytoin in the body (see below).

How to use: As anticonvulsants (see page 47).

Precautions: Tell your doctor if you think you could be pregnant, plan to become pregnant or are breastfeeding, or if you have heart or breathing problems, or if you have liver or kidney problems.

Side effects: Side effects are common and include drowsiness, clumsiness, unsteadiness, dizziness, nausea, visual disturbances, excitement and restlessness.

Warnings: As anticonvulsants (see page 47). Check with your doctor immediately if you develop a rash.

Interactions: As anticonvulsants (see page 47).

Available preparations: Tablets, liquid

Brand names: Mysoline

Phenytoin

General information: Phenytoin is used for most types of epilepsy and also for trigeminal neuralgia (facial nerve pain).

How to use: As anticonvulsants (see page 47).

Precautions: Tell your doctor if you think you could be pregnant, plan to become pregnant or are breastfeeding, or you have heart problems, liver or kidney problems, diabetes or porphyria.

Side effects: Side effects are common and include nausea, vomiting, confusion, headache, dizziness, trembling, nervousness, insomnia, increased hair growth and redness, bleeding and swelling of the gums.

Warnings: As anticonvulsants (see page 47). In addition, check with your doctor immediately if you experience sore throat, fever, mouth sores, any unusual bleeding or bruising, rash, yellowing of the skin or eyes or dark urine. Your doctor will want to check the levels of this drug in your blood from time to time. Phenytoin is safe and effective, but small changes in dosage can lead to large changes in the level of the drug in the blood. These blood tests are therefore very important.

Interactions: As anticonvulsants (see page 47).

Available preparations: Tablets, capsules, liquid

Brand names: Epanutin

Topiramate

General information: Topiramate is used for certain types of epilepsy.

How to use: As anticonvulsants (see page 47).
Precautions: Tell your doctor if you think you could be pregnant, plan to become pregnant or are breastfeeding, or if you have liver or kidney problems.
Side effects: Side effects are relatively rare with this drug, but the following can occur: stomach pain, nausea, loss of appetite and weight loss, mood changes, poor memory, inability to concentrate, confusion, clumsiness, unsteadiness, tingling in hands and feet, dizziness, drowsiness, blurred or double vision.
Warnings: As anticonvulsants (see page 47).
Interactions: As anticonvulsants (see page 47).
Available preparations: Tablets
Brand names: Topamax

Valproate

General information: Valproate is used for certain types of epilepsy.

How to use: As anticonvulsants (see page 47).
Precautions: Tell your doctor if you think you could be pregnant, plan to become pregnant or are breastfeeding, or if you have liver problems.
Side effects: Side effects are relatively uncommon with this drug, but the following may occur: temporary hair loss, increase in appetite and weight gain, nausea and indigestion. Drowsiness is rare.
Warnings: As anticonvulsants (see page 47). In addition, check with your doctor immediately if you experience sore throat, fever, mouth sores, any unusual bleeding or bruising, rash, yellowing of the skin or eyes or dark urine.
Interactions: As anticonvulsants (see page 47).
Available preparations: Tablets, capsules, liquid
Brand names: Convulex, Epilim

Vigabatrin

General information: Vigabatrin is used for certain types of epilepsy, particularly in those who do not respond to other anticonvulsants.

How to use: As anticonvulsants (see page 47).
Precautions: Tell your doctor if you think you could be pregnant, plan to become pregnant or are breastfeeding, or if you have liver or kidney problems.
Side effects: Drowsiness, dizziness, nervousness, irritability, agitation, depression, headache, trembling, clumsiness, unsteadiness, visual disturbances.
Warnings: As anticonvulsants (see page 47). In addition, check with your doctor immediately if you experience any visual changes.
Interactions: As anticonvulsants (see page 47).
Available preparations: Tablets, powder
Brand names: Sabril

DRUGS USED FOR PARKINSON'S DISEASE

Parkinson's disease is caused by degenerative changes in part of the brain. This leads to an imbalance between two neurotransmitters - dopamine and acetylcholine - in the brain. These neurotransmitters are responsible for transmitting messages in the parts of the brain responsible for movement. Well co-ordinated movement depends on dopamine and acetylcholine being in perfect balance. In Parkinson's disease, however, there is a relative lack of dopamine in comparison with acetylcholine and this leads to the disturbances in movement which are a well-known feature of Parkinson's disease. Several drugs are used to treat Parkinson's disease and they all work by helping to restore the balance between acetylcholine and dopamine. They either boost the levels, or mimic the actions, of dopamine or reduce the levels of acetylcholine.

How to use: Take the medicine exactly as prescribed by the doctor. If you miss a dose, take it as soon as you remember. Do not stop taking the medicine without checking with your doctor because symptoms may recur.

Precautions, side effects, warnings and interactions: See also individual drugs. Note that pregnancy and breastfeeding are not mentioned in relation to these drugs. This is because Parkinson's disease is mainly a disease of old age. However, some of these drugs can be used for conditions other than Parkinson's disease, for example, to relieve side effects caused by certain antipsychotic drugs, and in these circumstances, the normal warnings about pregnancy and breastfeeding apply.

Drugs with an anticholinergic action

Benzhexol

General information: Benzhexol is used for Parkinson's disease and also for Parkinson-like symptoms induced by some antipsychotics (see page 40).

How to use: As drugs used for Parkinson's disease (see above).
Precautions: Tell your doctor if you have any of the following conditions: heart problems, liver or kidney problems, peptic ulcer, glaucoma, difficulties passing urine, prostate problems or constipation.
Side effects: Dry mouth, constipation, blurred vision, increased palpitations, dizziness, lightheadedness, drowsiness, insomnia, nervousness, problems in passing urine.
Warnings: Do not drink alcohol because this will increase the sedative effect of the medicine. Do not drive or take part in any activity that requires you to be alert until you know how you react to the medicine. You will be asked to attend for eye examinations (because prolonged use of this drug may cause glaucoma). Do not miss your appointments.
Interactions: Other sedative medicines (eg drugs used for anxiety, insomnia, antidepressants and antihistamines) increase the effects of benzhexol. Several over-the-

counter medicines (eg remedies for coughs, colds, hayfever and travel sickness) contain sedatives, so always tell your pharmacist if you are taking benzhexol.
Available preparations: Tablets, liquid
Brand names: Broflex

Benztropine

General information: Benztropine is used for Parkinson's disease and also for some of the Parkinson-like symptoms induced by some antipsychotics (see page 40).

How to use: As drugs used for Parkinson's disease (see page 52).
Precautions, side effects, warnings, interactions: As benzhexol (see page 52).
Available preparations: Tablets, injection
Brand names: Cogentin

Biperiden

General information: Biperiden is used for Parkinson's disease and also for Parkinson-like symptoms induced by some antipsychotics (see page 40).

How to use: As drugs used for Parkinson's disease (see page 52).
Precautions, side effects, warnings, interactions: As benzhexol (see page 52).
Available preparations: Tablets, injection
Brand names: Akineton

Orphenadrine

General information: Orphenadrine is used for Parkinson's disease and also for Parkinson-like symptoms induced by some antipsychotics (see page 40).

How to use: As drugs used for Parkinson's disease (see page 52).
Precautions, side effects, warnings, interactions: As benzhexol (see page 52).
Available preparations: Tablets, liquid
Brand names: Biorphen, Disipal

Procyclidine

General information: Procyclidine is used for Parkinson's disease and also for Parkinson-like symptoms induced by some antipsychotics (see page 40).

How to use: As drugs used for Parkinson's disease (see page 52).
Precautions, side effects, warnings, interactions: As benzhexol (see page 52).
Available preparations: Tablets, liquid, injection
Brand names: Arpicolin, Kemadrin

Drugs which boost levels or mimic actions of dopamine

Amantadine

General information: Amantadine is used for Parkinson's disease. It is also used in the treatment and prevention of respiratory infections caused by influenza A virus (see page 269).

How to use: As drugs used for Parkinson's disease (see page 52).
Precautions: Tell your doctor if you have epilepsy, heart, kidney or liver problems or peptic ulcer.
Side effects: Side effects with this drug are not common, but the following may occur: nervousness, agitation, inability to concentrate, insomnia, dizziness, convulsions, gastrointestinal disturbances, rashes, swelling of hands, legs and feet.
Warnings: Do not drive or take part in any activity that requires you to be alert until you know how you react to the medicine. Do not drink a lot of alcohol (no more than a glass of wine or a pint of beer each day).
Interactions: There are no potentially serious interactions with amantadine. However, always check with your doctor or pharmacist if you are taking other medication.
Available preparations: Capsules, syrup
Brand names: Symmetrel

Apomorphine

General information: Apomorphine is used for Parkinson's disease, where other drugs have not provided adequate control of the disease. The drug is started in hospital and given by injection.

How to use: As drugs used for Parkinson's disease (see page 52).
Precautions: Tell your doctor if you have epilepsy, heart, breathing or kidney problems or a history of mental illness.
Side effects: Side effects are quite common and may include the following: nausea and vomiting, muscle spasms and clumsiness, dizziness and falls, confusion, hallucinations, drowsiness, restlessness, trembling.
Warnings: Do not drink alcohol because this will increase the sedative effect of the medicine. Do not drive or take part in any activity which requires you to be alert until you know how you react to the medicine.
Interactions: There are no important interactions with this drug.
Available preparations: Injection
Brand names: Britaject

Bromocriptine

General information: Bromocriptine is used for Parkinson's disease and also for various hormonal disorders (see page 190).

How to use: As drugs for Parkinson's disease (see page 52).
Precautions: Tell your doctor if you have problems with your circulation, a stomach ulcer or a history of mental illness.

Side effects: Side effects are quite common, and include: nausea, vomiting, constipation, dizziness, headache, abnormal movements, drowsiness, confusion.

Warnings: Do not drink alcohol because this will increase the sedative effect of the medicine. Dizziness (which may lead to falls) can sometimes be a problem during the first few days of using this medicine. Do not drive or take part in any activity that requires you to be alert until you know how you react to the medicine.

Interactions: Bromocriptine interacts with a few other drugs. This includes some ingredients, such as ephedrine, phenylephrine, pseudoephedrine and phenyl-propanolamine, which are found in certain over-the-counter cough and cold medicines. Tell your pharmacist if you are taking bromocriptine.

Available preparations: Tablets, capsules

Brand names: Parlodel

Cabergoline

General information: Cabergoline is used for Parkinson's disease and also for various hormonal disorders (see page 191).

How to use: As drugs for Parkinson's disease (see page 52).

Precautions, side effects, warnings, interactions: As bromocriptine (see page 54). In addition, tell your doctor if you have liver problems. Stomach pain and dyspepsia are common side effects.

Available preparations: Tablets

Brand names: Cabaser

Co-beneldopa

General information: Co-beneldopa is used for Parkinson's disease. It contains levodopa in combination with benserazide. Benserazide increases the level of levodopa in the brain. This means that the same dose of levodopa can be used without increasing the risk of side effects.

How to use: See drugs for Parkinson's disease (see page 52).

Precautions, side effects, warnings, interactions: As levodopa (see page 56).

Available preparations: Tablets, capsules

Brand names: Madopar, Madopar CR

Co-careldopa

General information: Co-careldopa is used for Parkinson's disease. It contains levodopa in combination with carbidopa. Carbidopa increases the level of levodopa in the brain. This means that the same dose of levodopa can be used without increasing the risk of side effects.

How to use: As drugs for Parkinson's disease (see page 52).

Precautions, side effects, warnings, interactions: As levodopa (see page 56).

Available preparations: Tablets

Brand names: Sinemet, Sinemet LS, Sinemet-Plus, Sinemet CR, Half Sinemet CR

Entacapone

General information: Entacapone is used in Parkinson's disease when either co-beneldopa or co–careldopa do not produce an adequate response. Entacapone prolongs the response to levodopa in the brain by interfering with enzymes that break down levodopa.

How to use: As drugs for Parkinson's disease (see page 52).
Precautions: Tell your doctor if you have or have had liver disease or phaeocromocytoma.
Side effects: The most common side effects are related to an increase in the action of levodopa and include abnormal movements and confusion. Other side effects include diarrhoea, nausea, vomiting and abdominal pains.
Warnings: Do not drive or take part in any activity that requires you to be alert until you know how you react to the medicine.
Interactions: Levodopa interacts with several drugs, in particular with monamine oxidase inhibitors (MAOIs).
Available preparations: Tablets
Brand names: Comtess

Levodopa

General information: Levodopa is used for Parkinson's disease.

How to use: As drugs for Parkinson's disease (see page 52).
Precautions: Tell your doctor if you have or have had glaucoma, lung disease or breathing problems, skin cancer, stomach ulcer, heart problems, diabetes, kidney problems or severe mental illness.
Side effects: Side effects are common and include upset stomach, vomiting, insomnia, agitation, dizziness (which may lead to falls), abnormal movements, confusion, vivid dreams, drowsiness, headache. Levodopa may cause your urine to be reddish in colour.
Warnings: Do not drive or take part in any activity that requires you to be alert until you know how you react to the medicine.
Interactions: Levodopa interacts with several drugs, in particular with monamine oxidase inhibitors (MAOIs). In addition, do not take any vitamin or mineral supplements without checking with your doctor or pharmacist. This is because iron and vitamin B6 can reduce the effect of levodopa.
Available preparations: Tablets
Brand names: None

Lysuride

General information: Lysuride is used for Parkinson's disease.

How to use: As drugs for Parkinson's disease (see page 52).
Precautions: Tell your doctor if you have or have had heart or circulatory problems, tumour of the pituitary gland, mental illness, porphyria.
Side effects: Side effects are quite common and include nausea, vomiting, dizziness, drowsiness and lethargy, hallucinations, abnormal movements and confusion.

Warnings: Do not drink alcohol because this will increase the sedative effect of the medicine. Dizziness (which may lead to falls) can sometimes be a problem during the first few days of using this medicine. Do not drive or take part in any activity that requires you to be alert until you know how you react to the medicine.

Interactions: Lysuride interacts with very few drugs. However, always check with your doctor or pharmacist before taking other medicines.

Available preparations: Tablets

Brand names: Revanil

Pergolide

General information: Pergolide is used for Parkinson's disease. It binds to dopamine receptors and so mimics the effects of dopamine.

How to use: See drugs for Parkinson's disease (see page 52).

Precautions: Tell your doctor if you have or have ever had heart or circulatory problems or mental illness.

Side effects: Side effects are quite common and include confusion, abnormal movements, dizziness, hallucinations, stomach pain, nausea, heartburn, insomnia, constipation, diarrhoea, rash, runny nose.

Warnings: Do not drink alcohol because this will increase the sedative effect of the medicine. Dizziness (which may lead to falls) can sometimes be a problem during the first few days of using this medicine. Do not drive or take part in any activity that requires you to be alert until you know how you react to the medicine.

Interactions: Pergolide interacts with very few drugs. However, always check with your doctor or pharmacist before taking other medicines.

Available preparations: Tablets

Brand names: Celance

Ropinirole

General information: Ropinirole is used for Parkinson's disease. It acts on the dopamine receptor to mimic the effect of dopamine.

How to use: See drugs used for Parkinson's disease (see page 52).

Precautions: Tell your doctor if you have or have had liver or kidney problems, heart problems or severe mental illness.

Side effects: Side effects are quite common and include nausea, drowsiness, swelling of the legs, stomach pain, vomiting, abnormal movements, hallucinations and confusion.

Warnings: Do not drink alcohol because this will increase the sedative effect of the medicine. Dizziness (which may lead to falls) can sometimes be a problem during the first few days of using this medicine. Do not drive or take part in any activity that requires you to be alert until you know how you react to the medicine.

Interactions: Always check with your doctor or pharmacist before taking other medicines.

Available preparations: Tablets

Brand names: Requip

Selegeline

General information: Selegeline is used for Parkinson's disease. It works by interfering with dopamine breakdown, so boosting levels of the neurotransmitter.

How to use: As drugs used for Parkinson's disease (see page 52).

Precautions: Tell your doctor if you have or have had heart problems or mental illness.

Side effects: Side effects are common and include: dizziness, nausea, vomiting, confusion, agitation, dry mouth, difficulty in passing urine and rash.

Warnings: Do not drive or take part in any activity that requires you to be alert until you know how you react to the medicine.

Interactions: Selegeline interacts with antidepressants and pethidine. Always check with your doctor or pharmacist before taking other medicines.

Available preparations: Tablets, liquid

Brand names: Eldepryl, Zelapar

DRUGS FOR ALZHEIMER'S DISEASE

Drugs for Alzheimer's disease have not been available for very long. Like most other drugs which act on the nervous system, they work by altering the levels of chemical neurotransmitters – in this case, by inhibiting an enzyme called acetylcholinesterase that breaks down the neurotransmitter acetylcholine and thus enhances its action. Antipsychotic drugs (see page 40) may be used in low doses to deal with restlessness or difficulty in sleeping.

Donepezil

General information: Donepezil is used to treat signs of dementia in Alzheimer's disease.

How to use: Take the medicine exactly as prescribed by the doctor. If you miss a dose, take it as soon as you remember. Do not stop taking the medicine without checking with your doctor because symptoms may recur.

Precautions: Tell your doctor if you have or have had heart problems, stomach ulcer, asthma or any other lung disease.

Side effects: Side effects are quite common and include nausea, vomiting, diarrhoea, tiredness, insomnia, muscle cramps, headache and dizziness.

Warnings: Your underlying condition as well as taking this drug may make it inadvisable to drive and take part in other activities that require you to be alert.

Interactions: Donepezil may interact with other drugs. Check with your doctor or pharmacist before taking any other medicines.

Available preparations: Tablets

Brand names: Aricept

Rivastigmine

General information: Rivastigmine is used for signs of dementia in Alzheimer's disease.

How to use: Take the medicine exactly as prescribed by the doctor. If you miss a dose, take it as soon as you remember. Do not stop taking the medicine without checking with your doctor because symptoms may recur.

Precautions: Tell your doctor if you have or have had heart problems, liver or kidney problems, stomach ulcer, asthma or any other lung disease.

Side effects: Side effects are quite common and include nausea, vomiting, diarrhoea, heartburn, weight loss, drowsiness, insomnia, agitation and confusion, trembling, headache, sweating.

Warnings: Your underlying condition as well as taking this drug may make it inadvisable to drive and take part in other activities that require you to be alert.

Interactions: Rivastigmine may interact with other drugs. Check with your doctor or pharmacist before taking any other medicines.

Available preparations: Capsules

Brand names: Exelon

ANALGESICS (PAINKILLERS)

Analgesics are drugs that help to relieve pain. There are three main groups of analgesics: non-opioid analgesics (eg paracetamol, nefopam), opioid analgesics (eg morphine, pethidine) and non-steroidal anti-inflammatory drugs (NSAIDs). Aspirin is strictly an NSAID, but because it is commonly used as an alternative to paracetamol for most types of pain (including headache, toothache, period pain and rheumatic pain), it is covered in this section. Other NSAIDs, which tend to be used for rheumatic pain, arthritis and muscular aches and pains, are found in the musculoskeletal section (see page 146).

Non-opioid analgesics

Both aspirin and paracetamol are used in the treatment of a wide variety of painful conditions, and products containing these drugs are obtainable over the counter as well as on prescription. Nefopam is a stronger painkiller than either aspirin or paracetamol and is therefore used in more severe pain such as that associated with surgery, cancer, injury or severe toothache. Aspirin works by blocking the production of chemical transmitters known as prostaglandins. Prostaglandins stimulate pain receptors and the signals generated are passed to the brain. Aspirin is an effective analgesic and it reduces inflammation and brings down temperature when there is a fever. Paracetamol is also thought to act by blocking the action of prostaglandins, but it does this only in the central nervous system while aspirin has an effect in both the central and peripheral nervous systems. Nefopam appears to have an action on pain receptors in the brain, but its precise mode of action is unclear.

How to use: Take the medicine exactly as prescribed by the doctor. If you miss a dose, take it as soon as you remember. However, if it is almost time for your next dose, skip the missed dose. Do not take double the dose. Unless the medicine has been prescribed for long term use (eg aspirin for prevention of blood clots), it can safely be stopped at any time.

Precautions, side effects, warnings, interactions: See individual drugs.

Aspirin

General information: Aspirin is used for mild to moderate pain and reduction of fever and inflammation in a variety of medical conditions such as headache, muscle and joint pain, period pain and toothache. It is also used to help prevent blood from clotting (see page 104) and to reduce the risk of a second heart attack or stroke.

How to use: As non-opioid analgesics (see page 59).
Precautions: Tell your doctor (or your pharmacist if buying aspirin over the counter) if you are pregnant, planning to become pregnant or are breastfeeding, or if you have or have had asthma, allergies, liver or kidney problems, stomach ulcer, haemophilia or any other blood clotting disorder, or glucose-6-phosphate dehydrogenase (G6PD) deficiency.
Side effects: Stomach irritation, particularly heartburn, is quite common with aspirin. This can be avoided or reduced by taking the medicine with food or milk. Other possible side effects include allergic reactions such as rash and breathlessness or wheezing.
Warnings: Never give aspirin to a child under the age of 12 years. A large number of over-the-counter remedies contain aspirin. Do not take any of these if you have been prescribed aspirin by your doctor. Aspirin increases the risk of bleeding so if you need any surgery, tell your doctor or dentist that you are taking aspirin.
Interactions: Aspirin can influence the effects of anticoagulants (eg warfarin) and drugs used for gout. Always check with your doctor or pharmacist before taking other medicines.
Available preparations: Tablets, soluble tablets, suppositories
Brand names: An enormous variety of aspirin preparations is available over the counter.
Combination preparations: Benoral (a mixture of aspirin and paracetamol, known as benorylate)

Paracetamol

General information: Paracetamol is used for mild to moderate pain and reduction of fever and inflammation in a variety of medical conditions such as headache, muscle and joint pain, period pain and toothache.

How to use: As non-opioid analgesics (see page 59).
Precautions: Tell your doctor (or your pharmacist if buying paracetamol over the counter) if you think you have liver or kidney problems.
Side effects: Side effects are rare, but rash may occur.

Warnings: Never give paracetamol to a baby under the age of 3 months unless advised by your doctor. Never take more than the prescribed dose (or follow the instructions on the packet if bought over the counter), because this can lead to liver damage and occasionally to kidney damage. Prolonged and excessive alcohol intake can increase the effects of paracetamol on the liver. An enormous number of over-the-counter products (eg analgesics, cold, cough and flu remedies) contain paracetamol. Do not take any of these if you have been prescribed paracetamol by your doctor.

Interactions: Paracetamol can influence the effects of some drugs (eg anticoagulants, zidovudine). Always check with your doctor or pharmacist before taking other medicines.

Available preparations: Tablets, soluble tablets, liquid, suppositories. Paracetamol is also found in several combination preparations with other analgesics. These preparations include paracetamol with codeine (co-codamol), paracetamol with dihydrocodeine (co-dydramol) and paracetamol with dextropropoxyphene (co-proxamol). Paracetamol is also made in combination with methionine. Methionine has no analgesic activity, but it helps to prevent liver toxicity if paracetamol is taken in overdose.

Brand names: An enormous variety of preparations containing paracetamol, either alone or in combination with other ingredients. is available over the counter.

Combination preparations available on prescription only include: Fortagesic (paracetamol, pentazocine), Kapake (co-codamol), Solpadol (co-codamol), Tylex (co-codamol).

Nefopam

General information: Nefopam is used for moderate pain.

How to use: As non-opioid analgesics (see page 59).

Precautions: Tell your doctor if you are pregnant, planning to become pregnant or are breastfeeding, or if you have heart problems, liver or kidney problems, problems passing urine, or epilepsy.

Side effects: Side effects are quite common and include nausea, nervousness, problems passing urine, dry mouth, dizziness, blurred vision, palpitations, drowsiness, headache, insomnia, sweating.

Warnings: Do not drink alcohol because this will increase the sedative effect of the medicine. Do not drive or take part in any activity that requires you to be alert until you know how you react to the medicine.

Interactions: Nefopam interacts with antidepressants (including tricyclics and monoamine oxidase inhibitors).

Available preparations: Tablets, injection

Brand names: Acupan

Opioid analgesics

The opioid analgesics, as the name suggests, were originally derived from opium. They are the most powerful painkillers available and are generally reserved for severe pain associated with chronic conditions such as cancer. They are sometimes given to reduce the pain of a heart attack and following severe injury or surgery. There are 17 of these drugs available and which one is prescribed depends on the severity of the pain, and your response to the drug in terms of its effectiveness and side effects. Opioid analgesics work by stimulating pain receptors in the brain. These receptors interpret the message of pain coming from a part of the body that is injured or diseased.

How to use: Opioids are often prescribed to be taken as needed, particularly for very severe pain. Follow the instructions your doctor has given you and check again if you feel you need more than the prescribed dose to relieve pain. Pain is easier to control if the drug is taken regularly. If you miss a dose, take it as soon as you remember. However, if it is almost time for your next dose, skip the missed dose. Do not take double the dose. Check with your doctor if you want to stop taking the drug, because stopping abruptly can cause withdrawal symptoms.

Precautions: Tell your doctor if you are pregnant, planning to become pregnant or breastfeeding, or if you have or have had breathing problems or lung disease, heart problems, prostate problems, thyroid disease or liver or kidney problems.

Side effects: The frequency and severity of side effects – particularly the level of sedation they cause – varies between the different drugs. Nausea and vomiting are common with most of them, especially in the early days, and other drugs are sometimes given to counteract these effects. Other side effects include constipation, drowsiness, breathing difficulties, difficulty in passing urine, dizziness, confusion, rashes, headache, sweating, palpitations, euphoria, hallucinations and mood changes. In addition, these drugs can cause dependence.

Warnings: Do not drink alcohol because this will increase the sedative effect of the medicine. Do not drive or take part in any activity that requires you to be alert until you know how you react to the medicine.

Interactions: Other sedative medicines (eg drugs used for anxiety, insomnia, antidepressants and antihistamines) increase the effects of opioid analgesics. Always check with your doctor or pharmacist before taking any other medicines.

Buprenorphine

General information: Buprenorphine is used for severe pain and premedication before surgery. Vomiting is a particular problem with this drug.

Available preparations: Tablets, injection
Brand names: Temgesic

Codeine

General information: Codeine is used for mild to moderate pain. Constipation is a particular problem with this drug, but other side effects are less than those of some of the stronger drugs in this group.

Available preparations: Tablets, liquid, injection
Brand names: None

Dextromoramide

General information: Dextromoramide is used for severe pain. It tends to be less sedating than morphine.

Available preparations: Tablets, suppositories
Brand names: Palfium

Dextropropoxyphene

General information: Dextropropoxyphene is used for mild to moderate pain.

Available preparations: Capsules. Also contained in combination preparations with paracetamol (see page 60).
Brand names: Doloxene

Diamorphine

General information: Diamorphine is used for severe pain. It tends to cause less nausea than morphine.

Available preparations: Tablets, injection

Dihydrocodeine

General information: Dihydrocodeine is used for moderate to severe pain.

Available preparations: Tablets, liquid, injection
Brand names: DF118, DHC Continus

Dipipanone

General information: Dipipanone is used for moderate to severe pain.

Available preparations: Tablets
Brand names: Diconal

Fentanyl

General information: Fentanyl is used for severe pain due to cancer. This drug has a long duration of action and you may experience side effects for up to 72 hours after stopping it.

Available preparations: Patches
Brand names: Durogesic

Hydromorphone

General information: Hydromorphone is used for severe pain in cancer.

Available preparations: Capsules
Brand names: Palladone, Palladone SR

Meptazinol

General information: Meptazinol is used for moderate to severe pain, including post-operative pain and pain in childbirth. It is also used as premedication before surgery.

Available preparations: Tablets, injection
Brand names: Meptid

Methadone

General information: Methadone is used for severe pain and in the treatment of dependence on drugs such as heroin. It is less sedating than morphine.

Available preparations: Tablets, liquid, injection

Morphine

General information: Morphine is considered to be the most powerful opioid analgesic, although it frequently causes nausea and vomiting. It is the gold standard by which all the others are judged. It is used for severe pain and as premedication before surgery.

Available preparations: Tablets, liquid, injection
Brand names: Cyclimorph, Morcap SR, MST, MXL, Oramorph, Oramorph SR, Sevredol, Zomorph

Nalbuphine

General information: Nalbuphine is used for severe pain. It is as effective as morphine, but may lead to fewer side effects.

Available preparations: Injection
Brand names: Nubain

Pentazocine

General information: Pentazocine is used for moderate to severe pain, but it is prescribed infrequently because it has a particular risk of causing hallucinations.

Available preparations: Tablets, capsules, suppositories, injection
Brand names: Fortral

Pethidine

General information: Pethidine is used for moderate to severe pain, including that associated with childbirth.

Available preparations: Tablets, injection
Brand names: Pamergan P100

Phenazocine

General information: Phenazocine is used for severe pain.

Available preparations: Tablets
Brand names: Narphen

Tramadol

General information: Tramadol is used for moderate to severe pain.

Available preparations: Tablets, soluble tablets, capsules, sachets
Brand names: Tramake Insts, Zamadol, Zamadol SR, Zydol, Zydol SR

DRUGS USED IN MIGRAINE

Drugs can be used two ways in migraine. Firstly, they can be used to treat an attack once it has come on, and secondly, drugs can be used to prevent attacks from occurring.

Drugs used in the treatment of migraine attacks include analgesics such as aspirin and paracetamol (see page 60). Migraine is often accompanied by symptoms of sickness and some preparations used to treat migraine contain an ingredient (eg buclizine, domperidone, metoclopramide) which helps to relieve nausea and vomiting. Other drugs used in migraine treatment include ergotamine and the $5HT_1$ agonists (eg sumatriptan).

Drugs used to prevent migraine attacks include the beta-blockers (eg propranolol, metoprolol, nadolol and timolol – see pages 82-86), clonidine (see page 69), methysergide (see page 69), pizotifen (see page 70), the tricyclic antidepressants (see page 32) and valproate (see page 51).

Analgesic combinations

General information: Combination preparations for migraine contain an analgesic (aspirin, paracetamol, codeine) with a drug to combat nausea and vomiting.

Available preparations: Tablets, sachets
Brand names: Domperamol (paracetamol with domperidone); Migraleve (paracetamol, codeine, buclizine), Migravess (aspirin, metoclopramide), Paramax (paracetamol, metoclopramide)

Dihydroergotamine

General information: A nasal spray containing this drug has recently become available for the treatment of migraine attacks.

Uses, precautions, side effects, warnings and interactions: As ergotamine (see below). In addition, the nasal spray may cause a runny or stuffy nose.
Available preparations: Nasal spray
Brand names: Migranal

Ergotamine

General information: Ergotamine is used in the treatment of migraine attacks when analgesics fail to work. It can help the pain, but has no effect on any of the other symptoms. It must be used early on in an attack – if used later, the drug can make the nausea and vomiting worse. One of the features of migraine is that the blood vessels in the scalp dilate and ergotamine works by narrowing these blood vessels.

How to use: Use this medicine at the first sign of a migraine attack. Take the medicine exactly as prescribed. Read the label on your medicine very carefully and do not exceed the stated dose. You must not exceed a certain number of doses in 24 hours and a certain number of doses in one week.
Precautions: Tell your doctor if you are pregnant, planning to become pregnant or are breastfeeding, or if you have or have had heart or circulatory problems, liver or kidney problems, thyroid disease, high blood pressure or a stroke.
Side effects: Common side effects with ergotamine include upset stomach and vomiting.
Warnings: As how to use (see above).
Interactions: Ergotamine interacts with some antibiotics (eg erythromycin) and with $5HT_1$ agonists (eg sumatriptan).
Available preparations: Tablets, inhaler, suppositories
Brand names: Cafergot, Lingraine, Medihaler-Ergotamine, Migril

Isometheptene

General information: Isometheptene is used in the treatment of migraine attack.

How to use: Use this medicine at the first sign of a migraine attack. Take the medicine exactly as prescribed. Read the label very carefully and do not exceed the stated dose.

Precautions: Tell your doctor if you are pregnant, planning to become pregnant or are breastfeeding, or if you have or have had heart or circulatory problems, liver or kidney problems, thyroid disease, diabetes, porphyria, high blood pressure or a stroke.

Side effects: Dizziness, rashes

Warnings: As how to use (see page 66).

Interactions: Isometheptene can interact with a number of other drugs, including antidepressants and those used in high blood pressure and other heart conditions.

Available preparations: Capsules

Brand names: Midrid

Naratriptan

General information: Naratriptan is a $5HT_1$ agonist and is used in the treatment of migraine attack. It mimics the effect of the neurotransmitter 5-hydroxytryptamine and this helps to narrow the blood vessels in the scalp and so to reduce the pain of migraine.

How to use: The medicine should be used at the first sign of a migraine attack. Take it exactly as prescribed. Usually only one dose is needed, although the dose may be repeated after 4 hours if your doctor says so.

Precautions: Tell your doctor if you are pregnant, planning to become pregnant or are breastfeeding, or if you have a heart condition or high blood pressure or liver problems.

Side effects: Pain or tightness in the chest or throat, tingling feeling, flushing, feeling of warmth or heaviness, nausea and vomiting, dizziness.

Warnings: Stop the medicine and call your doctor if you experience pain and tightness in the chest or any allergic symptoms such as difficulty in breathing, wheezing, rash, swelling, redness or itching of the eye lids, face or lips.

Interactions: Naratriptan interacts with antidepressants, lithium and ergotamine.

Available preparations: Tablets

Brand names: Naramig

Rizatriptan

General information: Rizatriptan is a $5HT_1$ agonist (see naratriptan) and is used in the treatment of migraine attack.

How to use: The medicine should be used at the first sign of a migraine attack. Take it exactly as prescribed. Usually only one dose is needed, although the dose may be repeated if your doctor says so.

Precautions, side effects, warnings, interactions: As naratriptan (see above).

Available preparations: Tablets, wafers

Brand names: Maxalt

Sumatriptan

General information: Sumatriptan is a $5HT_1$ agonist (see naratriptan) and is used in the treatment of migraine attack.

How to use: The medicine should be used at the first sign of a migraine attack. Take it exactly as prescribed. Usually only one dose is needed, although the dose may be repeated if your doctor says so.
Precautions, side effects, warnings, interactions: As naratriptan (see page 67).
Available preparations: Tablets, nasal spray, injection
Brand names: Imigran

Tolfenamic acid

General information: Tolfenamic acid is a non-steroidal anti-inflammatory drug (NSAID) used in the treatment of migraine attack.

How to use: The medicine should be used at the first sign of a migraine attack. Take it exactly as prescribed. Usually only one dose is needed, although the dose may be repeated after 1–2 hours if your doctor says so.
Precautions: Tell your doctor if you think you are pregnant, planning to become pregnant or breastfeeding, or if you have or have had asthma, haemophilia or other blood clotting disorder, stomach ulcer or liver or kidney problems.
Side effects: These may include nausea, vomiting, heartburn, indigestion, wheezing, breathlessness or rash.
Warnings: Stop taking the medicine and call the doctor if you experience rash or breathing problems.
Interactions: Tolfenamic acid interacts with a wide range of drugs including aspirin, other NSAIDs, oral anticoagulants, lithium, corticosteroids and drugs used for high blood pressure.
Available preparations: Tablets
Brand names: Clotam

Zolmitriptan

General information: Zolmitriptan is a $5HT_1$ agonist (see naratriptan) and is used in the treatment of migraine attack.

How to use: The medicine should be used at the first sign of a migraine attack. Take it exactly as prescribed. Usually only one dose is needed, although the dose may be repeated after 2 hours if your doctor says so.
Precautions, side effects, warnings, interactions: As naratriptan (see page 67).
Available preparations: Tablets
Brand names: Zomig

Drugs used to prevent migraine

Brand names: Drugs used to prevent migraine attacks include the beta-blockers (eg propranolol, metoprolol, nadolol and timolol – see pages 82-86), clonidine (see below), methysergide (see below), pizotifen (see page 70), the tricyclic antidepressants (see page 32) and valproate (see page 51).

Clonidine

General information: Clonidine is used to prevent migraine attacks, but is prescribed far less frequently than it was a few years ago. It is also used – again infrequently – in hypertension (high blood pressure), menopausal flushing and vascular headache.

How to use: Take the medicine exactly as prescribed by your doctor. If you miss a dose, take it as soon as you remember. However, if it is almost time for your next dose, skip the missed dose. Do not take double the dose. Do not stop taking the medicine without checking with your doctor.

Precautions: Tell your doctor if you are pregnant, planning to become pregnant or are breastfeeding, or if you have or have had circulatory problems, depression or porphyria.

Side effects: These may include dry mouth, drowsiness, dizziness, nausea, rash and restlessness.

Warnings: Do not drink alcohol because this will increase the sedative effect of the medicine. Do not drive or take part in any activity that requires you to be alert until you know how you react to the medicine.

Interactions: Clonidine interacts with antidepressants and beta-blockers. Always check with your doctor or pharmacist before taking other medicines.

Available preparations: Tablets

Brand names: Dixarit

Methysergide

General information: Methysergide is used to prevent severe migraine attacks, but only under hospital supervision and is now used very rarely.

How to use: Take the medicine exactly as prescribed by your doctor. If you miss a dose, take it as soon as you remember. However, if it is almost time for your next dose, skip the missed dose. Do not take double the dose. Do not stop taking the medicine without checking with your doctor.

Precautions: Tell your doctor if you are pregnant, planning to become pregnant or are breastfeeding, or if you have or have had heart problems, lung disease or breathing problems, liver or kidney problems, prostate trouble or problems passing urine.

Warnings: Do not drink alcohol because this will increase the sedative effect of the medicine. Do not drive or take part in any activity that requires you to be alert until you know how you react to the medicine.

Available preparations: Tablets

Brand names: Deseril

Pizotifen

General information: Pizotifen is used to prevent migraine attacks.

How to use: Take the medicine exactly as prescribed by your doctor. If you miss a dose, take it as soon as you remember. However, if it is almost time for your next dose, skip the missed dose. Do not take double the dose. Do not stop taking the medicine without checking with your doctor.

Precautions: Tell your doctor if you are pregnant, planning to become pregnant or are breastfeeding, or if you have or have had glaucoma, kidney problems, prostate trouble or problems passing urine.

Warnings: Do not drink alcohol because this will increase the sedative effect of the medicine. Do not drive or take part in any activity that requires you to be alert until you know how you react to the medicine.

Available preparations: Tablets, liquid

Brand names: Sanomigran

DRUGS USED IN NAUSEA AND DIZZINESS

Drugs used to suppress nausea and vomiting are known as anti-emetics. These drugs are used in the prevention and treatment of travel sickness and several products are available over the counter for this purpose. Anti-emetics are also used in the vomiting associated with chronic disease such as cancer and the sickness caused by various drugs such as opioid analgesics (see page 62) and anti-cancer drugs. Anti-emetics are only very rarely prescribed to treat pregnancy sickness.

Drugs used as anti-emetics include chlorpromazine, perphenazine, prochlorperazine and trifluoperazine – drugs which are also used in the treatment of schizophrenia (see page 40). Other drugs include various antihistamines, some of which are available over the counter, and also domperidone and metoclopramide. In recent years, a new group of drugs – the $5HT_3$ antagonists – has been developed. These drugs are used principally in the treatment of vomiting caused by anti-cancer drugs and after surgery.

Nausea and vomiting are caused by stimulation of an area of the brain called the vomiting centre. The vomiting centre receives signals from various parts of the body (eg the blood, the intestine, the middle ear) and if the vomiting centre detects a problem, you may be physically sick. Anti-emetic drugs work – in slightly different ways – to suppress the signals received by the vomiting centre and so to prevent you from being sick.

Betahistine

General information: Betahistine is used for the treatment of nausea and dizziness and hearing loss associated with Ménière's disease.

How to use: Take the medicine as prescribed. If you miss a dose, take it as soon as you remember. However, if it is almost time for your next dose, skip the missed dose. Do not take double the dose. Do not stop taking the medicine without asking your doctor because symptoms may recur.

Precautions: Tell your doctor if you are pregnant, planning to become pregnant or breastfeeding, or if you have or have had asthma, stomach ulcer or phaeocromocytoma.

Side effects: Side effects are uncommon, but the following may occur: nausea, indigestion, headache, rash.

Warnings: None

Interactions: None

Available preparations: Tablets

Brand names: Serc

Cinnarizine

General information: Cinnarizine is an antihistamine used in the treatment of travel sickness and the nausea and dizziness associated with inner ear (vestibular) disorders, such as Ménière's disease.

How to use: If taking the medicine for travel sickness, take 2 hours before your journey and repeat every 8 hours if necessary. Stop taking the medicine at the end of the journey. If taking the medicine on a longer term basis (eg for dizziness caused by an inner ear disorder), take any missed dose as soon as you remember. However, if it is almost time for your next dose, skip the missed dose. Do not take double the dose.

Precautions: Tell your doctor if you are pregnant, planning to become pregnant or breastfeeding, or if you have or have had glaucoma, prostate problems or liver problems.

Side effects: Drowsiness, occasional dry mouth and blurred vision. Allergic skin reactions may occur. Tremor and shakiness may occur in elderly people if they are taking the medicine for a long period of time.

Warnings: Do not drink alcohol because this will increase the sedative effect of the medicine. Do not drive or take part in any activity that requires you to be alert until you know how you react to the medicine.

Interactions: Other sedative medicines (eg drugs used for anxiety, insomnia, antidepressants and other antihistamines) increase the effects of antihistamines. Several over-the-counter medicines (eg remedies for coughs, colds, hayfever and travel sickness) contain sedatives, so always tell your pharmacist if you are taking antihistamines.

Available preparations: Tablets

Brand names: Stugeron

Cyclizine

General information: Cyclizine is an antihistamine used in the treatment of travel sickness and the nausea and dizziness associated with inner ear disorders such as Ménière's disease.

Use, precautions, side effects, warnings, interactions: As cinnarizine (see above).

Available preparations: Tablets, injection

Brand names: Valoid

Dimenhydrinate

General information: Dimenhydrinate is an antihistamine used in the treatment of travel sickness and the nausea and dizziness associated with inner ear disorders such as Ménière's disease.

Use, precautions, side effects, warnings, interactions: As cinnarizine (see above). For travel sickness, take the first dose 30 minutes before your journey.
Available preparations: Tablets
Brand names: Dramamine

Domperidone

General information: Domperidone is used in nausea and vomiting, including that induced by drugs such as anti-cancer drugs. It is also used to relieve symptoms of heartburn, stomach pain, bloating and a persistent feeling of fullness after meals.

How to use: Take the medicine as prescribed. If you miss a dose, take it as soon as you remember. However, if it is almost time for your next dose, skip the missed dose. Do not take double the dose. You can stop taking this medicine as soon as you feel better.
Precautions: Tell your doctor if you are pregnant, planning to become pregnant or breastfeeding, or if you have or have had kidney problems.
Side effects: Side effects are rare, but the following may occur: breast enlargement and milk production, muscle spasms, reduced sexual ability, rash.
Warnings: None
Interactions: There are a few possible interactions with domperidone. Check with your doctor or pharmacist before taking any other medicine.
Available preparations: Tablets, liquid, suppositories
Brand names: Motilium

Granisetron

General information: Granisetron is a $5HT_3$ receptor antagonist used in the treatment of nausea and vomiting induced by chemotherapy, radiotherapy, or following surgery.

How to use: Take the medicine as prescribed. If you miss a dose, take it as soon as you remember. However, if it is almost time for your next dose, skip the missed dose. Do not take double the dose. You can stop taking this medicine as soon as you feel better.
Precautions: Tell your doctor if you are pregnant, planning to become pregnant or breastfeeding.
Side effects: Side effects are not common, but the following may occur: constipation, headache, rash and other allergic reactions.
Warnings: None

Interactions: None reported, but check with your doctor or pharmacist before taking any other medicines.
Available preparations: Tablets, liquid, injection
Brand names: Kytril

Hyoscine

General information: Hyoscine is used in travel sickness, irritable bowel syndrome (see page 116) and also as premedication before surgery.

How to use: Hyoscine comes in the form of a patch for travel sickness. Use exactly as prescribed by the doctor. Always wash your hands after handling the patch, wash the application site after removing the patch and use only one patch at a time.
Precautions: Tell your doctor if you are pregnant, planning to become pregnant or are breastfeeding, or if you have or have had glaucoma, prostate problems, heart problems or liver or kidney problems.
Side effects: Drowsiness is the most common side effect. Other side effects include dry mouth, dizziness, blurred vision, problems passing urine.
Warnings: Do not drink alcohol because this will increase the sedative effect of the medicine. Do not drive or take part in any activity that requires you to be alert until you know how you react to the medicine.
Interactions: Other sedative medicines (eg drugs used for anxiety, insomnia antidepressants and other antihistamines) increase the effects of antihistamines. Several over-the-counter medicines (eg remedies for coughs, colds, hayfever and travel sickness) contain sedatives, so always tell your pharmacist if you are taking hyoscine.
Available preparations: Skin patch. However, tablets are available over the counter.
Brand names: Scopoderm TTS

Meclozine

General information: Meclozine is an antihistamine used in the treatment of travel sickness.

Use, precautions, side effects, warnings, interactions: As cinnarizine (see page 71). For travel sickness, take the first dose the night before or one hour before your journey.
Available preparations: Tablets
Brand names: Sea Legs

Metoclopramide

General information: Metoclopramide is used in nausea and vomiting, including that induced by drugs such as anti-cancer drugs. It is also used to relieve symptoms of heartburn caused by hiatus hernia.

How to use: As domperidone (see page 72).

Precautions: As domperidone (see page 72).

Side effects: Drowsiness is the most common side effect with this drug. Other side effects include involuntary movements of the limbs or eyes and spasm of the neck face and jaw muscles, restlessness, diarrhoea and depression.

Warnings: Do not drink alcohol because this will increase the sedative effect of the medicine. Do not drive or take part in any activity that requires you to be alert until you know how you react to the medicine.

Interactions: A few drugs interact with metoclopramide. Check with your doctor or pharmacist before taking other medicines.

Available preparations: Tablets, capsules, liquid, injection

Brand names: Gastrobid, Gastromax, Maxolon, Maxolon SR

Ondansetron

General information: Ondansetron is a $5HT_3$ receptor antagonist used in the treatment of nausea and vomiting induced by chemotherapy, radiotherapy, or following surgery.

How to use: Take the medicine as prescribed. If you miss a dose, take it as soon as you remember. However, if it is almost time for your next dose, skip the missed dose. Do not take double the dose. You can stop taking this medicine as soon as you feel better.

Precautions: Tell your doctor if you are pregnant, planning to become pregnant or are breastfeeding, or if you have or have had severe liver problems.

Side effects: Side effects are not common, but the following may occur: constipation, headache, sensation of warmth or flushing, hiccups, rash and other allergic reactions. Involuntary movements may occur, but only rarely.

Warnings: None

Interactions: None

Available preparations: Tablets, liquid, suppositories, injection

Brand names: Zofran

Promethazine

General information: Promethazine is an antihistamine used in the treatment of travel sickness and the nausea and dizziness associated with inner ear disorders such as Ménière's disease.

Use, precautions, side effects, warnings, interactions: As cinnarizine (see page 71). For travel sickness, take the first dose the night before or one to two hours before your journey.

Available preparations: Tablets, liquid, injection

Brand names: Avomine, Phenergan

Tropisetron

General information: Tropisetron is a $5HT_3$ receptor antagonist used in the treatment of nausea and vomiting induced by chemotherapy, radiotherapy, or following surgery.

How to use: Take the medicine as prescribed. If you miss a dose, take it as soon as you remember. However, if it is almost time for your next dose, skip the missed dose. Do not take double the dose. You can stop taking this medicine as soon as you feel better.

Precautions: Tell your doctor if you are pregnant, planning to become pregnant or breastfeeding.

Side effects: Side effects are not common, but the following may occur: constipation, diarrhoea, headache, dizziness. Allergic reactions, such as chest tightness, flushing, breathing difficulties and rash may occur.

Warnings: None

Interactions: None

Available preparations: Capsules, injection

Brand names: Navoban

DRUGS FOR OBESITY

More than half of the UK population is now overweight and the number is increasing year by year. This is occurring in spite of the variety of reduced fat and low calorie foods and drinks. Indeed, as a nation our calorie intake has fallen since the 1950s, yet we are still growing fatter. Many theories have been put forward to help explain this, such as the ready availability of high-fat, high-sugar food that is all too easy to eat to excess. However, the most significant factor is likely to be lack of regular physical exercise. The healthiest way to lose weight is by a combination of a reduced calorie diet and increase in exercise.

Drugs have been used for obesity, but they have something of a chequered history, with several being withdrawn from the market because of serious side effects. Moreover, if the drug is stopped, there is a likelihood that weight will eventually be put on again. At the moment there are two drugs on the UK market prescribable for obesity, but there are several others in the pipeline.

Orlistat

General information: Orlistat is a newly introduced drug for obesity. It works by inhibiting the enzymes in the gut which absorb fat and therefore reduces fat absorption.

How to use: Take as prescribed. This drug should be taken immediately before, during or up to one hour after each main meal. If you miss a meal, or you eat a meal containing no fat, miss the dose.

Precautions: Tell your doctor if you are pregnant, planning to become pregnant or are breastfeeding, or if you have diabetes or liver or gastrointestinal problems.

Side effects: Common side effects include: increase in number, softness and urgency of bowel movements (possibly incontinence), fat in the faeces, wind and bloating. Other effects include: abdominal pain, wind, infection of the respiratory and urinary tracts, teeth and gum discomfort.
Warnings: None
Interactions: Orlistat interacts with several other drugs including some of those used for diabetes and cholesterol lowering.
Available preparations: Capsules
Brand names: Xenical

Phentermine

General information: Phentermine is available for the treatment of obesity, but is rarely prescribed because of the risk of serious side effects and because weight relapse often occurs.

Precautions: Tell your doctor if you are pregnant, planning to become pregnant or are breastfeeding, or if you have heart disease, including high blood pressure, glaucoma, thyroid problems, epilepsy, history of psychiatric disorders.
Side effects: Dry mouth, headaches and euphoria may occur, and it is possible to become dependent on this drug. Other side effects include insomnia, restlessness, agitation, nausea, vomiting, dizziness, depression, hallucinations, palpitations, constipation and increased frequency of passing urine. Tell your doctor immediately if you have any breathing difficulties while taking this medicine.
Warnings: Do not drink alcohol because this will increase the sedative effect of the medicine. Do not drive or take part in any activity which requires you to be alert until you know how you react to the medicine.
Interactions: Phentermine interacts with several other drugs, including antidepressants and drugs used for high blood pressure. Do not take any other medicines without checking with your doctor or pharmacist.
Available preparations: Capsules
Brand names: Duromine, Ionamin

The Cardiovascular System

THE CARDIOVASCULAR SYSTEM consists of the heart and blood vessels. The heart is situated in the centre of the chest, from where it pumps blood through the blood vessels; its main function is to supply oxygen to the body and get rid of waste (which is mostly carbon dioxide). The heart consists of four chambers – two ventricles and two atria. To make sure that blood flows in only one direction, the ventricles have an inlet and an outlet valve. With each beat of the heart, blood from the body tissues, depleted in oxygen and laden with carbon dioxide, enters the right atrium and progresses to the right ventricle. The right ventricle contracts, driving blood to the lungs where it offloads carbon dioxide and picks up oxygen. The oxygen-rich blood then flows to the left atrium and then into the left ventricle. This in turn contracts and sends blood to the rest of the body. The heart beat is set by and controlled by a pacemaker, called the sinoatrial node.

The rest of the cardiovascular system is composed of the blood vessels: the arteries, capillaries and veins. Strong and flexible, the arteries carry blood away from the heart and bear the highest blood pressure. The veins carry blood back to the heart, but they transport blood more slowly than the arteries and under lower pressure. The capillaries are tiny blood vessels that act as bridges in the body tissues between the arteries and the veins. Capillaries allow nutrients and oxygen to pass from the blood into the tissues, and waste products to pass from the tissues back into the blood.

An average-sized adult has about five litres (nearly nine pints) of blood in his or her body. The blood consists of two basic parts: the cells and the plasma. The red cells carry oxygen round the body, the white cells help to fight infection and the platelets help with the blood clotting process. Together these cells make up about 40 per cent of your blood and they are all made in the bone marrow. The rest of the blood is made up of plasma. Plasma carries nutrients, antibodies, hormones and waste material.

What can go wrong

Coronary heart disease is the most common problem. It is caused by the build up of fatty deposits in the arteries which lead to narrowing or the eventual blockage of the blood vessels that supply the heart (atherosclerosis). This reduces the supply of blood – and consequently of oxygen – to the heart, causing pain called angina, particularly when the heart is working hard, for example during exercise. Narrow arteries are also prone to blood clots and if a blood clot forms in the heart, this can lead to a heart attack (technically known as a myocardial infarction). If a blood clot forms in the brain, this can cause a stroke.

Another heart problem is arrhythmia or irregular heart beat. The contraction of the heart is controlled by an electrical discharge or current. Various problems can occur with this electrical flow, resulting in arrhythmias which range from the harmless to life-threatening. Arrhythmias can occur in otherwise healthy hearts, but their most common causes are coronary heart disease, abnormal heart valve function, heart failure and an overactive thyroid gland.

Heart (or cardiac) failure is a serious condition in which the quantity of blood pumped by the heart is insufficient to meet the body's demands for oxygen and nutrients. People with heart failure feel tired and weak when performing physical activity because their muscles are not getting enough oxygen. Heart failure also leads to fluid retention (oedema), the location of which depends on which side of the heart is most affected. Left-sided heart disease tends to cause build up of fluid in the lungs (pulmonary oedema), whilst right-sided disease leads to fluid build up in the feet, ankles and legs. Left- and right-sided heart failure commonly occur together, producing symptoms of breathlessness together with signs of fluid retention (oedema).

High blood pressure (hypertension) is a very common, but symptomless, condition, in which there is abnormally high blood pressure in the arteries. This accelerates the development of problems such as heart failure, heart attack, stroke and kidney damage. Blood pressure, especially in developed countries, increases with age, and this is taken into account in setting the normal range. The vast majority of patients have so-called essential hypertension where no underlying cause can be found. They often have relatives with high blood pressure, and the condition is also associated with obesity, alcohol, and possibly high salt consumption in the Western diet. As the disease develops, the smaller blood vessels lose their flexibility and the heart has to work hard and pump blood at higher pressure. About 10 per cent of patients may have underlying causes, including diabetes, kidney disease and other rarer conditions. Some women on the contraceptive pill may experience a rise in blood pressure, as may some women in pregnancy. Kidney disease leads to a rise in blood pressure by causing the retention of salt and water, which leads to a consequent increase in blood volume.

Common conditions and drugs used to treat them

Heart failure – diuretics, ACE inhibitors, digoxin

Irregular heart beat (arrhythmia) – anti-arrhythmics (eg amiodarone, disopyramide, flecainide), digoxin and some beta-blockers (eg atenolol, propranolol)

High blood pressure (hypertension) – diuretics, beta-blockers, ACE inhibitors, calcium channel blockers

Angina – nitrates, calcium channel blockers, beta-blockers

Blood clots – anticoagulants (eg warfarin), and anti-platelet drugs (eg aspirin, dipyridamole)

High cholesterol (and other lipid) levels – lipid-lowering drugs (eg fibrates and statins)

DIURETICS

Often called water tablets, diuretics help to get rid of excess fluid. By getting rid of fluid, they help to control two conditions – heart failure and high blood pressure (hypertension). Reducing the amount of fluid helps to reduce the amount of blood in the circulation. A decrease in blood volume reduces the workload of the heart and also lowers the pressure of the blood in the arteries.

There are several types of diuretics in common use: loop diuretics, thiazides, potassium-sparing diuretics and various combinations of potassium-sparing diuretics with other diuretics, and also diuretics with potassium. They all reduce body fluid, and they all achieve this by acting on the kidney. However, the different types of diuretics work at different places in the kidney, influencing the speed and strength of their action. Loop diuretics, for example, are powerful, fast acting drugs. Potassium-sparers have a mild action, and thiazides fall in between the two.

Thiazides can be used for either hypertension or heart failure, while loop diuretics tend to be used more for heart failure. Potassium-sparing diuretics are used for various conditions in which fluid retention occurs, such as heart failure. However, they are sometimes given with thiazides and loop diuretics to help reduce the loss of potassium that can occur with these drugs.

How to use: Take the medicine exactly as prescribed by the doctor. Most diuretics are prescribed to be taken once daily in the morning. Try not to miss this dose. However, if you do miss this dose and remember late in the day, take it anyway, but bear in mind that you may need to get up in the night to pass urine. Return to your normal dose schedule the next morning. Do not stop taking diuretics without asking your doctor, because this may cause your underlying condition to get worse.

Precautions: Tell your doctor if you are pregnant, planning to become pregnant or are breastfeeding, or if you have or have had severe liver or kidney problems, gout, diabetes, Addison's disease, prostate problems or porphyria.

Side effects: All diuretics – but particularly the loop diuretics – increase the frequency of urination, but this should decrease after you have taken the medicine for a few weeks. Side effects of the different diuretics vary somewhat, but are generally related to loss of water and potassium. They may include dizziness, due to low blood pressure (particularly on standing up, which may lead to falls), upset stomach, muscle cramps, lethargy and tiredness, and rash. Impotence may occur with thiazides. Potassium-sparing diuretics avoid the possibility of potassium loss, but the opposite may occur, with rising potassium levels in the blood leading to muscle weakness. Your potassium levels should therefore be monitored while taking diuretics. Always remember to attend any appointments. Note also that loop diuretics may affect your hearing.

Warnings: Limit alcohol consumption to one glass of wine or half a pint of beer a day, unless you are taking other medicines where alcohol avoidance is recommended.

Interactions: Diuretics interact with a few other drugs. For example, they may interact with lithium to increase blood lithium levels. Diuretics and corticosteroids may interact to increase potassium loss. If excessive potassium is lost, the toxicity of digoxin is increased. Always check with your doctor or pharmacist before taking other medicines. In particular, be aware that non-steroidal anti-inflammatory drugs (NSAIDs), some of which are available over the counter, can reduce the beneficial effects of some diuretics.

Loop diuretics

Bumetanide

Available preparations: Tablets, injection
Brand names: Burinex
Combination preparations: Burinex K (bumetanide, potassium)

Ethacrynic acid

Available preparations: Injection
Brand names: Edecrin

Frusemide

Available preparations: Tablets, liquid, injection
Brand names: Lasix
Combination preparations: Diumide-K Continus (frusemide, potassium), Lasikal (frusemide, potassium)

Torasemide

General information: Torasemide is used for high blood pressure as well as fluid retention.

Available preparations: Tablets
Brand names: Torem

Thiazide diuretics

Bendrofluazide

Available preparations: Tablets
Brand names: None
Combination preparations: Neonaclex K (bendrofluazide, potassium)

Chlorothiazide

Available preparations: Tablets
Brand names: Saluric

Chlorthalidone

General information: In addition to the customary uses for thiazide diuretics, Chlorthalidone is also used for the disorder called diabetes insipidus (see page 175).

Available preparations: Tablets
Brand names: Hygroton

Cyclopenthiazide

Available preparations: Tablets
Brand names: Navidrex

Hydrochlorothiazide

Available preparations: Tablets
Brand names: HydroSaluric

Indapamide

Use, precautions, side effects, warnings, interactions: As diuretics (see page 79). In addition, tell your doctor if you have had a stroke or parathyroid problems.
Available preparations: Tablets
Brand names: Natrilix, Natrilix SR

Mefruside

Available preparations: Tablets
Brand names: Baycaron

Metolazone

Available preparations: Tablets
Brand names: Metenix 5

Polythiazide

Available preparations: Tablets
Brand names: Nephril

Xipamide

Available preparations: Tablets
Brand names: Diurexan

Potasssium-sparing diuretics

Amiloride

General information: Amiloride is used for fluid retention caused by various problems, including heart conditions. It is also used to conserve potassium in people taking thiazide or loop diuretics.

Available preparations: Tablets
Brand names: None
Combination preparations: Burinex A (co-amilofruse: amiloride, frusemide); Navispare (co-amilozide: amiloride, hydrochlorothiazide)

Potassium canrenoate

General information: Potassium canrenoate is used for fluid retention caused by liver failure, heart failure and hyperaldosteronism.

Available preparations: Tablets, capsules, liquid
Brand names: Spiroctan-M

Spironolactone

General information: Spironolactone is used for fluid retention caused by cirrhosis of the liver, heart failure, severe kidney disease and hyperaldosteronism.

Available preparations: Tablets, capsules, liquid
Brand names: Aldactone, Spiroctan, Lasilactone (spironolactone, frusemide)

Triamterene

General information: Triamterene is used for fluid retention caused by various problems including heart conditions. It is also used to conserve potassium in people taking thiazide or loop diuretics.

Available preparations: Capsules
Brand names: Dytac
Combination preparations: Dyazide (co-triamterzide: triamterene, hydrochlorothiazide), Dytide (triamterene, benzthiazide), Frusene (triamterene with frusemide), Kalspare (triamterene, chlorthalidone)

BETA-BLOCKERS

Beta-blockers are used in a wide variety of heart and circulatory conditions: high blood pressure (hypertension), angina, arrhythmias and following heart attacks (to help prevent further attacks). They are also used in other conditions, such as anxiety (see page 29), migraine (see page 65), thyroid disease (see page 171) and glaucoma (see page 228).

These drugs block the transmission of chemical messages at various sites in the body – sites which contain receptors called beta receptors. A natural body chemical which acts at beta receptors, noradrenaline plays a part in controlling the heart and blood vessels. For example, it makes the heart beat faster and more strongly. Beta-blockers oppose this action of noradrenaline at beta receptors, causing the heart rate to slow down and the force of the heart beat to decrease. This action helps to lower blood pressure, and also, by reducing the requirement of the heart for oxygen, helps in the treatment of angina. In addition, beta-blockers interrupt the conduction of the electric current through the heart, which helps in the treatment of certain arrhythmias.

There are 15 different beta-blockers, and although all of them work in much the same way, there are some differences in the range of activities and side effects they have. Some beta-blockers (eg atenolol, betaxolol, bisoprolol, metoprolol) work more specifically on the heart than others and are known as cardioselective beta-blockers. One of the problems with beta-blockers is that they can cause breathing difficulties by blocking beta receptors in the smooth airways of the lungs. Using a cardioselective beta-blocker is thought to reduce the risk of such problems, but doctors generally avoid prescribing beta-blockers to patients with asthma and other breathing difficulties.

Some beta-blockers (eg acebutolol, celiprolol, oxprenolol, pindolol) have the capacity to stimulate as well as block beta receptors. Such drugs tend to slow the heart rate less than other beta-blockers. Certain beta-blockers are water-soluble while others are fat-soluble (ie they dissolve in the body fat). Atenolol, celiprolol, nadolol and sotalol are the most water-soluble beta-blockers; they are less likely to enter the brain than the fat-soluble drugs. The relevance of this is that the water-soluble drugs tend to cause less sleep disturbances and nightmares as a result.

How to use: Take the medicine exactly as prescribed by the doctor. If you miss a dose, take it as soon as you remember. However, if it is almost time for your next dose, skip the missed dose. Do not take double the dose. Do not stop taking the medicine without asking your doctor because this may cause your underlying condition to get worse.

Precautions: Tell your doctor if you are pregnant, planning to become pregnant or are breastfeeding, or if you have asthma or other lung disease, diabetes or kidney problems.

Side effects: Side effects with beta-blockers are usually temporary and go away with prolonged use. They include upset stomach, excessive tiredness, sleep disturbances, cold hands and feet, headache and rash. If you develop shortness of breath or wheezing, you should stop the drug immediately and call your doctor, who will prescribe a different drug.

Warnings: None. Alcohol is not a problem with these drugs.

Interactions: Beta-blockers interact with several other drugs (eg anti-arrhythmics, antidepressants, anti-psychotics and other cardiovascular drugs) which may lead to increased or reduced effects of the drug. Always check with your doctor or pharmacist before taking any other medication.

Acebutolol

General information: Acebutolol is used for hypertension, angina and arrhythmias.

Available preparations: Tablets, capsules
Brand names: Sectral
Combination preparations: Secadrex (acebutolol, hydrochlorothiazide)

Atenolol

General information: Atenolol is used for hypertension, angina, arrhythmias and as a preventative measure following heart attacks.

Available preparations: Tablets, liquid, injection
Brand names: Tenormin
Combination preparations: Beta-Adalat (atenolol, nifedipine), Kalten (atenolol, amiloride, hydrochlorothiazide), Tenben (atenolol, bendrofluazide), Tenif (atenolol, nifedipine), Tenoret 50 (atenolol, chlorthalidone)

Betaxolol

General information: Betaxolol is used for hypertension. It is also used for glaucoma (see page 229).

Available preparations: Tablets
Brand names: Kerlone

Bisoprolol

General information: Bisoprolol is used for hypertension and angina.

Available preparations: Tablets
Brand names: Emcor, Monocor
Combination preparations: Monozide 10 (bisoprolol, hydrochlorothiazide)

Carvedilol

General information: Carvedilol is used for hypertension and angina. It is also used for heart failure (but under hospital supervision only).

Available preparations: Tablets
Brand names: Eucardic

Celiprolol

General information: Celiprolol is used for hypertension.

Available preparations: Tablets
Brand names: Celectol

Esmolol

General information: Esmolol is used for various types of arrhythmias (irregular heart beat) and for hypertension which may occur following an operation.

Available preparations: Injection
Brand names: Brevibloc

Labetalol

General information: Labetalol is used for hypertension.

Available preparations: Tablets, injection
Brand names: Trandate

Metoprolol

General information: Metoprolol is used for hypertension, angina and arrhythmias. It is also used for prevention of migraine attacks (see page 65) and in thyroid disease (see page 171).

Available preparations: Tablets, injection
Brand names: Betaloc, Betaloc SA, Lopressor, Lopressor SR
Combination preparations: Co-Betaloc and Co-Betaloc SA (metoprolol, hydrochlorothiazide)

Nadolol

General information: Nadolol is used for hypertension, angina and arrhythmias. It is also used for prevention of migraine attacks (see page 65) and in thyroid disease (see page 171).

Available preparations: Tablets
Brand names: Corgard
Combination preparations: Corgaretic (nadolol, bendrofluazide)

Oxprenolol

General information: Oxprenolol is used for hypertension, angina and arrhythmias. It is also used for symptoms of anxiety (see page 29).

Available preparations: Tablets
Brand names: Trasicor, Slow Trasicor
Combination preparations: Trasidrex (co-prenozide: oxprenolol, cyclopenthiazide)

Pindolol

General information: Pindolol is used for hypertension and angina.

Available preparations: Tablets
Brand names: Visken
Combination preparations: Viskaldix (pindolol, clopamide)

Propranolol

General information: Propranolol is used for hypertension, angina, arrhythmias, after heart attacks and in phaeocromocytoma. It is also used for prevention of migraine attacks (see page 65) and for symptoms of anxiety (see page 29).

Available preparations: Tablets, capsules, liquid, injection
Brand names: Inderal, Half Inderal LA, Inderal LA
Combination preparations: Inderetic and Inderex (propranolol, bendrofluazide)

Sotalol

General information: Sotalol is used for various arrhythmias.

Available preparations: Tablets, injection
Brand names: Betacardone, Sotacor

Timolol

General information: Timolol is used for hypertension, angina and as a preventative measure after heart attacks. It is also used for prevention of migraine attacks (see page 65) and glaucoma (see page 232).

Available preparations: Tablets
Brand names: Betim, Blocadren
Combination preparations: Moducren (timolol, co-amilozide: amiloride, hydrochlorothiazide), Prestim (timolol, bendrofluazide)

ANGIOTENSIN-CONVERTING ENZYME (ACE) INHIBITORS AND SIMILAR DRUGS

Angiotensin-converting enzyme (ACE) inhibitors (eg captopril, enalapril, lisinopril) are used mainly in the treatment of hypertension and heart failure. They are also sometimes prescribed for people who have diabetes in order to protect the kidneys. Diuretics are often prescribed with ACE inhibitors.

As their name suggests, ACE inhibitors work by inhibiting the enzyme called angiotensin-converting enzyme. This enzyme causes the production of the chemical angiotensin, a substance which causes the blood vessels to constrict and the blood pressure to rise. If the production of angiotensin is prevented, the blood vessels will consequently widen (dilate) and the blood pressure will fall. ACE inhibitors cause the blood vessels to dilate, leading to a reduction in the heart's workload – it does not have to pump with quite such force – which is useful in the treatment of both heart failure and hypertension. They also cause a small loss of salt and water from the body.

A relatively new group of drugs – the angiotensin-II-receptor antagonists (eg losartan, valsartan) work in a similar way to the ACE inhibitors in that they prevent the effect of angiotensin. Included in this section, these drugs have similar characteristics to the ACE inhibitors, except that they do not commonly cause the persistent dry cough which is often such a nuisance with ACE inhibitors.

How to use: Take the medicine exactly as prescribed by the doctor. If you have not had one of these drugs before, you should take the first dose lying down, ideally at bedtime, because there is a risk of a fall in blood pressure. If you miss a dose, take it as soon as you remember. However, if it is almost time for your next dose, skip the missed dose. Do not take double the dose. Do not stop taking the medicine without asking your doctor because this may cause your underlying condition to get worse.

Precautions: Tell your doctor if you are pregnant, planning to become pregnant or are breastfeeding, or if you have or have had kidney or liver problems, porphyria or coronary artery disease.

Side effects: Dizziness and/or fainting, loss of taste or taste changes, loss of appetite, persistent dry cough, runny nose, sore throat, mouth sores, upset stomach, nausea, vomiting, diarrhoea, constipation, heartburn, chest pain, palpitations, mood changes, rash. Tell your doctor if you develop a rash or other allergic symptoms, such as swollen mouth, lips and tongue, and breathing difficulties, or a cough, sore throat, fever or chest pain.

Warnings: Do not drink excessive alcohol (eg more than a glass of wine or half a pint of beer a day) while you are taking ACE inhibitors because this will increase the risk of adverse effects. Do not drive or take part in any activity that requires you to be alert until you know how you react to the medicine. Do not use salt substitutes while taking ACE inhibitors. Many salt substitutes contain potassium and this could lead to a rise in blood levels of potassium if you are also taking an ACE inhibitor. Your potassium levels will often be monitored while you are taking these drugs.

Interactions: ACE inhibitors interact with a number of other drugs including non-steroidal anti-inflammatory drugs (NSAIDs), potassium-sparing diuretics, lithium and cyclosporin. Check with your doctor or pharmacist before taking any other medication.

Candesartan

General information: Candesartan is an angiotensin-II receptor antagonist used for hypertension.

Available preparations: Tablets
Brand names: Amias

Captopril

General information: Captopril is an ACE inhibitor used for hypertension, heart failure and in diabetic kidney disease.

Available preparations: Tablets
Brand names: Capoten
Combination preparations: Capozide (captopril, hydrochlorothiazide)

Cilazapril

General information: Cilazapril is an ACE inhibitor used for hypertension and heart failure.

Available preparations: Tablets
Brand names: Vascace

Enalapril

General information: Enalapril is an ACE inhibitor used for hypertension, heart failure and prevention of heart failure and heart attack in people with a poorly functioning left ventricle.

Available preparations: Tablets, wafers
Brand names: Innovace
Combination preparations: Innozide (enalapril, hydrochlorothiazide)

Fosinopril

General information: Fosinopril is an ACE inhibitor used for hypertension and heart failure.

Available preparations: Tablets
Brand names: Staril

Irbesartan

General information: Irbesartan is an angiotensin-II receptor used for hypertension.

Available preparations: Tablets
Brand names: Aprovel

Lisinopril

General information: Lisinopril is an ACE inhibitor used for hypertension, heart failure, following heart attacks and in diabetic kidney disease.

Available preparations: Tablets
Brand names: Carace, Zestril
Combination preparations: Carace Plus and Zestoretic (lisinopril, hydrochlorothiazide)

Losartan

General information: Losartan is an angiotensin-II receptor antagonist used for hypertension.

Available preparations: Tablets
Brand names: Cozaar
Combination preparations: Cozaar-Comp (losartan, hydrochlorothiazide)

Moexipril

General information: Moexipril is an ACE inhibitor used in hypertension.

Available preparations: Tablets
Brand names: Perdix

Perindopril

General information: Perindopril is an ACE inhibitor used in hypertension and heart failure.

Available preparations: Tablets
Brand names: Coversyl

Quinapril

General information: Quinapril is an ACE inhibitor used in hypertension and heart failure.

Available preparations: Tablets
Brand names: Accupro
Combination preparations: Accuretic (quinapril, hydrochlorothiazide)

Ramipril

General information: Ramipril is an ACE inhibitor used in hypertension, heart failure and as a preventative measure following heart attacks.

Available preparations: Capsules
Brand names: Tritace

Trandolapril

General information: Trandolapril is an ACE inhibitor used in hypertension and as a preventative measure following heart attacks.

Available preparations: Capsules
Brand names: Gopten, Odrik
Combination preparations: Tarka (trandolapril, verapamil)

Valsartan

General information: Valsartan is an angiotensin-II receptor antagonist used in hypertension.

Available preparations: Capsules
Brand names: Diovan

ALPHA-BLOCKERS AND OTHER VASODILATORS

Vasodilators are drugs that dilate, or widen, the blood vessels. Those discussed in this section include the alpha-blockers and a miscellaneous variety of other drugs including clonidine, hydralazine and methyldopa. Most of these drugs cause vasodilatation (widening of the blood vessels); they are used in the treatment of hypertension, and some are used in heart failure and other conditions.

Alpha-blockers (eg doxazosin, indoramin, prazosin, terazosin) work by blocking alpha receptors in the small blood vessels. Stimulating these receptors causes constriction of the blood vessels, so blocking the receptors has a dilating effect which enlarges the blood vessels. This helps to control blood pressure. The other drugs included in this section have a variety of mechanisms of action, but they all act as vasodilators.

How to use: Take the medicine exactly as prescribed by the doctor. If you miss a dose, take it as soon as you remember. However, if it is almost time for your next dose, skip the missed dose. Do not take double the dose. Do not stop taking the medicine without asking your doctor because this may cause your underlying condition to get worse.

Precautions: Tell your doctor if you are pregnant, planning to become pregnant or are breastfeeding, or if you have or have had kidney or liver problems.

Side effects: These drugs may cause dizziness and fainting, drowsiness, depression, weakness, headache, urinary incontinence, stuffy nose, dry mouth, rashes.

Warnings: Do not drink excessive alcohol (eg more than a glass of wine or half a pint of beer a day) while you are taking these medicines because this will increase the risk of adverse effects. Do not drive or take part in any activity that requires you to be alert until you know how you react to the medicine.

Interactions: These medicines interact with various cardiovascular and other drugs. Check with your doctor or pharmacist before taking any other medicines.

Clonidine

General information: Clonidine is a vasodilator used in hypertension. It is also used in the treatment of migraine (see page 69). However, it is used much less frequently than in the past.

How to use: As alpha-blockers and other vasodilators (see above).
Precautions, warnings: As alpha-blockers and other vasodilators. In addition, tell your doctor if you have or have had circulatory problems or depression.
Side effects: These may include dry mouth, drowsiness dizziness, nausea, rash, restlessness.
Interactions: Clonidine interacts with antidepressants and beta-blockers. Check with your pharmacist or doctor before taking any other medicines.
Available preparations: Tablets, injection
Brand names: Catapres

Doxazosin

General information: Doxazosin is an alpha–blocker used in hypertension. It is also used in benign prostatic hyperplasia (see page 197).

Use, precautions, side effects, warnings, interactions: As alpha–blockers and other vasodilators (see above).
Available preparations: Tablets
Brand names: Cardura

Hydralazine

General information: Hydralazine is a vasodilator used in hypertension (usually in combination with a thiazide diuretic and a beta–blocker).

How to use: As alpha–blockers and other vasodilators (see page 90).
Precautions, warnings and interactions: As alpha–blockers and other vasodilators (see page 90). In addition, tell your doctor if you have or have had heart disease, stroke, porphyria, systemic lupus erythmatosus.
Side effects: Dizziness may occur when getting up – rising slowly will help this. The following may also occur: rapid heart beat, headache, fluid retention, nausea and vomiting, diarrhoea, flushing (feeling of warmth), rash.
Available preparations: Tablets, injection
Brand names: Apresoline

Indoramin

General information: Indoramin is an alpha–blocker used in hypertension. It is also used in benign prostatic hyperplasia (see page 197).

Use, precautions, side effects, warnings, interactions: See alpha–blockers and other vasodilators. In addition, tell your doctor if you have Parkinson's disease or epilepsy.
Available preparations: Tablets
Brand names: Baratol

Methyldopa

General information: Methyldopa is a vasodilator used in hypertension (usually with a diuretic). It is sometimes prescribed in late pregnancy to treat high blood pressure, as it does not affect the unborn child.

How to use: As alpha–blockers and other vasodilators (see page 90).
Precautions: Tell your doctor if you have or have had depression, porphyria, phaeocromocytoma or liver or kidney disease.
Side effects: Drowsiness and depression are the most common side effects, but headaches, dry mouth, fluid retention, stuffy nose and rash may occur.
Warnings and interactions: As alpha–blockers and vasodilators (see page 90).
Available preparations: Tablets, liquid, injection
Brand names: Aldomet

Minoxidil

General information: Minoxidil is a vasodilator used in hypertension (usually with a diuretic and a beta-blocker). It is also used externally (in the form of a lotion) for the treatment of baldness in men (see page 222).

How to use: As alpha-blockers and other vasodilators (see page 90).
Precautions: Tell your doctor if you are pregnant, planning to become pregnant or are breastfeeding, or if you have or have had kidney problems, heart disease or porphyria.
Side effects: Fluid retention and increased hair growth are the most common side effects, but rapid heart beat and palpitations, weight gain, upset stomach, breast tenderness and rash may occur.
Warnings and interactions: As alpha-blockers and other vasodilators (see page 90).
Available preparations: Tablets
Brand names: Loniten

Moxonidine

General information: Moxonidine is a vasodilator used in hypertension.

How to use: As alpha-blockers and other vasodilators (see page 90).
Precautions: Tell your doctor if you are pregnant or are breastfeeding, or if you have or have had heart or circulatory problems, liver or kidney problems, depression, Parkinson's disease or glaucoma.
Side effects: Dry mouth, headache, drowsiness, dizziness, nausea and sleep disturbance may occur.
Warnings and interactions: As alpha-blockers and other vasodilators (see page 90).
Available preparations: Tablets
Brand names: Physiotens

Prazosin

General information: Prazosin is an alpha-blocker used in hypertension and heart failure. It is also used in benign prostatic hyperplasia (see page 197) and Raynaud's syndrome.

Use, precautions, side effects, warnings, interactions: As alpha-blockers and other vasodilators (see page 90).
Available preparations: Tablets
Brand names: Hypovase

Terazosin

General information: Terazosin is an alpha-blocker used in hypertension. It is also used in benign prostatic hyperplasia (see page 197).

Use, precautions, side effects, warnings, interactions: As alpha-blockers and other vasodilators (see page 90).
Available preparations: Tablets
Brand names: Hytrin

NITRATES

Used in medical treatments for over a hundred years, nitrates are prescribed for angina or occasionally heart failure. There are four types – glyceryl trinitrate, isosorbide mononitrate, isosorbide dinitrate and pentaerythritol tetranitrate; angina sufferers will no doubt be familiar with the small white tablets (glyceryl trinitrate) that are placed under the tongue to relieve chest pain. Glyceryl trinitrate may be used with other anti-angina medicines, but sometimes it may be the only medicine you have to take, particularly if your symptoms occur very infrequently.

Nitrates are vasodilators and work by relaxing the muscle in the walls of the arteries, which helps the arteries to dilate (widen). Dilated arteries reduce the workload of the heart so less oxygen is required, thus helping to control the symptoms of angina.

How to use: Nitrates come in a variety of types of preparations: ordinary tablets, tablets which dissolve under the tongue, slow- or modified-release tablets, aerosol spray, skin patches and an ointment. All are used somewhat differently so you need to follow the instructions given with your medicine very carefully. It is often best to take the first dose while you are sitting down, because nitrates can cause an initial rapid fall in blood pressure which may cause fainting. If you miss a dose, take it as soon as you remember. However, if it is almost time for your next dose, skip the missed dose. Do not take double the dose. Do not stop taking the medicine without asking your doctor because this may cause your underlying condition to get worse.

Precautions: Tell your doctor if you have or have had glaucoma, thyroid disease, severe liver or kidney problems.

Side effects: Throbbing headache, flushing, dizziness and rapid heartbeat may occur.

Warnings: Do not drink an excessive amount of alcohol while you are taking these medicines because this will increase the risk of adverse effects – particularly dizziness. Do not drive or take part in any activity that requires you to be alert until you know how you react to the medicine.

Interactions: Nitrates interact with some cardiovascular and other drugs. Ask your doctor or pharmacist before using other medicines.

Glyceryl trinitrate

General information: Glyceryl trinitrate is used in angina.

Available preparations: Tablets, modified-release tablets, oral sprays, skin patches, ointment
Brand names: Tablets: none; Modified-release tablets: Suscard, Sustac; Sprays: Coro-Nitro Pump Spray, Glytrin Spray, Nitrolingual Pump Spray, Nitromin; Skin patches: Deponit, Minitran, Nitro-Dur, Transiderm-Nitro; Ointment: Percutol

Isosorbide dinitrate

General information: Isosorbide dinitrate is used in angina.

Available preparations: Tablets, modified-release tablets, skin spray
Brand names: Tablets: Isordil, Sorbichew, Sorbitrate; Modified-release tablets: Cedocard Retard, Isoket Retard, Isordil Tembids, Sorbid SA; Skin spray: Isocard

Isosorbide mononitrate

General information: Isosorbide mononitrate is used in angina.

Available preparations: Tablets, modified-release tablets
Brand names: Tablets: Elantan, Ismo, Isotrate, Monit, Mono-Cedocard; Modified-release tablets: Elantan LA, Imdur, Isib 60XL, Ismo Retard, MCR-50, Modisal XL, Monit SR, Monomax SR, Monosorb XL-60
Combination products: Imazin XL (aspirin, isosorbide mononitrate)

Pentaerythritol tetranitrate

General information: Pentaerythritol is used in angina.

Available preparations: Tablets
Brand names: Mycardol

CALCIUM CHANNEL BLOCKERS

Like nitrates (see page 93), calcium channel blockers are used to treat angina. Some are also used to treat high blood pressure and one (verapamil) is used additionally to treat arrhythmias (irregular heart beat).

Calcium entry into smooth muscle cells is essential for muscle contraction and calcium channel blockers interfere with this. By interfering in this way, these drugs relax the blood vessels and encourage them to dilate (widen). This helps in the treatment of angina by allowing more oxygen to get to the heart. Dilation of the blood vessels also helps in high blood pressure by reducing the resistance in the arteries. Verapamil also blocks the entry of calcium into the conducting tissue of the heart, making it effective in the treatment of arrhythmias.

How to use: Take the medicine exactly as prescribed by the doctor. If you miss a dose, take it as soon as you remember. However, if it is almost time for your next dose, skip the missed dose. Do not take double the dose. Do not stop taking the medicine without asking your doctor because this may cause your underlying condition to get worse.

Precautions: Tell your doctor if you are pregnant, planning to become pregnant, or are breastfeeding or if you have or have had kidney problems, heart failure or diabetes.

Side effects: These drugs can produce a variety of side effects, particularly headache, dizziness, flushing, and ankle and leg swelling. Upset stomach, tiredness, rash and dry mouth may also occur. Slow heart beat is a possibility with diltiazem and constipation may occur with verapamil.

Warnings: Do not drink an excessive amount of alcohol (eg more than a glass of wine or half a pint of beer a day) while you are taking these medicines because this will increase the risk of adverse effects. Do not drive or take part in any activity that requires you to be alert until you know how you react to the medicine. Avoid grapefruit juice if you are taking felodipine, isradipine, lacidipine, lercanidipine, nicardipine, nifedipine, nimodipine, nisoldipine and verapamil.

Interactions: Calcium channel blockers interact with a number of other medicines, including certain cardiovascular drugs, some antibiotics, anticonvulsants, theophylline and cyclosporin. Ask your doctor or pharmacist before taking any other medicines.

Amlodipine

General information: Amlodipine is used in angina and hypertension.

Available preparations: Tablets
Brand names: Istin

Diltiazem

General information: Diltiazem is used in angina and hypertension.

Available preparations: Tablets, modified-release tablets and capsules
Brand names: Tablets: Tildiem; Modified-release tablets: Adizem-SR, Adizem-XL, Angitil SR, Calcicard CR, Dilcardia SR, Dilzem SR, Dilzem XL, Slozem, Tildiem LA, Tildiem Retard, Viazem XL, Zemtard

Felodipine

General information: Felodipine is used in angina and hypertension.

Available preparations: Tablets
Brand names: Plendil

Isradipine

General information: Isradipine is used in hypertension.

Available preparations: Tablets
Brand names: Prescal

Lacidipine

General information: Lacidipine is used in hypertension.

Available preparations: Tablets
Brand names: Motens

Lercanidipine

General information: Lercanidipine is used in hypertension.

Available preparations: Tablets
Brand names: Zanidip

Nicardipine

General information: Nicardipine is used in angina and hypertension.

Available preparations: Capsules
Brand names: Cardene, Cardene SR

Nifedipine

General information: Nifedipine is used in angina and hypertension.

Available preparations: Capsules, modified-release tablets and capsules
Brand names: Capsules: Adalat; Modified-release preparations: Adalat LA, Adalat Retard, Adipine MR, Angiopine 40 LA, Cardilate MR, Coracten, Coroday MR, Fortipine LA 40, Hypolar Retard 20, Nifedipress MR, Nifedotard 20 MR, Nifelease, Nivaten Retard, Slofedipine XL, Tensipine MR, Unipine XL

Nimodipine

General information: Nimodipine is used to treat symptoms resulting from a ruptured blood vessel in the brain (haemorrhage). It increases blood flow to damaged tissue.

Available preparations: Tablets, injection
Brand names: Nimotop

Nisoldipine

General information: Nisoldipine is used in angina and hypertension.

Available preparations: Slow-release tablets
Brand names: Syscor MR

Verapamil

General information: Verapamil is used in angina, hypertension and arrhythmias (irregular heart beat).

Available preparations: Tablets, modified-release tablets and capsules
Brand names: Tablets: Cordilox, Securon; Modified-release preparations: Securon SR, Half Securon SR, Univer, Verapress MR; **Combination preparations:** Tarka (verapamil and trandolapril, an ACE inhibitor). This preparation is used for hypertension in those who have been stabilised on the two ingredients separately.

POTASSIUM CHANNEL ACTIVATORS

Nicorandil

General information: Nicorandil is the first – and, so far, the only – one of a new group of drugs known as potassium channel activators. As a vasodilator, it has properties similar to nitrates and calcium channel blockers and is used in angina.

How to use: As calcium channel blockers (see page 94).
Precautions: Tell your doctor if you are pregnant, plan to become pregnant or are breastfeeding.
Side effects: The most common side effects are headache, flushing and dizziness. Nausea, vomiting and weakness may occur.
Warnings: As calcium channel blockers (see page 95).
Interactions: None reported so far, but this is a relatively new drug. Check with your pharmacist or doctor before taking any other medicines.
Available preparations: Tablets
Brand names: Ikorel

LIPID-LOWERING DRUGS

The blood contains several types of fat (lipid), including various types of cholesterol and also triglycerides. Despite its reputation, cholesterol is an essential substance in the body. Made in the liver, it is the starting point for the production of several other body chemicals, including certain hormones and it is essential for the health of cell membranes. It is only when cholesterol levels rise too high that problems can develop. Accumulation of cholesterol and other fat deposits along the walls of the arteries (a process known as atherosclerosis) gradually decreases blood flow to the heart, brain and other parts of the body. Lowering your blood level of cholesterol may therefore help to prevent angina, heart attacks and stroke. Cholesterol can sometimes be reduced by decreasing the amount of fat in your diet, but some people – either those with both particularly high levels of cholesterol and other fats and other risk factors for heart disease (eg diabetes or hypertension), or those with an inherited tendency to high levels of fat in the blood (hyperlipidaemia), may require extra help. In such circumstances, lipid–lowering drugs are prescribed.

There are several types of lipid-lowering drugs, including the statins (eg pravastatin, simvastatin), the fibrates (eg bezafibrate), anion–exchange resins, nicotinic acid, and fish oils.

How to use: Lipid-lowering drugs are normally used in conjunction with a low fat diet. It is therefore important to follow any dietary advice you have been given. Take the medicine exactly as prescribed by the doctor. If you miss a dose, take it as soon as you remember. However, if it is almost time for your next dose, skip the missed dose. Do not take double the dose. Do not stop taking the medicine without asking your doctor because this may cause your underlying condition to get worse.

Precautions, side effects, warnings, interactions: See individual groups of drugs listed below.

STATINS

Statins are the newest group of lipid-lowering drugs. They reduce cholesterol by inhibiting an enzyme that produces cholesterol in the liver. They are used to lower lipid levels in the blood in those who have not responded to dietary changes.

How to use: As lipid-lowering drugs (see page 97).

Precautions: Tell your doctor if you are pregnant, planning to become pregnant or are breastfeeding, or if you have or have had liver disease.

Side effects: Side effects are not common, but the following may occur: headache, stomach pain, nausea, vomiting and rash. Muscle problems may occasionally occur with this drug. Tell your doctor immediately if you experience any muscle pain, cramps, weakness or tenderness.

Warnings: You will be asked to attend for various tests to monitor blood cholesterol level and liver function. Keep your appointments. Alcohol is not a particular problem with these drugs, but excessive intake may not be helpful to your condition.

Interactions: Atorvastatin may interact with other drugs such as anticoagulants (eg warfarin) and cyclosporin. Check with your pharmacist or doctor before taking any other medication.

Atorvastatin

Available preparations: Tablets
Brand names: Lipitor

Cerivastatin

Available preparations: Tablets
Brand names: Lipobay

Fluvastatin

Available preparations: Capsules
Brand names: Lescol

Pravastatin

Available preparations: Tablets
Brand names: Lipostat

Simvastatin

Available preparations: Tablets
Brand names: Zocor

FIBRATES

Fibrates are used to lower lipid levels in the blood in those who have not responded to a low-fat diet. They are particularly effective in reducing blood fat, including both triglycerides and cholesterol. The fibrates alter the way in which fats are absorbed from the blood into the liver cells, and can therefore reduce the level of fats in the blood.

How to use: As lipid-lowering drugs (see page 97). Take this medicine with food.

Precautions: Tell your doctor if you are pregnant, planning to become pregnant or are breastfeeding, or if you have or have had liver, kidney or gall bladder disease or alcoholism.

Side effects: Common side effects include nausea, loss of appetite and stomach pain. The following may also occur: headache, rash, dizziness, hair loss and muscular pain. Tell your doctor if you experience any muscle pain/cramps.

Warnings: None. Alcohol is not a particular problem with these drugs but excessive intake may not be helpful to your condition.

Interactions: Fibrates may interact with anticoagulants (eg warfarin) and with other lipid-lowering drugs. Check with your doctor or pharmacist before taking other medicines.

Bezafibrate

Available preparations: Tablets
Brand names: Bezalip, Bezalip Mono

Ciprofibrate

Available preparations: Tablets
Brand names: Modalim

Clofibrate

Available preparations: Capsules
Brand names: Atromid S

Fenofibrate

Available preparations: Capsules
Brand names: Lipantil

Gemfibrozil

Available preparations: Tablets, capsules
Brand names: Lopid

ANION-EXCHANGE RESINS

Anion-exchange resins are used to lower lipid levels in those who have not responded to dietary changes. Anion-exchange resins act via the bile, which is produced by the liver and released into the small intestine via the bile duct. Bile contains a large amount of cholesterol which normally is reabsorbed in the intestine. Anion-exchange resins combine with bile salts in the intestine and prevent this reabsorption, so reducing cholesterol levels in the blood.

How to use: As lipid-lowering drugs (see page 97).

Precautions: Tell your doctor if you are pregnant, planning to become pregnant or are breastfeeding, or if you have or have had gall bladder disease.

Side effects: Upset stomach, nausea, constipation and diarrhoea may occur. Occasionally this drug increases the tendency to bleeding. Tell your doctor if you notice any unusual bleeding (such as bleeding from the gums or rectum).

Warnings: None. Alcohol is not a particular problem with these drugs, but excessive intake may not be helpful to your condition.

Interactions: These drugs interfere with the absorption of fat-soluble vitamins (vitamins A, D, E and K) and also folic acid. You may be given supplements if you take these drugs for a long period. Anion-exchange resins also reduces the absorption of many other drugs; it may be necessary to take them at set times in relation to the rest of your drug therapy (including any over-the-counter medicines). Check this with your doctor or pharmacist.

Cholestyramine

Available preparations: Powder
Brand names: Questran, Questran Light

Colestipol

Available preparations: Granules
Brand names: Colestid

MISCELLANEOUS

Acipimox

General information: Acipimox is used to lower lipid levels in the blood in those who have not responded to a low-fat diet.

How to use: As lipid-lowering drugs (see page 97). Take this medicine with food.
Precautions: Tell your doctor if you are pregnant, planning to become pregnant or are breastfeeding, or if you have or have had a stomach ulcer or kidney problems.
Side effects: Possible side effects include flushing, itching, rashes and other allergic reactions, heartburn, nausea, diarrhoea and headache.
Warnings and interactions: None reported, but check with your doctor or pharmacist before taking other medicines.
Available preparations: Capsules
Brand names: Olbetam

Fish oils

General information: Fish oils are used to lower one particular type of fat in the blood (known as triglycerides) in those who have high levels in the blood. Fish oils are rich in various fatty acids (eg eicoapentaenoic acid and docosahexanoic acid) and the preparation below has been formulated to have significant amounts of these substances.

How to use: As lipid-lowering drugs (see page 97). Take this medicine with food.
Side effects: Nausea and belching may occur occasionally.
Precautions, warnings and interactions: No special instructions.
Available preparations: Capsules, liquid
Brand names: Maxepa

Ispaghula

General information: Ispaghula is a form of soluble dietary fibre. Soluble fibre helps to lower cholesterol levels and ispaghula is used in those with mild to moderately high levels of blood cholesterol. Ispaghula is also used for constipation (see page 127).

How to use: As lipid-lowering drugs (see page 97). Drink plenty of water when you take this medicine. Do not take immediately before bedtime.
Precautions: Tell your doctor if you have or have had any form of gastrointestinal obstruction or diabetes.
Side effects: Bloating and wind may occur, particularly at the start of treatment.
Warnings and interactions: No special instructions.
Available preparations: Granules
Brand names: Fybozest Orange

Nicotinic acid

General information: Nicotinic acid is a form of the B vitamin, niacin, and is used to lower lipid levels in the blood in those who have not responded to a low-fat diet.

How to use: As lipid-lowering drugs (see page 97). Take this medicine with food.
Precautions: Tell your doctor if you are pregnant, plan to become pregnant or are breastfeeding, or have or have had diabetes, stomach ulcer or liver disease.
Side effects: Side effects can be troublesome with this drug, particularly if it is used

in high dosage, and include flushing, dizziness, headache, palpitations, nausea, vomiting and rashes.

Warnings and interactions: None, but check with your doctor or pharmacist before taking other medicines.

Available preparations: Tablets

Brand names: None

DRUGS AFFECTING BLOOD CLOTTING

The fact that blood clots is in itself a good thing. Indeed, those whose blood does not clot normally can suffer from uncontrolled bleeding or severe bruising – particularly after an accident or injury. Sometimes, however, the opposite problem occurs and the blood clots too readily or in the wrong parts of the body, such as blood vessels. A blood clot (known as a thrombus) is potentially dangerous because it restricts the flow of blood through a blood vessel. Formation of a blood clot is known as thrombosis, and when it prevents blood flow it is known as an embolism.

Blood clots forming in the deep veins of the legs are a particular risk. They may occur after operations and childbirth, in women taking the contraceptive pill and in many types of serious illness, such as major burns, trauma and severe infections. They are a risk to life because fragments of the clot may break off and lodge in the arteries of the lungs (pulmonary embolism), where they may cause chest pain, cough or even collapse and death. Blood clots forming in arteries are associated with atheroma and are a cause of heart attacks (coronary thrombosis) or strokes (blood clot in the arteries of the brain).

Three main types of drugs are used to prevent and/or dissolve unwanted blood clots. These are anticoagulants, antiplatelet drugs and thrombolytic drugs. Anticoagulants are often referred to as drugs that thin the blood. This is not strictly true, but they do prevent blood clots from forming in the veins by interfering with the normal blood clotting process. However, anticoagulants do not dissolve clots that have already formed.

Heparin is used to prevent blood clots after surgery and in kidney dialysis. It is given by injection and its administration is strictly supervised in hospital. Given in low dosage, heparin is also used for the prevention of deep-vein thrombosis in patients at high risk. It does not interfere with surgery or cross the placenta in pregnancy, and patients can administer it themselves. However, the oral anticoagulant, warfarin, is often prescribed by general practitioners for longer term use.

Antiplatelet drugs (eg aspirin, clopidogrel, dipyridamole, ticlopidine) are, like anticoagulants, used to prevent clots from forming. However, antiplatelet drugs prevent clots from forming in the arteries while anticoagulant drugs prevent the formation of clots in the veins. A clot in an artery is caused by platelets (a type of blood cell) sticking together; anti-platelet drugs, as their name suggests, work by preventing platelets clumping together to form clots.

Thrombolytic drugs (eg streptokinase) actually dissolve blood clots that have already formed. They are often used in people who have just suffered a heart attack. Like heparin, these drugs are given by injection and their administration is supervised in hospital.

ANTICOAGULANTS

Oral anticoagulants are used to prevent blood clots from forming or growing larger. They work by antagonising the effects of vitamin K, a vitamin essential for blood clotting. Unlike heparin and similar drugs, they can be taken by mouth. However, their effects may take a week or more to develop, so they are often given together with heparin at first. Warfarin, in particular, is often prescribed for patients with certain types of irregular heart beat (arrhythmia) or after a heart attack or heart valve replacement surgery. It is also used for patients with deep-vein thrombosis or pulmonary embolism.

Precautions: Tell your doctor if you are pregnant, planning to become pregnant or are breastfeeding, or if you have or have had stomach ulcer, high blood pressure, liver or kidney disease or recent surgery.

Side effects: Increased tendency to bleed is the greatest risk with warfarin. Tell your doctor immediately if you experience unusual bleeding or bruising, black or bloody stools or dark urine. Other side effects include rash, hair loss, diarrhoea, nausea and vomiting.

Warnings: Do not drink excessive amounts of alcohol because this may increase the adverse effects of the drug. Do not increase the consumption of foods or vitamin supplements containing vitamin K (eg green leafy vegetables) without consulting your doctor. You will be asked to attend for regular blood tests. Do not miss your appointments.

Interactions: Anticoagulants interact with a wide variety of other drugs. Do not take any other medicine – including those available over the counter – without asking your doctor or pharmacist. Be particularly careful not to take aspirin unless it has been prescribed by your doctor.

Nicoumalone

Available preparations: Tablets
Brand names: Sinthrome

Phenindione

Available preparations: Tablets
Brand names: Dindevan

Warfarin

Available preparations: Tablets
Brand names: None

ANTIPLATELET DRUGS

Aspirin

General information: Discovered more than 100 years ago, aspirin is one of our oldest medicines. Traditionally, it has been used for pain relief (see page 60), but in recent years it has started to be used in small doses for the prevention of blood clotting. It is used in those who have had heart attacks and strokes to help prevent recurrence.

How to use: Take the medicine as prescribed. For prevention, aspirin should be taken regularly. Stick carefully to the prescribed dose. Do not stop taking it without asking your doctor. Note that the dose for prevention of heart attack and stroke is different from that for pain. If you need a painkiller, do not increase your dose of aspirin or you will interfere with blood clotting. Take an alternative painkiller.
Precautions, side effects, warnings, interactions: As analgesics (see page 60).
Available preparations: Tablets
Brand names (for prevention of blood clotting): Angettes 75, Caprin, Disprin CV, Nu-Seals Aspirin

Clopidogrel

General information: Clopidogrel is a newly introduced antiplatelet drug used for reduction of stroke or heart attack in people with atherosclerosis.

How to use: Take the medicine exactly as prescribed by the doctor. If you miss a dose, take it as soon as you remember. However, if it is almost time for your next dose, skip the missed dose. Do not take double the dose. Do not stop taking the medicine without asking your doctor because this may cause your underlying condition to get worse.
Precautions: Tell your doctor if you are pregnant, planning to become pregnant or are breastfeeding, or if you have or have had any bleeding disorder, peptic ulcer, liver or kidney disorder.
Side effects: Stomach upset, skin reactions and bleeding episodes may occur. Report any unusual bleeding to your doctor.
Interactions: Clopidogrel interacts with several other drugs, including aspirin, NSAIDs and anticoagulants. These interactions increase the risk of bleeding episodes.
Available preparations: Tablets
Brand names: Plavix

Dipyridamole

General information: Dipyridamole is used with oral anticoagulants to reduce the risk of blood clots after heart valve replacement.

How to use: Take the medicine exactly as prescribed by the doctor. If you miss a dose, take it as soon as you remember. However, if it is almost time for your next dose, skip the missed dose. Do not take double the dose. Do not stop taking the medicine without asking your doctor because this may cause your underlying condition to get worse.

Precautions: Tell your doctor if you are pregnant, planning to be pregnant or are breastfeeding, or if you have or have had low blood pressure, migraine or angina.

Side effects: Side effects are not common, but the following can occur: dizziness, upset stomach, throbbing headache and rash.

Interactions: Dipyridamole interacts with anticoagulants (eg warfarin) and if you take both drugs, the dosage may need adjustment.

Precautions: Tell your doctor if you have or have had low blood pressure, migraine or angina.

Available preparations: Tablets, capsules, injection

Brand names: Persantin, Persantin Retard

Combination preparations: Assantin Retard (dipyridamole, aspirin)

Ticlopidine

General information: Ticlopidine is a newly introduced antiplatelet drug, which stops platelets sticking to each other. It is used to prevent thrombosis in patients with a history of stroke and other cardiovascular disorders. A full blood count should be done every 2 weeks for the first 3 months of treatment. This drug is for specialist use only and is available under special arrangements.

How to use: Exactly as prescribed.

Side effects: Ticlopidine may cause skin rash, diarrhoea, haemorrhagic complications and other blood disorders.

Interactions: Ticlopidine interacts with anticoagulants, other antiplatelet drugs and NSAIDs (eg ibuprofen). Check with your doctor or pharmacist before taking any other medicines.

Available preparations: Tablets

Brand names: Ticlid

ANTI-ARRHYTHMICS

Anti-arrhythmics are used to treat irregular heart beat (arrhythmias). There are several types of arrhythmias and more than 15–20 drugs (including specialist ones) used in their treatment. These include digoxin (see page 109), verapamil (see page 96), certain beta-blockers (see page 82) and the drugs listed below in this section.

Each drug works in a slightly different way, but all basically act by altering the conduction of the electrical current through the heart (see page 78) and restoring the heart's normal rhythm.

How to use: Take the medicine exactly as prescribed by the doctor. If you miss a dose, take it as soon as you remember. However, if it is almost time for your next dose, skip the missed dose. Do not take double the dose. Do not stop taking the medicine without asking your doctor because this may cause your underlying condition to get worse.

Precautions, side effects, warnings and interactions: See individual drugs listed below.

Amiodarone

General information: Amiodarone is used in the treatment of arrhythmias, especially when other drugs have not worked for a particular patient. It should always be started in hospital or under specialist supervision, and its use is limited because of unpleasant side effects.

How to use: As anti-arrhythmic drugs (see page 105).
Precautions: Tell your doctor if you are pregnant, planning to become pregnant or are breastfeeding, or if you have or have had thyroid disease or liver or kidney problems.
Side effects: Side effects can be serious with amiodarone, particularly if it is used long term, and include damage to the eyes (eg corneal deposits and coloured haloes), lungs and liver, and also thyroid problems. More rarely, you could experience nausea, vomiting, a metallic taste in the mouth, increased sensitivity of the skin to sunlight, grey skin colour, rash and excessive tiredness. Sometimes it may also cause other arrhythmias.
Warnings: Tell your doctor if you experience any of the above side effects, particularly if they are severe. While taking this drug you will be asked to attend for various tests. Keep all your appointments.
Interactions: Amiodarone can interact with many drugs. Ask your doctor or pharmacist before taking any other medication.
Available preparations: Tablets, injection
Brand names: Cordarone X

Disopyramide

General information: Disopyramide is used in the treatment of arrhythmias.

How to use: As anti-arrhythmic drugs (see page 105).
Precautions: Tell your doctor if you are pregnant, planning to become pregnant or are breastfeeding, or if you have or have had glaucoma, an enlarged prostate, diabetes, heart failure, or liver or kidney problems.
Side effects: Side effects which may occur include dry mouth, blurred vision, problems with passing urine, constipation, dizziness.
Warnings: Do not drink an excessive amount of alcohol (eg more than a glass of wine or half a pint of beer a day) while you are taking this medicine because this will increase the risk of adverse effects. Do not drive or take part in any activity that requires you to be alert until you know how you react to the medicine.
Interactions: Disopyramide interacts with a variety of other drugs including some antibiotics, antidepressants, antihistamines, anti-psychotics, beta-blockers, calcium channel blockers and diuretics. Check with your doctor or pharmacist before taking any other medicines.
Available preparations: Tablets (slow-release only), capsules
Brand names: Dirythmin SA, Rythmodan, Rythmodan SR

Flecainide

General information: Flecainide is used in the treatment of arrhythmias. It should be started in hospital.

How to use: As anti-arrhythmic drugs (see page 105).

Precautions: Tell your doctor if you are pregnant, planning to become pregnant or are breastfeeding, or if you have or have had heart failure, liver or kidney problems or have a pacemaker.

Side effects: Dizziness and visual disturbances may occur. More rarely, nausea, vomiting, jaundice, and tingling of the hands and feet may be experienced, and the skin may become sensitive to sunlight. Sometimes this drug can cause other arrhythmias.

Warnings: Do not drink excessive amount of alcohol (eg more than a glass of wine or half a pint of beer a day) while you are taking these medicines because this will increase the risk of adverse effects. Do not drive or take part in any activity that requires you to be alert until you know how you react to the medicine.

Interactions: Flecainide interacts with a number of other medicines including antidepressants, antihistamines, antipsychotics, beta-blockers, calcium channel blockers and diuretics. Check with your doctor or pharmacist before taking any other medicine.

Available preparations: Tablets, injection

Brand names: Tambocur

Mexiletine

General information: Mexiletine is used in the treatment of arrhythmias.

How to use: As anti-arrhythmic drugs (see page 105).

Precautions: Tell your doctor if you are pregnant, planning to become pregnant or are breastfeeding, or if you have had liver disease.

Side effects: Nausea, vomiting, constipation, palpitations, drowsiness, confusion, trembling, numbness and other arrhythmias may occur.

Warnings: Do not drink an excessive amount of alcohol (eg more than a glass of wine or half a pint of beer a day) while you are taking this medicine because this will increase the risk of adverse effects. Do not drive or take part in any activity that requires you to be alert until you know how you react to the medicine.

Interactions: Mexiletine interacts with a number of other medicines. Check with your pharmacist or doctor before taking any other medicine.

Available preparations: Tablets, capsules, injection

Brand names: Mexitil, Mexitil PL

Moracizine

General information: Moracizine is used in the treatment of arrhythmias. Treatment is often initiated in hospital.

How to use: As anti-arrhythmic drugs (see page 105).

Precautions: Tell your doctor if you are pregnant, planning to become pregnant or are breastfeeding, or if you have or have had heart failure, liver or kidney problems.

Side effects: Upset stomach, dizziness, headache, tiredness or other arrhythmias may occur. If you develop chest pain or breathing difficulty, tell your doctor immediately.

Warnings: Do not drink an excessive amount of alcohol (eg more than a glass of wine or half a pint of beer a day) while you are taking this medicine because this will increase the risk of adverse effects. Do not drive or take part in any activity that requires you to be alert until you know how you react to the medicine.

Interactions: Moracizine interacts with a number of other medicines. Check with your doctor or pharmacist before taking any other medicines.

Available preparations: Tablets

Brand names: Ethmozine

Procainamide

General information: Procainamide is used in the treatment of arrhythmias.

How to use: As anti-arrhythmic drugs (see page 105).

Precautions: Tell your doctor if you are pregnant, planning to become pregnant or are breastfeeding or if you have or have had heart failure, liver or kidney problems or systemic lupus erythmatosus (SLE). SLE is a condition with symptoms of fever, malaise, joint swelling and light sensitive skin.

Side effects: Upset stomach, rash and other arrhythmias. This drug causes symptoms of lupus in some people. Tell your doctor if you experience any of the following: muscle pain or weakness, chest pain, fever or skin rash.

Interactions: Procainamide interacts with a number of other medicines. Check with your doctor or pharmacist before taking any other medicines.

Warnings: Do not drink an excessive amount of alcohol (eg more than a glass of wine or half a pint of beer a day) while you are taking this medicine because this will increase the risk of adverse effects. Do not drive or take part in any activity that requires you to be alert until you know how you react to the medicine.

Available preparations: Tablets, injection

Brand names: Pronestyl

Propafenone

General information: Propafenone is used in the treatment of arrhythmias. Treatment is initiated in hospital with this drug.

How to use: As anti-arrhythmic drugs (see page 105).

Precautions: Tell your doctor if you are pregnant, planning to become pregnant or are breastfeeding or if you have or have had heart failure, liver or kidney problems, breathing problems or lung disease.

Side effects: These may include dry mouth, blurred vision, dizziness, nausea and vomiting, diarrhoea, headache, bitter taste and rash.

Warnings: Do not drink an excessive amount of alcohol (eg more than a glass of

wine or half a pint of beer a day) while you are taking this medicine because this will increase the risk of adverse effects. Do not drive or take part in any activity that requires you to be alert until you know how you react to the medicine.
Interactions: Propafenone interacts with a number of other medicines. Check with your doctor or pharmacist before taking any other medicines.
Available preparations: Tablets
Brand names: Arythmol

Quinidine

General information: Quinidine is used in the treatment of arrhythmias.

How to use: As anti-arrhythmic drugs (see page 105).
Precautions: No special instructions, but this drug should be started under the supervision of a hospital consultant.
Side effects, warnings, interactions: As procainamide (see page 108).
Available preparations: Tablets
Brand names: Kinidin Durules

INOTROPIC DRUGS

Inotropic drugs increase the force with which the heart beats. They help the heart work better and so are used to treat heart failure and arrhythmias. Two drugs – digoxin and xamoterol – are included in this section.

How to use: Take the medicine exactly as prescribed by the doctor. If you miss a dose, take it as soon as you remember. However, if it is almost time for your next dose, skip the missed dose. Do not take double the dose. Do not stop taking the medicine without asking your doctor because this may cause your underlying condition to get worse.

Precautions, side effects, warnings, interactions: See individual drugs listed below.

Digoxin

General information: Digoxin is used in heart failure and arrhythmias (irregular heart beat), especially atrial fibrillation. Widely used in the past, particularly for heart failure, it is not used as much now. When it is prescribed for heart failure, a diuretic is generally used as well.

How to use: As inotropic drugs (see above).
Precautions: Tell your doctor if you are pregnant, planning to become pregnant or are breastfeeding or if you have or have had Wolff-Parkinson-White syndrome (a particular type of heart rhythm irregularity), liver or kidney problems or thyroid disease.
Side effects: Loss of appetite, nausea, vomiting, diarrhoea, tiredness, drowsiness, irregular heartbeat, confusion. Contact your doctor if you experience any side

effects with this medicine. This is because side effects are often caused by levels of digoxin being too high in the blood. Side effects with this drug are more common if you are over 65 or if your blood potassium levels are low. Your doctor may prescribe a potassium supplement, particularly if you are taking a diuretic as well. This is because diuretics can lower your blood potassium levels. The therapeutic dose for digoxin is close to the toxic dose, so it is very important to tell your doctor about any side effects.

Warnings: You may have to attend for regular blood tests. Do not miss your appointments.

Interactions: Digoxin interacts with several other medicines, including anti-arrhythmics and calcium channel blockers. Check with your pharmacist or doctor before taking any other medicines.

Available preparations: Tablets, liquid, injection

Brand names: Lanoxin, Lanoxin PG

Xamoterol

General information: Xamoterol is used in mild (but not severe) heart failure. Treatment will be started in hospital

How to use: As inotropic drugs (see page 109).

Precautions: Tell your doctor if you are pregnant, planning to become pregnant or are breastfeeding, or if you have kidney disease.

Side effects: Upset stomach, headache, dizziness, breathing problems, palpitations, chest pain, muscle cramps, rash.

Warnings: You will have to attend for regular monitoring. Do not miss your appointments.

Interactions: There are no important interactions with xamoterol, but check with your doctor or pharmacist before taking any other medication.

Available preparations: Tablets

Brand names: Corwin

The Gastrointestinal System

EXTENDING FROM THE MOUTH to the anus, the gastrointestinal system is responsible for digesting your food, absorbing the nutrients into the bloodstream and eliminating the undigestible parts of food from the body. It also breaks down medicines – at least those you take by mouth – and absorbs drugs into the blood. The gastrointestinal system consists of the digestive tract – the mouth, throat, oesophagus, stomach, small intestine, large intestine and rectum – and also a number of organs that lie outside of the digestive tract, such as the liver, pancreas and gall bladder.

Food enters the gastrointestinal system through the mouth and is propelled through the oesophagus to the stomach by waves of rhythmic contractions and relaxations called peristalsis. Digestion begins in the mouth through the action of the teeth and the saliva and continues in the stomach. A hollow, muscular bag, the stomach produces several substances that aid digestion. The first is hydrochloric acid, which kills bacteria in food; the second is pepsin, which starts to break down protein; and the third is intrinsic factor, which is essential for the absorption of vitamin B12.

Food stays in the stomach for up to five hours, where it is thoroughly mixed with the gastric juice. At regular intervals, the muscular contractions of the stomach push a small amount of the semi-digested food into the small intestine where digestion continues. The first part of the small intestine is known as the duodenum, and below the duodenum are the jejunum and ileum. Enzymes – from the pancreas and the intestinal wall – and various other substances such as bile acids, produced by the liver and stored in the gall bladder, continue the work of digestion, and by this time the food has the consistency of soup. Absorption of nutrients takes place throughout the small intestine, but mainly in the jejunum and ileum; it is helped by the fact that the small intestine has a vast surface area. Inside, it is not just a smooth tube, but is made up of folds known as villi and microvilli, which are richly supplied with blood vessels that help to carry the nutrients into the bloodstream. Nutrients are taken immediately to the liver where they are further processed and made ready for use by the rest of the body.

Unabsorbed food components are propelled along to the large intestine, which consists of the colon, rectum and anus. Further digestion and absorption, particularly of minerals, takes place here, but the main function of the large intestine is to absorb water from the food mixture to produce the faecal matter.

What can go wrong

Problems can occur almost anywhere in the gastrointestinal tract. Indigestion, or dyspepsia, as it is often called, is a common condition arising from excessive acid production and irritation of the stomach lining. The main symptom is pain in the upper abdomen, and the condition may be exacerbated by overeating (particularly fatty and spicy foods), coffee, alcohol, smoking and anxiety. It is also common in pregnancy. Sometimes the stomach contents flow upwards into the oesophagus. This happens when the muscle dividing the oesophagus from the stomach (the oesophageal sphincter) is not working properly. Another condition, known as hiatus hernia, is the protrusion of a part of the stomach from its normal position upwards through the diaphragm. Both these conditions can cause symptoms of heartburn – a burning sensation in the centre of the chest.

Normally a coating of mucus protects the linings of the stomach and duodenum from damage by the stomach acid and other digestive juices. Should this mucus layer break down – for example from the use of drugs such as aspirin and ibuprofen – damage can occur that leads to a peptic ulcer. Peptic ulcer can occur in the stomach, the duodenum or the jejunum, and although the cause is not fully understood, it seems that the majority of people with ulcer are also infected with the bacterium known as *Helicobacter pylori*.

Any part of the wall of the digestive tract can become inflamed and this can lead to severe pain and diarrhoea. There are two main types of inflammatory bowel disease (IBD) – Crohn's disease, which can affect any part of the digestive tract, but mainly affects the small intestine, and ulcerative colitis, which affects the large intestine. Other conditions that affect the intestine include irritable bowel syndrome (IBS) and diverticulitis. Irritable bowel syndrome is a disorder of bowel movement which results in abdominal pain together with constipation and/or diarrhoea. Diverticulitis is another inflammatory condition, which occurs with the development of sac-like protrusions (diverticula) in the digestive tract. The most common site for diverticula is the large intestine and if one or more of these become inflamed or infected, diverticulitis occurs.

Two of the most common disorders affecting the gastrointestinal system are diarrhoea and constipation. By the time unabsorbed food – the faecal matter – reaches the rectum it should be quite dry. However, if waste material moves through your colon too fast, leaving insufficient time to absorb water, diarrhoea occurs. The most common causes of diarrhoea are viral infection and food poisoning, but a number of illnesses (eg Crohn's disease, ulcerative colitis, cancer) can cause this condition. The opposite problem, constipation, occurs if movement in the colon is too slow. Far too much water is absorbed, leaving hard, dry faeces that are difficult to get rid of. Constipation may be caused by other illnesses and also by various drugs (eg codeine and other opioid analgesics), but the most common cause is lack of fibre. Eating wholemeal bread and wholegrain cereals with plenty of fruit and vegetables is the best way to treat constipation.

Common conditions and drugs used to treat them

Indigestion and gastro-oesophageal reflux disease – antacids, alginates, histamine H2 antagonists

Peptic ulcer – antacids, histamine H2 antagonists, proton pump inhibitors, misoprostol, sucralfate. Triple therapy with antibiotics is also used to eradicate the bacterium, *Helicobacter pylori*, associated with peptic ulcer.

Irritable bowel syndrome – bulk laxatives, anti-diarrhoeals, antispasmodics

Diarrhoea – codeine, loperamide oral rehydration therapy

Crohn's disease and ulcerative colitis – aminosalicylates (eg sulphasalazine, mesalazine) and corticosteroids

Constipation – laxatives

Piles (haemorrhoids) – various creams, ointments and suppositories containing local anaesthetics and/or soothing ingredients

Pancreatic disease, including cystic fibrosis – pancreatin

Gall bladder disease – bile acids (eg chenodeoxycholic acid, ursodeoxycholic acid)

ANTACIDS

Antacids are used for symptoms of indigestion and acid reflux. Doctors prescribe them occasionally for peptic ulcer, but since the advent of histamine H2 antagonists and proton pump inhibitors, antacids are used for ulcers less frequently. There are two main groups of antacids – those containing aluminium and those containing magnesium – as well as sodium bicarbonate and a range of others which are found largely in over-the-counter remedies for indigestion and heartburn. Most antacids prescribed by doctors contain aluminium or magnesium or a mixture of the two. Some of the branded products also contain other ingredients such as dimethicone, which helps to relieve flatulence and is used on its own in preparations for infant colic. Alginates (see below) are useful in treating symptoms of gastro-oesophageal reflux and hiatus hernia, and are added to several antacid mixtures.

How they work: All antacids combine with stomach acid and neutralise it. They therefore help to reduce symptoms caused by excessive stomach acid. Both aluminium- and magnesium-containing antacids work quite quickly – within 15 minutes – and their effects last for two to four hours. Sodium bicarbonate also works quickly, but its effect soon wears off – within 30–60 minutes.

How to use: The dose is usually prescribed to be taken three to four times a day. This is best taken about one hour after meals because the movements of the stomach will have slowed sufficiently to allow the antacid to remain in the stomach for a reasonable length of time. Taken just before a meal, antacids are rapidly emptied from the stomach and their effect does not last so long. If you miss a dose, just take the next dose as usual. Unless the antacid is prescribed for a long term condition, it is quite safe to stop taking it whenever you feel better.

Precautions: Tell your doctor if you are pregnant or plan to become pregnant or if you are breastfeeding, if you have or have had kidney problems, heart disease or bone disease, or if you are on a low-sodium diet.

Side effects: The most common side effect of aluminium salts is constipation, while magnesium salts tend to cause diarrhoea. This is why the two salts are often combined in one preparation.

Warnings: None

Interactions: Antacids interact with a large number of other drugs by altering their absorption. Common ones include antibiotics, oral anticoagulants, digoxin, phenytoin, corticosteroids and antipsychotics. Antacids may also break up the enteric coating on other tablets, and this may lead to stomach irritation.

Alginates

General information: Alginates are used in indigestion, particularly for that caused by gastro-oesophageal reflux. They form a raft or barrier between the stomach contents and the oesophagus and help to protect the lining of the oesophagus from the irritant action of the stomach acid.

Available preparations: Tablets, liquid (all in combination with antacids)
Brand names: Algicon, Gastrocote, Gaviscon, Gaviscon Advance, Gaviscon Infant, Topal, and a range of over-the-counter remedies contain antacids with alginates.

Aluminium hydroxide

General information: Aluminium hydroxide is used in indigestion. It is also used to reduce high phosphate levels in the blood (hypophosphataemia).

Available preparations: Tablets, capsules, liquid
Brand names: Alu-Cap
Combination preparations: Altacite Plus (aluminium, magnesium, simethicone), Asilone (aluminium, dimethicone), Diovol (aluminium, magnesium, dimethicone), Maalox (aluminium, magnesium), Maalox Plus (aluminium, magnesium, dimethicone), Maalox TC (aluminium, magnesium), Mucaine (aluminium, magnesium, oxethazaine), Mucogel (aluminium, magnesium), and a range of over-the-counter remedies contain antacid combinations.

Dimethicone

General information: Dimethicone is used for gripes, colic or wind in infants.

Available preparations: Liquid
Brand names: Dentinox, Infacol

Magnesium carbonate

General information: Magnesium carbonate is used in indigestion.

Available preparations: Liquid
Brand names: None, but a range of over-the-counter remedies contain magnesium carbonate.

Magnesium trisilicate

General information: Magnesium trisilicate is used in indigestion.

Available preparations: Tablets, liquid, powder

Brand names: None, but a range of over-the-counter remedies contain magnesium trisilicate.

Sodium bicarbonate

General information: Sodium bicarbonate is sometimes used to treat indigestion, but it is not recommended because of its short duration of action and also because of its high sodium content.

Available preparations: Tablets
Brand names: None, but a range of over-the-counter remedies contain sodium bicarbonate.

ANTISPASMODICS

Antispasmodics, although not used much nowadays, are available for the treatment of a number of conditions affecting the gastrointestinal tract, including irritable bowel syndrome and diverticular disease as well as – very occasionally – symptoms of indigestion.

How they work: Antispasmodics reduce both gastrointestinal motility and production of acid in the stomach. They work by relaxing the muscle that surrounds the digestive tract and so relax the gut.

How to use: Take the medicine exactly as prescribed by the doctor. If you miss a dose, take it as soon as you remember. However, if it is almost time for your next dose, skip the missed dose. Do not take double the dose. Do not stop taking the medicine without asking your doctor because this may cause your underlying condition to get worse.

Precautions, side effects, warnings, interactions: see individual drugs listed below.

Alverine

General information: Alverine is used for irritable bowel syndrome and diverticular disease. It is also used for severe period pain (dysmenorrhoea: see page 178).

How to use: As antispasmodics (see above).
Precautions: Tell your doctor if you are pregnant, plan to become pregnant or are breastfeeding, or if you have or have had intestinal obstruction.
Side effects: Side effects are rare, but nausea, headache, dizziness and rash may occur.
Warnings: None
Interactions: None reported.
Available preparations: Capsules
Brand names: Spasmonal
Combination preparations: Alvercol (alverine with sterculia – a bulk laxative).

Dicyclomine

General information: Dicyclomine is used for some types of indigestion and for irritable bowel syndrome and diverticular disease.

How to use: As antispasmodics (see page 115).
Precautions: Tell your doctor if you are pregnant, plan to become pregnant or are breastfeeding, or if you have or have had glaucoma, enlarged prostate or hiatus hernia.
Side effects: Dry mouth, blurred vision, constipation, diarrhoea, drowsiness, difficulty in passing urine may occur.
Warnings: Do not drink alcohol while you are taking this medicine because this will increase the risk of adverse effects. Do not drive or take part in any activity that requires you to be alert until you know how you react to the medicine.
Interactions: Antispasmodics interact with a number of other medicines. Check with your doctor or pharmacist before taking any other medicine.
Available preparations: Tablets, liquid
Brand names: Merbentyl
Combination preparations: Kolanticon (dicyclomine with antacids)

Hyoscine

General information: Hyoscine is used for some types of indigestion and for irritable bowel syndrome, diverticular disease and period pain (dysmenorrhoea).

How to use: As antispasmodics (see page 115).
Precautions, side effects, warnings, interactions: As dicyclomine (see above).
Available preparations: Tablets, injection
Brand names: Buscopan

Mebeverine

General information: Mebeverine is used for irritable bowel syndrome and diverticular disease.

How to use: As antispasmodics (see page 115).
Precautions, side effects, warnings, interactions: As alverine (see page 115).
Available preparations: Tablets, liquid
Brand names: Colofac
Combination preparations: Fybogel Mebeverine (mebeverine with ispaghula – a bulk laxative).

Peppermint oil

General information: Peppermint oil is used for colic and distension, particularly in irritable bowel syndrome.

How to use: As antispasmodics (see page 115). In addition, do not break or chew the capsules, because peppermint oil will be released and could cause irritation of the mouth or oesophagus.

Precautions, side effects, warnings, interactions: As alverine (see page 115).
Available preparations: Capsules,.
Brand names: Colpermin (contains peanut oil), Mintec

Propantheline

General information: Propantheline is used for some types of indigestion, and for irritable bowel syndrome and diverticular disease.

How to use: As antispasmodics (see page 115).
Precautions, side effects, warnings, interactions: As dicyclomine (see page 116).
Available preparations: Tablets
Brand names: Probanthine

Cisapride

General information: Cisapride stimulates movement in the oesophagus, stomach and intestine by increasing the contraction of the muscles in the stomach and gut wall. It is useful in a number of conditions, including gastro-oesophageal reflux, indigestion, and conditions where stomach emptying is slowed or delayed for some reason.

How to use: Take the medicine exactly as prescribed by the doctor. If you miss a dose, take it as soon as you remember. However, if it is almost time for your next dose, skip the missed dose. Do not take double the dose. Do not stop taking the medicine without asking your doctor because this may cause your underlying condition to get worse.
Precautions: Tell your doctor if you are pregnant, planning a pregnancy or are breastfeeding, or have or have had liver, kidney or heart problems.
Side effects: Side effects are mainly gastrointestinal and include nausea, diarrhoea and abdominal cramps. Dizziness, tremor and increased urinary frequency may also occur.
Warnings: Take care with driving and other similar activities until you have found out how the drug affects you, because it can cause dizziness.
Interactions: Cisapride interacts with several other drugs, including some antibiotics, antidepressants, and the antihistamines astemizole and terfenadine. Check with your doctor or pharmacist before taking any other medicines.
Available preparations: Tablets, liquid
Brand names: Prepulsid

ULCER-HEALING DRUGS

Two main groups of drugs are used in the treatment of peptic ulcer. These are: histamine H2 antagonists (eg cimetidine, ranitidine) and proton pump inhibitors (eg omeprazole, lansoprazole). Other drugs used include bismuth chelate, sucralfate, misoprostol and carbenoxolone. Antacids are also used (see page 113), but with the advent of more powerful drugs they are used in the treatment of ulcers much less frequently than previously. Some of these drugs (eg omeprazole, lansoprazole, ranitidine, bismuth chelate) are used in conjunction with various antibiotics (eg amoxycillin, clarithromycin, metronidazole, tetracycline) to eradicate the bacterium known as *Helicobacter pylori*, which is thought to cause peptic ulcer in many people.

How they work: Histamine H2 antagonists, proton pump inhibitors and misoprostol work by reducing the output of acid from the stomach. This reduces stomach irritation and erosion, and helps ulcers to heal. Misoprostol has an additional action in that it helps to increase the production of the mucus lining in the stomach and small intestine. Bismuth chelate and sucralfate work by forming a protective coat round the ulcer. They have no effect on acid production, but the protective coat prevents acid getting to the ulcers and so allows healing to take place.

How to use: Take the medicine exactly as prescribed by the doctor. If you are being treated for *Helicobacter pylori* it is particularly important to follow the regime exactly. If you miss a dose, take it as soon as you remember. However, if it is almost time for your next dose, skip the missed dose. Do not take double the dose. Do not stop taking the medicine without asking your doctor because this may cause your underlying condition to get worse.

Precautions, side effects, warnings, interactions: See individual drugs listed below.

Histamine H2 antagonists

Histamine H2 antagonists are used to treat peptic ulcers and reflux oesophagitis. They work by binding to histamine H2 receptors and result in reduced production of stomach acid. This reduces acid erosion and stomach irritation, and helps the ulcer to heal. These drugs are different in their actions to the classical antihistamines (see page 284).

How to use: As ulcer-healing drugs (see above).

Precautions: Tell your doctor if you are pregnant, planning to become pregnant or are breastfeeding, or if you have or have had liver or kidney problems.

Side effects: Side effects are uncommon, but the following may occur: diarrhoea, headache, dizziness and rash. Breast enlargement (men only) and impotence may occur, but these side effects are quite rare.

Warnings: Take care with driving and other similar activities until you have found out how the drug affects you, because it can cause dizziness.

Interactions: None of these drugs is involved in significant interactions apart from cimetidine (see below).

Cimetidine

General information: Cimetidine was the first of this group to be introduced and is now available over the counter in pharmacies as well as on prescription. Like all H2 antagonists it is a safe drug, but, unlike the other four drugs in this group, cimetidine is involved in significant interactions with other drugs.

Use, precautions, side effects, warnings: As histamine H2 antagonists (see page 118).
Interactions: Cimetidine interacts with a number of drugs, including oral anticoagulants (eg warfarin), anticonvulsants (eg phenytoin), theophylline, cyclosporin beta-blockers and benzodiazepines. In some cases the dose of these other drugs may need to be altered. Check with your pharmacist or doctor before taking cimetidine if you are taking other medicines, both prescribed and over the counter.
Available preparations: Tablets, liquid, injection
Brand names: Dyspamet, Tagamet
Combination preparations: Algitec (cimetidine and alginate)

Famotidine

Available preparations: Tablets
Brand names: Pepcid

Nizatidine

Available preparations: Capsules, injection
Brand names: Axid

Ranitidine

Available preparations: Tablets, liquid, injection
Brand names: Zantac

Ranitidine bismuth citrate

Available preparations: Tablets
Brand names: Pylorid

Proton pump inhibitors

Proton pump inhibitors are used to treat peptic ulcer and reflux oesophagitis. They work by acting on the acid pump in the stomach and reducing acid production. This in turn reduces acid erosion and stomach irritation and helps ulcers to heal.

How to use: As ulcer-healing drugs (see page 118).

Precautions: Tell your doctor if you are pregnant, planning a pregnancy or are breastfeeding, or if you have or have had liver problems.

Side effects: Side effects are uncommon and usually mild, but the following may occur: headache, diarrhoea, rash, dizziness, nausea, constipation.

Interactions: Proton pump inhibitors interact with a number of other drugs, including oral anticoagulants (eg warfarin) and anticonvulsants (eg phenytoin). However, significant interactions have been more frequently reported with omeprazole than the other drugs in this group. This may be in part because omeprazole is the oldest of these drugs and there is less experience with the newer drugs.

Lansoprazole

Available preparations: Capsules, liquid
Brand names: Zoton
Combination preparations: HeliClear: for eradication of *Helicobacter pylori* in patients with duodenal ulcer (lansoprazole, with two antibiotics – clarithromycin and amoxycillin)

Omeprazole

Available preparations: Capsules
Brand names: Losec

Pantoprazole

Available preparations: Tablets, injection
Brand names: Protium

Rabeprazole

Available preparations: Tablets
Brand names: Pariet

Miscellaneous drugs for ulcer-healing

Bismuth chelate

General information: Bismuth chelate is used to treat peptic ulcers. It works by forming a protective coat round the ulcer. It has no effect on acid production, but the protective coat prevents acid getting to the ulcers and so allows healing to take place. Bismuth chelate may be given in combination with antibiotics (typically amoxycillin and metronidazole) for the eradication of *Helicobacter pylori* (an infection which often occurs with ulcers and is thought to be involved in causing them).

How to use: As ulcer-healing drugs (see page 118).
Precautions: Tell your doctor if you are pregnant, planning a pregnancy or are breastfeeding, or if you have or have had kidney problems.

Side effects: Bismuth may darken the tongue and cause black stools. Nausea and vomiting may also occur.
Warnings and interactions: None
Available preparations: Tablets, liquid
Brand names: De-Nol, De-Noltab

Carbenoxolone

General information: Carbenoxolone is a derivative of liquorice. It can be used for ulceration and inflammation of the oesophagus, but the danger of unpleasant side effects with this drug means that it is used very rarely these days.

How to use: As ulcer-healing drugs (see page 118).
Precautions: Tell your doctor if you are pregnant, planning a pregnancy or are breastfeeding, or if you have or have had heart problems or liver or kidney problems.
Side effects: Carbenoxolone can cause serious side effects – notably sodium and water retention, which can lead to high blood pressure and heart failure. It can also cause muscle damage.
Warnings: You will be asked to attend for blood tests while taking this medicine. Do not miss your appointments.
Interactions: Carbenoxolone interacts with several other medicines. Check with your doctor or pharmacist before taking any other medication.
Available preparations: Tablets, liquid
Brand names: Pyrogastrone

Misoprostol

General information: Misoprostol is used mainly in the prevention and treatment of ulcers caused by non-steroidal anti-inflammatory drugs (NSAIDs). It works by reducing acid production in the stomach and also helps to increase the production of the mucus lining in the stomach and small intestine.

How to use: As ulcer-healing drugs (see page 118).
Precautions: Tell your doctor if you are pregnant, planning a pregnancy or are breastfeeding, or if you have or have had heart or circulatory problems or a stroke.
Side effects: Gastrointestinal side effects are common with this drug and may include diarrhoea, abdominal pain, indigestion, flatulence, nausea and vomiting. Rash, dizziness and vaginal bleeding may occur, but these are rare side effects.
Warnings: It is particularly important that you do not become pregnant while taking this drug. This is because misoprostol causes the uterine muscle to contract and cause abortion. Use adequate contraception.
Interactions: Misoprostol interacts with few drugs, but check with your doctor or pharmacist before taking any other medicines.
Available preparations: Tablets
Brand names: Cytotec
Combination preparations: Arthrotec (misoprostol and diclofenac); Napratec (misoprostol and naproxen)

Sucralfate

General information: Sucralfate is used to treat peptic ulcers. It works by forming a protective coat round the ulcer. It has no effect on acid production, but the protective coat prevents acid from getting to the ulcers and so allows healing to take place.

How to use: As ulcer-healing drugs (see page 118).
Precautions: Tell your doctor if you are pregnant, planning to become pregnant or are breastfeeding, or if you have or have had kidney problems.
Side effects: Gastrointestinal effects are the most common and include constipation, diarrhoea, nausea and indigestion. Rash, dizziness, headache, drowsiness, dry mouth and back pain may also occur.
Warnings: Avoid alcohol because it may counteract the effects of the drug.
Interactions: Sucralfate interacts with several drugs including oral anticoagulants (eg warfarin) and anticonvulsants (eg phenytoin). Antibacterial drugs should not be taken at the same time as sucralfate – leave a gap of two hours.
Available preparations: Tablets, liquid
Brand names: Antepsin

DRUGS FOR DIARRHOEA

Drugs have a very limited place in the treatment of diarrhoea, unless it is diarrhoea caused by a more serious illness (eg inflammatory bowel disease, bowel cancer). The best treatment for acute diarrhoea – which normally lasts no more than a couple of days – is to drink plenty of fluid and to avoid food for about 24 hours. In adults this is often all that is needed. However, particular care must be taken with babies, children and frail, elderly people who can soon get dehydrated if they have severe diarrhoea.

A variety of preparations containing a mixture of sodium and potassium salts, and glucose, is available to prevent dehydration in episodes of diarrhoea. Known as oral rehydration solutions, these preparations are dissolved in water to make a drink and replace lost salts and water.

Sometimes drugs (eg codeine, loperamide) are used, particularly in cases where diarrhoea is socially inconvenient (eg when travelling), but they are not a substitute for oral rehydration therapy.

How they work: All these drugs work by reducing the activity of the muscles in the gut, so enabling the absorption of water and stopping the diarrhoea. The main reason why doctors do not recommend them is that in slowing muscular activity in the gut, these drugs cause bacteria and viruses to stay longer in the gut where they can cause damage. In addition, some anti-diarrhoeal drugs can cause sedation and people can easily become dependent on them. None of these preparations is recommended for use in young children.

Precautions, side effects, warnings, interactions: see individual drugs listed below.

Codeine

General information: Codeine is used in the treatment of diarrhoea. It is also used in the treatment of severe pain (see page 63).

Precautions, side effects, warnings, interactions: As opioids (see page 62).
Available preparations: Tablets
Brand names: None
Combination preparations: Diarrest (codeine, dicyclomine, sodium and potassium salts)

Co-phenotrope

General information: Co-phenotrope used in the treatment of diarrhoea. This preparation is a mixture of diphenoxylate and atropine.

Precautions, side effects, warnings, interactions: As opioids (see page 62).
Available preparations: Tablets
Brand names: Lomotil

Kaolin and Morphine

General information: Kaolin and morphine mixture is used in the treatment of diarrhoea.

Precautions, side effects, warnings, interactions: As opioids (see page 62).
Available preparations: Liquid
Brand names: None, but some preparations available over the counter.

Loperamide

General information: Loperamide is used in the treatment of diarrhoea.

Precautions, side effects, warnings, interactions: As opioids (see page 62).
Available preparations: Capsules, liquid
Brand names: Imodium

Oral rehydration solutions

General information: Oral rehydration solutions are used to replace the salts and water lost in diarrhoea. Follow the directions on the packet very carefully if you use one of these products, making sure that the dose you use and the amount of water is suitable for the age of the person you are treating.

Brand names: Diocalm Junior, Dioralyte, Dioralyte Relief, Electrolade, Rehidrat

DRUGS FOR INFLAMMATORY BOWEL DISEASE

Inflammatory bowel conditions such as Crohn's disease and ulcerative colitis can be treated with drugs that help to reduce the inflammation and associated symptoms of pain, diarrhoea and general malaise. Two main groups of drugs are used in these conditions – corticosteroids and aminosalicylates. Both groups of drugs work by dampening down the process of inflammation in the gut and allowing ulcerated and damaged tissue to recover.

Corticosteroids

Treatment for inflammatory bowel disease is a matter for specialists, but in general, steroids are used to bring the disease under control. In localised gastrointestinal disease they can be given as suppositories, foam or enemas, but in severe disease they can be given by mouth. Foams are particularly useful in patients who cannot retain enemas. Prednisolone is preferred to hydrocortisone as it has a more powerful anti-inflammatory effect and causes less fluid retention. Budesonide is not so well absorbed from the gut into the bloodstream, and what is absorbed is broken down in the liver. It is therefore a useful drug, achieving a more localised anti-inflammatory effect with fewer side effects.

How to use: Take the medicine exactly as prescribed by the doctor. If you miss a dose, take it as soon as you remember. However, if it is almost time for your next dose, skip the missed dose. Do not take double the dose. Do not stop taking the medicine without asking your doctor because this may cause your underlying condition to get worse.

Precautions, side effects, warnings, interactions: See individual drugs listed below.

Budesonide

Available preparations: Capsules, enema
Brand names: Budenofalk, Entocort

Hydrocortisone

Available preparations: Rectal foam
Brand names: Colifoam

Prednisolone

Available preparations: Suppositories, enema, rectal foam
Brand names: Predenema, Predfoam, Predsol

Aminosalicylates

Aminosalicylates act on the lining of the colon. They are not as useful as corticosteroids in terminating an attack, but they are useful in preventing relapses of ulcerative colitis. These drugs are absorbed in the small intestine, so, because they have to be delivered to the colon, they are either coated in a resin or combined with other compounds. This ensures that they reach the large bowel.

How to use: Take the medicine exactly as prescribed by the doctor. If you miss a dose, take it as soon as you remember. However, if it is almost time for your next dose, skip the missed dose. Do not take double the dose. Do not stop taking the medicine without asking your doctor because this may cause your underlying condition to get worse.

Precautions: Tell your doctor if you are pregnant, planning to become pregnant or breastfeeding, or if you have or have had liver or kidney problems.

Side effects: Diarrhoea and other gastrointestinal disturbances, nausea, headache, rash and other allergic reactions.

Warnings: Tell your doctor immediately if you experience sore throat, fever, mouth sores, any unusual bleeding or bruising, or rash.

Interactions: None reported.

Balsalazide

Available preparations: Capsules
Brand names: Colazide

Mesalazine

Precautions, side effects, warnings, interactions: As aminosalicylates (see above). In addition, tell your doctor if you have any blood clotting disorder.
Available preparations: Tablets, enema, suppositories
Brand names: Asacaol, Pentasa, Salofalk

Olsalazine

Available preparations: Tablets, capsules
Brand names: Dipentum

Sulphasalazine

General information: Sulphasalazine is a mixture of 5-aminosalicylate and sulphapyridine (a sulphonamide). It is used in the treatment of Crohn's disease as well as ulcerative colitis, and also in rheumatoid arthritis (see page 153). Because it contains a sulphonamide drug, the side effects, precautions and warnings are different from those of the other drugs in this group.

How to use: Take the medicine exactly as prescribed by the doctor. If you miss a dose, take it as soon as you remember. However, if it is almost time for your next dose, skip the missed dose. Do not take double the dose. Do not stop taking the medicine without asking your doctor because this may cause your underlying condition to get worse.
Precautions: Tell your doctor if you are pregnant, planning to become pregnant or

are breastfeeding, or if you have or have had liver or kidney problems, or glucose 6-phosphate (G6PD) deficiency, or if you wear contact lenses.

Side effects: Nausea, vomiting, loss of appetite, ringing in the ears, headache, joint pain, fever, rash and other allergic symptoms. Urine may be coloured orange. Staining of soft contact lenses may occur. Long term use leads to a decreased sperm count, which is reversible on stopping the drug.

Warnings: Tell your doctor immediately if you experience sore throat, fever, mouth sores, any unusual bleeding or bruising or rash.

Available preparations: Tablets, liquid, enema, suppositories

Brand names: Salazopyrin

LAXATIVES

Laxatives are used in the treatment of constipation. If you are constipated, this means that you are not passing faeces as often as usual and your faeces are hard and dry. Constipation is often quite harmless, but it can be a sign of a more serious disorder, particularly if it continues for longer than a few days and it occurs in someone over 40. The best way to treat constipation is to increase the fibre content of your diet, by eating wholemeal bread, wholegrain cereals, beans and peas and fruit and vegetables. It is also important to include plenty of fluid in your diet and to have plenty of exercise.

Laxatives should never be used as a first resort in constipation and are only justified when:

- Straining to pass faeces might worsen a condition such as angina or piles;
- You have a temporary illness that causes constipation (eg one that keeps you in bed and perhaps leads to poor appetite);
- You have been treated for worms; laxatives may be used to expel any worms left after treatment;
- The gastrointestinal tract needs to be cleared for surgery or examination;
- An elderly person develops constipation due to immobility;
- Other drugs have caused constipation (eg opioid analgesics such as morphine).

Many people abuse laxatives and this can lead to various problems. For example, it is possible to become too dependent on laxatives for normal bowel function and the bowel may cease to work properly on its own. In addition, excessive use of laxatives can lead to diarrhoea and loss of salts and water from the body.

There are three different groups of laxatives: bulk-forming laxatives, stimulant laxatives and osmotic laxatives. In addition, liquid paraffin, although a traditional laxative, is now very rarely prescribed because it can cause serious side effects, particularly when it is used for long periods of time.

Bulk-forming laxatives

Bulk forming laxatives (eg bran, ispaghula) absorb or retain water in themselves and increase the mass of faeces in the bowel, which makes the faeces softer and easier to pass. They work in just the same way as high-fibre diets — so they take a few days to work – and to some extent are safer than other laxatives. However, unless you drink plenty of water with these medicines, they can cause intestinal obstruction.

How to use: Most of these preparations are in powder or granular form, so you need to stir them into plenty of water. If you miss a dose, take it as soon as you remember. You can stop taking the medicine as soon as your constipation has disappeared.

Precautions: Tell your doctor if you have or have had any intestinal obstruction or swallowing difficulty. These preparations are safe to use in pregnancy.

Side effects: Bloating or excess wind may occur. The faeces may become impacted in the intestine if you do not drink enough fluid with these preparations. If you miss a dose, take it when you remember. You can stop taking the medicine when your constipation has disappeared.

Warnings, interactions: None

Bran

Available preparations: Powder
Brand names: Trifyba

Ispaghula

Available preparations: Powder, granules
Brand names: Fybogel, Konsyl, Isogel, Regulan

Methylcellulose

Available preparations: Tablets
Brand names: Celevac

Sterculia

Available preparations: Granules
Brand names: Normacol, Normacol Plus

Stimulant laxatives

Stimulant laxatives (eg senna, bisacodyl) cause the intestinal muscle to contract, increasing the speed at which faeces pass through the intestine. Most take 8–12 hours to work. They should not be used for long periods of time, however, as they can destroy the nerves that supply the bowel.

How to use: They are usually prescribed to be taken at night and should work the following morning. If you miss a dose, take it as soon as you remember. You can stop taking the medicine as soon as your constipation has disappeared.

Precautions: Tell your doctor if you have or have had any intestinal obstruction.

Side effects: Griping, stomach pains may be experienced.

Warnings, interactions: None

Bisacodyl

Available preparations: Tablets, suppositories
Brand names: Dulco-Lax

Danthron

General information: This is a powerful laxative and its use is restricted to constipation in terminal illness and in those who have heart failure or who have had coronary thrombosis. It is probably used most often in elderly people. Danthron may turn the urine red.

Available preparations: Capsules, liquid
Brand names: None
Combination preparations: Co-danthrusate (danthron with docusate); Co-danthromer (danthron with poloxamer 188)

Docusate

Available preparations: Capsules, liquid, enema
Brand names: Dioctyl, Docusol, Fletcher's Enemette, Norgalax Micro-enema

Glycerol

Available preparations: Suppositories
Brand names: None

Senna

Available preparations: Tablets, granules, liquid
Brand names: Manevac, Senokot

Osmotic laxatives

Osmotic laxatives (eg lactulose and various magnesium and sodium salts) work by retaining water in the bowel, softening the faeces and making the faeces easier to pass.

How to use: Take as prescribed. If you miss a dose, take it as soon as you remember. You can stop using the medicine as soon as your constipation has disappeared.

Precautions: Tell your doctor if you have had severe abdominal pains or intestinal obstruction.

Side effects: See individual drugs listed below.

Warnings, interactions: None

Lactitol

General information: Lactitol is similar to lactulose (see below for further information).

Available preparations: Powder
Brand names: None

Lactulose

General information. Lactulose is used as a laxative and also used to prevent the brain disturbance associated with liver failure (hepatic encephalopathy). As a laxative it usually takes a couple of days to work from the start of treatment, so you should wait 48 hours before adjusting the dose. Most people who take it find it quite gentle, and it is considered to be safer than many other laxatives.

Precautions: Tell your doctor if you have had severe abdominal pain or intestinal obstruction.
Side effects: Stomach cramps are common at the start of treatment. Diarrhoea indicates that the dosage is too high for you.
Available preparations: Liquid and powder
Brand names: None; some preparations are available over the counter

Magnesium salts

General information: Magnesium salts have been used for many years as laxatives. They work quickly – in about four hours – and are only suitable for occasional use.

Precautions: Tell your doctor if you have or have had kidney problems.
Side effects: Colic
Available preparations: Liquid
Brand names: None; a wide range of preparations available over the counter

Phosphates

General information: Phosphates are available in the form of enemas to treat constipation. They are also used to clear the bowel before surgery and diagnostic examinations.

Precautions: Tell your doctor if you have any other serious gastrointestinal problems.
Available preparations: Suppositories, enema
Brand names: Carbalax, Fleet Ready-to-use Enema, Fletchers' Phosphate Enema

Sodium citrate

General information: Sodium citrate is available in the form of an enema to treat constipation. It has a rapid action and works in about four hours.

Precautions: Tell your doctor if you have any other serious gastrointestinal conditions.

Available preparations: Enemas

Brand names: Fleet Micro-enema, Micolette Micro-enema, Micralax Micro-enema, Relaxit Micro-enema

PREPARATIONS FOR PILES

Piles (haemorrhoids) are swollen veins in the lining of the anus and rectum. They may be external at the anus or internal in the rectum. Pregnant women are particularly prone to developing them, and they are made worse by constipation and straining to pass faeces.

There are many preparations available over the counter and on prescription for the treatment of piles. Only those available on prescription will be covered in this section. They tend to be a mixture of a corticosteroid (eg betamethasone, hydrocortisone, prednisolone) with astringents (eg zinc oxide, bismuth subgallate), lubricants, antiseptics and/or local anaesthetics (eg cinchocaine, lignocaine). They are suitable for occasional short-term use (usually no more than one to two weeks).

Available preparations: Creams, ointments, suppositories

Brand names:
Anugesic HC cream (hydrocortisone acetate, benzyl benzoate, bismuth oxide, Peru balsam, pramoxine, zinc oxide)
Anugesic HC suppositories (hydrocortisone acetate, benzyl benzoate, bismuth oxide, bismuth subgallate, Peru balsam, pramoxine, zinc oxide)
Anusol HC ointment and suppositories (hydrocortisone acetate, benzyl benzoate, bismuth oxide, bismuth subgallate, Peru balsam, pramoxine, zinc oxide)
Betnovate rectal ointment (betamethasone valerate, lignocaine, phenylephrine)
Perinal spray (hydrocortisone, lignocaine)
Proctocream HC (hydrocortisone, pramoxine)
Proctofoam HC (hydrocortisone, pramoxine)
Proctosedyl ointment and suppositories (hydrocortisone, cinchocaine)
Scheriproct ointment and suppositories (prednisolone, cinchocaine)
Ultraproct ointment and suppositories (flucortolone, cinchocaine)
Uniroid-HC ointment and suppositories (hydrocortisone, cinchocaine)
Xyloproct ointment and suppositories (hydrocortisone, aluminium acetate, lignocaine, zinc oxide)

DRUGS FOR GALL BLADDER CONDITIONS

The use of various surgical techniques has limited the use of drugs in gall bladder disease. Drugs are only suitable for patients who cannot be treated by any other means and who have mild symptoms. The two drugs used – chenodeoxycholic acid and ursodeoxycholic acid – are chemicals that occur naturally in bile and that act by increasing the amount of cholesterol held in solution in the bile. This helps gallstones made predominantly of cholesterol to dissolve. It can take up to 18 months for gallstones to dissolve and their progress is checked by regular ultrasound examination. Up to 50 per cent recur on stopping treatment.

How to use: Take the medicine exactly as prescribed by the doctor. If you miss a dose, take it as soon as you remember. However, if it is almost time for your next dose, skip the missed dose. Do not take double the dose. Do not stop taking the medicine without asking your doctor because this may cause your underlying condition to get worse.

Precautions: Tell your doctor if you are pregnant, planning to become pregnant or are breastfeeding, or if you have liver disease, peptic ulcer or inflammatory bowel disease.

Side effects: Diarrhoea is the most common side effect.

Warnings: None

Interactions: These drugs interact with various lipid-lowering drugs (eg cholestyramine, colestipol and the fibrate group – see page 97) and with oral contraceptives containing oestrogens.

Chenodeoxycholic acid

Available preparations: Capsules
Brand names: Chenofalk

Ursodeoxycholic acid

Available preparations: Tablets, capsules
Brand names: Destolit, Urdox, Ursofalk, Ursogal

PANCREATIN

Pancreatin is used to compensate for deficient production of pancreatic enzymes in people with cystic fibrosis, inflammation of the pancreas and pancreatic surgery, so it is a type of enzyme replacement therapy. Pancreatin helps in the digestion of fat, starch and protein, but does not cure the underlying disease.

How to use: Take the medicine exactly as prescribed by the doctor. Pancreatin should be taken just before or with meals. Do not stop taking the medicine without asking your doctor because this may cause your underlying condition to get worse.
Available preparations: Tablets, capsules, powder, granules
Brand names: Creon, Creon 10 000, Creon 25 000, Nutrizym GR, Nutrizym 10, Nutrizym 22, Pancrease, Pancrease HL, Pancrex, Pancrex V.

The Respiratory System

THE MAIN ROLE of the respiratory system is to bring oxygen to the lungs, transfer the oxygen to the blood and to every cell in the body, and expel the waste product called carbon dioxide. In short, the respiratory system effects an exchange of two gases – an exchange that is essential to life. Every day, your lungs move about 7,000 litres of air.

Air enters the respiratory system through the nose and mouth. It then passes down the back of the throat (pharynx) and through the voice box (larynx) into the windpipe (trachea). Inside the chest cavity, the trachea branches into two smaller tubes (the bronchi) to supply the lungs. Eventually these tubes divide into smaller and smaller tubes, known as bronchioles, which end ultimately in tiny, air-filled sacs. There are about 300 million of these sacs, known as alveoli, in the lungs. Each alveolus is surrounded by a dense network of tiny blood vessels called capillaries. The alveoli have extremely thin walls and this allows oxygen from the air you have breathed in to pass into the blood in the capillaries. Carbon dioxide, the waste gas, moves in the opposite direction from the capillaries to the alveoli and out through the lungs.

Breathing is usually automatic, controlled subconsciously by the respiratory centre in the brain. When oxygen levels are low or carbon dioxide levels high, the brain increases the speed and depth of breathing. Conversely, when carbon dioxide levels get too low, breathing slows down. The work of breathing is done primarily by the diaphragm, a large muscle separating the chest and stomach, and to a lesser extent by the muscles between the ribs (the intercostal muscles). When you breathe in, the diaphragm and the intercostal muscles contract. This causes the chest cavity to increase in volume and the pressure in the chest falls. As a result, air rushes into the lungs. When you breathe out, the diaphragm and the intercostal muscles relax, then pressure in the chest rises and air is forced out.

What can go wrong

The respiratory tract can, like any other part of the body, become infected and inflamed. If this happens, it can have serious consequences for breathing and thus for the exchange of the gases.

Asthma is a very common condition, characterised by wheezing, breathlessness, tightness in the chest and bouts of coughing – often at night. The airways are inflamed, with consequent swelling, build up of mucus and thickening of the muscles in the lung airways. The smooth muscle in the lung airways contracts readily in response to a range of stimuli, including allergens (eg pollens, house dust), changes in temperature or humidity or physical exercise. It may also occur following viral infections, in which the airways become narrower than normal as a result of build up of mucus, congestion and inflammation.

The causes of asthma are not completely understood. Some cases are believed to be due to chemicals at work; in five per cent of cases, asthma is precipitated by non-steroidal anti-inflammatory drugs (NSAIDs), including aspirin. Asthma – especially in the young – often has an allergic basis and runs in families, frequently accompanied by eczema and hayfever. Pollution may be a factor – patients sometimes report a worsening of symptoms after exposure to tobacco smoke and car fumes, for example. High concentrations of sulphuric acid, ozone and nitrogen dioxide have been linked with minor epidemics. Many allergens undoubtedly exist that trigger attacks in susceptible people. Common allergens include pollen, pets, especially cats, certain foods, such as dairy products and fizzy drinks, and the house dust mite – an invisible insect that forms part of general house dust, along with the skin cells shed from the occupants of a house. The house dust mite lives in large numbers on the mattresses and carpets of a home; it is actually their faeces which when inhaled trigger asthma in susceptible people.

Bronchitis is an inflammation of the lung airways. Acute bronchitis – which is commoner in smokers than non-smokers - is an infection due to common bacteria often following a flu-like illness or viral infection. Patients may have a fever and bring up green sputum, and there may be wheezing.

Chronic bronchitis, with emphysema (see below), forms part of a condition known as chronic obstructive airways disease. It results from scarring and damage to the lining of the airways as a result of smoking, air pollution and frequent chest infections. Patients tend to have a persistent cough and bring up phlegm in the morning (smoker's cough). Bronchitis often accompanies emphysema and can be a serious, chronic condition.

Emphysema, a condition in which the walls of the alveoli break down, making them less efficient in exchanging gases, is also quite a common condition. Like bronchitis, it is related to smoking. Both conditions cause shortness of breath and may eventually lead to respiratory failure and heart failure.

Cough is a symptom of many lung conditions – for example, asthma, emphysema and bronchitis - and it can also develop as a result of colds and flu. Essentially, coughing is a way in which the lungs are protected from any irritant material that gets into the airways and this includes excessive mucus. Coughs vary considerably in type and severity. They may be productive – that is, mucus is brought up from the lungs, or they may be dry and irritating, without any mucus. Coughs may develop over decades, particularly in smokers with chronic bronchitis, and the person may get so used to the cough that they are hardly aware of it.

Common conditions and drugs used to treat them

Asthma – bronchodilators (eg salbutamol, ipratropium) and corticosteroids (eg beclomethasone)

Chronic obstructive airways disease (chronic bronchitis and emphysema) – bronchodilators and, occasionally, corticosteroids and long term oxygen therapy

Coughs and colds – cough suppressants, expectorants and decongestants

Chest infections, such as acute bronchitis and pneumonia – antibiotics (see page 246)

Inhaler devices

Various inhaler devices are used to deliver drugs to the lungs. These include:

Inhalers (puffers). Inhalers, of which the main type is the pressurised metered dose inhaler (MDI), release a small amount of drug when a valve is pressed. Co-ordination is essential because you have to press the valve and breathe in at the same time; if an inhaler is not used properly, only a very small amount of drug will reach your lungs and the treatment will not be so effective. Many people, especially children and people with arthritis in their hands, may find inhalers difficult to use at first, so if you have any difficulty in using your inhaler, get your pharmacist or doctor to show you. In addition, large plastic devices called spacers are available on prescription to help you inhale the drug more efficiently. There are also other inhalers, known as breath controlled inhalers (eg Autohalers), which require no co-ordination and are easier to use.

Dry powder systems (eg accuhaler, clickhaler, diskhaler, rotahaler, turbohaler). Drugs from these systems are taken into the lungs as you breathe in from them. They are easy to use and suitable for people who have problems in using other inhalers. With some of these systems, the drug comes in the form of a capsule, which you put in a separate inhaler device. Once inside the inhaler, the capsule gets pierced and the drug is drawn into your lungs as you breathe in.

Nebulisers. Nebulisers are machines which deliver a higher dose of drug to the lungs, working faster than inhalers or other systems. They are very effective at relieving serious breathing problems in people with asthma and chronic obstructive airways disease. They require no co-ordination and can be used by people who are too breathless to use an inhaler. They work by pumping air through a liquid containing the drug. This turns the liquid into a fine mist which the person then inhales through a mask.

CHLOROFLUOROCARBON (CFC)-FREE INHALERS

Pressurised metered dose inhalers (MDIs) have traditionally used chlorofluorocarbon (CFC) gases as propellants. CFCs have been implicated in the depletion of the ozone layer, which shields the earth from harmful ultraviolet radiation from the sun. A reduction and eventual phase out of CFCs was agreed in 1987. As part of this agreement, pharmaceutical companies have developed new types of propellant known as hydrofluoralkanes (HFAs). HFAs are as safe as CFCs for patients, but do not deplete the ozone in the atmosphere.

Patients with asthma are being gradually changed over to CFC-free inhalers and there are some differences between the two. HFA-based inhalers have a different taste than their CFC counterparts. They make a different sound on pressing the valve and the spray may feel different in the mouth. These effects are solely due to the change in the propellant and do not change the way the medicine works.

There are three groups of bronchodilators – adrenoceptor stimulants (eg salbutamol), antimuscarinics (ipratropium) and theophylline-type drugs.

BRONCHODILATORS

Bronchodilators are used in the treatment of asthma and chronic obstructive airways disease (emphysema and chronic bronchitis). They open up the air passages in the lungs and help to relieve symptoms such as breathlessness, wheezing and coughing. They work by relaxing the muscles surrounding the bronchioles. When used in asthma, however, they do not prevent asthma attacks from happening, but they help the symptoms when they occur. For this reason bronchodilators are sometimes known as relievers. Corticosteroid drugs (see page 139) help to prevent asthma attacks, by dealing with the underlying inflammation, and are therefore known as preventers. If you suffer from asthma, the chances are that, unless your condition is very mild, you will be prescribed both a reliever and a preventer.

Bronchodilators are generally administered using an inhaler. This enables the drug to reach the lungs directly, rather than entering the bloodstream from the gastrointestinal tract – as it would if taken orally – and then having to travel to the lungs. As the inhaled drug is not travelling round in the bloodstream to other parts of the body – at least to any great extent – the severity of side effects is limited. Inhaling a drug means that it reaches the lungs directly, and little is absorbed from the lungs into the rest of the body.

ADRENOCEPTOR STIMULANTS

Adrenoceptor stimulants, as you might guess from their name, work by stimulating a type of receptor known as the adrenoceptor. One group of these drugs acts specifically at one type of adrenoreceptor – beta receptors – and these drugs are consequently known as beta stimulants. Beta stimulants have a generally opposite effect to beta-blockers, which are used in various heart and other conditions (see page 82). Alpha adrenoceptor stimulants have different actions and are used mainly as nasal decongestants (see page 143).

There are eight beta stimulant drugs available. All work in basically the same way: they bind to the beta receptors on the smooth muscle in the lung airways. This causes the muscles to relax, and so opens up the airways. However, there are some differences between the different beta stimulant drugs, particularly in their duration of action. Salbutamol and terbutaline are the most widely used from this group of drugs, and they work rapidly to relieve the symptoms of an asthma attack. The longer acting drugs (eg salmeterol) are not used for relief of asthma attacks – they do not act quickly enough. Instead, they are usually prescribed to be used on a twice-a-day basis to help control the symptoms.

How to use: Use the medicine exactly as prescribed by the doctor. Do not exceed the prescribed dose. If you miss a dose, take it as soon as you remember. However, if it is almost time for your next dose, skip the missed dose. Do not double the dose. Do not stop taking the medicine without asking your doctor because this may cause your underlying condition to get worse. If you are using both a beta stimulant and a corticosteroid at the same time, always use the beta stimulant first. This will help to open up your airways and so to increase the effectiveness of the steroid. For instructions on how to use inhalers (see page 134).

Precautions: Tell your doctor if you are pregnant, planning to become pregnant or are breastfeeding, or if you have or have had thyroid problems, kidney or heart problems or diabetes.

Side effects: Common side effects include tremor (especially in the hands), nervousness, headache, speeding of the heart and palpitations. Muscle cramps may occur, but this is rare.

Warnings. If your normal dose of medicine fails to give you at least three hours relief, consult your doctor immediately. Take care with driving and other similar activities until you know how the drug affects you. You may be asked to attend for monitoring while using these drugs – especially if you suffer from severe asthma. Keep your appointments.

Interactions: Other drugs may interact with beta stimulants, but interactions are not likely to be significant unless your condition is severe and you are using several drugs. Always check with your doctor or pharmacist before taking other medication.

Bambuterol

General information: Bambuterol is a short acting beta stimulant drug used in the treatment of asthma, chronic bronchitis and emphysema. In asthma, it is used as a 'reliever' to relieve the symptoms of an asthma attack.

Available preparations: Tablets
Brand names: Bambec

Eformoterol

General information: Eformoterol is a long acting beta stimulant drug used in the treatment of asthma, chronic bronchitis and emphysema. It is commonly used in conjunction with a short acting beta stimulant (eg salbutamol) and a corticosteroid, and should be used regularly as prescribed. Unlike salbutamol, it should not be used to relieve the symptoms of an asthma attack.

Available preparations: Inhaler (dry powder device), turbohaler
Brand names: Foradil, Oxis

Fenoterol

General information: Fenoterol is a short acting beta stimulant drug used in the treatment of asthma, chronic bronchitis and emphysema. In asthma, it is used as a 'reliever' to relieve the symptoms of an asthma attack.

Available preparations: Inhaler
Brand names: Berotec
Combination preparations: Duovent (fenoterol and ipratropium)

Orciprenaline

General information: Orciprenaline is a short acting beta stimulant drug used in the treatment of asthma, chronic bronchitis and emphysema. Used frequently up until a few years ago, orciprenaline has now been superseded by the other drugs listed in this section. It stimulates the heart more than the others do.

Available preparations: Inhaler, tablets, oral liquid
Brand names: Alupent

Reproterol

General information: Reproterol is a short acting beta stimulant drug used in the treatment of asthma, chronic bronchitis and emphysema. In asthma, it is used as a 'reliever' to relieve the symptoms of an asthma attack.

Available preparations: Inhaler
Brand names: Bronchodil

Salbutamol

General information: Salbutamol is a short acting beta stimulant drug used in the treatment of asthma, chronic bronchitis and emphysema. In asthma, it is used (in the form of an inhaler) as a 'reliever' to relieve the symptoms of an asthma attack.

Available preparations: Inhaler, various dry powder systems, nebuliser solution, tablets, oral liquid, injection
Brand names: Aerolin, Airomir, Asmasal, Salamol, Ventodiscs, Ventolin

Salmeterol

General information: Salmeterol is a long acting beta stimulant drug used in the treatment of asthma, chronic bronchitis and emphysema. It is commonly used in conjunction with a short acting beta stimulant (eg salbutamol) and a corticosteroid, and should be used regularly as prescribed. Unlike salbutamol, it should not be used to relieve the symptoms of an asthma attack.

Available preparations: Accuhaler, Diskhaler; Inhaler
Brand names: Servent

Terbutaline

General information: Terbutaline is a short acting beta stimulant drug used in the treatment of asthma, chronic bronchitis and emphysema. In asthma, it is used (in the form of an inhaler) as a 'reliever' to relieve the symptoms of an asthma attack.

Available preparations: Inhaler, turbohaler, nebuliser solution, tablets, oral liquid
Brand names: Bricanyl, Bricanyl SA, Monovent

Tulobuterol

General information: Tulobuterol is a long acting beta stimulant drug used in the treatment of asthma, chronic bronchitis and emphysema. In addition to the precautions (see page 136), tell your doctor if you have or have had kidney or liver problems.

Available preparations: Tablets, liquid
Brand names: Respacal

ANTIMUSCARINIC BRONCHODILATORS

Antimuscarinic (also called anticholinergic) bronchodilators work by inhibiting the action of the transmitter chemical – acetylcholine – at muscarinic receptors. Acetylcholine causes the airways to narrow, so by blocking the effects of acetylcholine, the airways can be made to widen. These drugs take longer to work than most of the beta stimulants (see page 135), and they have a longer duration of action. They are generally prescribed for long term rather than rapid relief, and tend to be used more commonly in chronic bronchitis than in asthma. Sometimes they work better than other bronchodilators (eg adrenoceptor stimulants) in very young children.

How to use: Use the medicine exactly as prescribed by the doctor. If you miss a dose, take it as soon as you remember. However, if it is almost time for your next dose, skip the missed dose. Do not take double the dose. Do not stop taking the medicine without asking your doctor because this may cause your underlying condition to get worse.

Precautions: Tell your doctor if you are pregnant, planning to become pregnant or are breastfeeding, or if you have glaucoma or an enlarged prostate gland.

Side effects: Side effects include dry mouth and throat, but these occur rarely.

Warnings: If your normal dose of medicine fails to give you at least three hours relief, consult your doctor immediately. Take care with driving and other similar activities until you know how this drug affects you.

Interactions: None significant

Ipratropium

General information: Ipratropium is an antimuscarinic bronchodilator used mainly in chronic bronchitis but occasionally also in asthma.

Available preparations: Various types of inhaler, nebuliser solution
Brand names: Atrovent, Respontin
Combination preparations: Combivent

Oxitropium

General information: Oxitropium is an antimuscarinic bronchodilator used mainly in chronic bronchitis, but occasionally also in asthma.

Available preparations: Various types of inhaler
Brand names: Oxivent

THEOPHYLLINE AND AMINOPHYLLINE

Theophylline and aminophylline (which is converted to theophylline in the body) are used in the treatment of chronic bronchitis and severe asthma. In asthma, these drugs are normally used in conjunction with adrenoceptor stimulants and corticosteroids, in other words when these latter drugs have failed to provide adequate relief and a further drug is needed. Many of the preparations are modified-release, long acting products where the drug is released slowly over a period; they are thus particularly useful for people whose symptoms are bad both in the night and first thing in the morning because they can be taken as a single night-time dose.

How to use: Use the medicine exactly as prescribed by the doctor. If you miss a dose, take it as soon as you remember. However, if it is almost time for your next dose, skip the missed dose. Do not take double the dose. Do not stop taking the medicine without asking your doctor because this may cause your underlying condition to get worse.

Precautions: Tell your doctor if you are pregnant, planning to become pregnant or are breastfeeding, or if you have or have had heart problems, liver problems, thyroid disease, epilepsy or porphyria.

Side effects: Side effects with these drugs are quite common and include nausea, headache, insomnia, palpitations and rapid heart beat.

Warnings: Avoid excessive intake of alcohol because it may increase the adverse effects of these drugs. You may be asked to attend for regular blood tests while taking this drug. Do not miss your appointments. It is important to stick to the same brand and tablet when using these preparations. Always check that you have the same preparation as previously before leaving the pharmacy.

Interactions: These drugs interact with a large number of other drugs. The important ones include certain antibiotics, certain antidepressants, calcium channel blockers and the ulcer healing drug, cimetidine. Check with your doctor or pharmacist before taking any other medicines.

Aminophylline

Available preparations: Tablets, injection
Brand names: Pecram, Phyllocontin Continus

Theophylline

Available preparations: Tablets, capsules, liquid
Brand names: Lasma, Nuelin, Nuelin SA, Slo-Phylin, Theo-Dur, Uniphyllin Continus

CORTICOSTEROIDS

Corticosteroid drugs, of which there are several, are used in a wide range of inflammatory conditions such as rheumatoid arthritis and inflammatory bowel disorders, and they are also used in asthma. In asthma, corticosteroids are used – by inhalation - to reduce the severity and frequency of attacks. Severe asthma is sometimes treated with corticosteroids given by mouth. Often described as 'preventers', corticosteroids do not give the rapid gratifying relief of symptoms that bronchodilators do, once an attack has started. However, it is the corticosteroids (either as tablets or puffers) that deal with the underlying inflammation, and this helps to reduce the severity and frequency of attacks. This is why you should continue with your steroids, or if your doctor has told you, increase the dose during an attack. Use your bronchodilator ('reliever') to control your breathlessness. This is important because if you suffer from asthma you will often have more than one type of inhaler and you must know which one to use if you have an attack.

How they work: It is not known exactly how these drugs work in asthma. However, corticosteroids are anti-inflammatories and therefore help to reduce inflammation in the airways. By reducing inflammation, they reduce mucus production and congestion.

How to use: Use the medicine exactly as prescribed by the doctor. The important thing with these medicines is to use them regularly and not just when your asthma is worse. If you miss a dose, take it as soon as you remember. However, if it is almost time for your next dose, skip the missed dose. Do not take double the dose. Do not stop taking the medicine without asking your doctor because this may cause your underlying condition to get worse. If your asthma is persistent, you should agree an asthma management plan with your doctor so that you can adjust the dose within agreed limits.

Precautions: Tell your doctor if you have ever had tuberculosis.

Side effects: Many people are concerned about using corticosteroids. However, when used by inhalation, the dose used is low and only a small proportion is absorbed into the rest of the body. Adverse side effects are therefore unlikely. However, irritation of the nasal passages and fungal infection of the mouth and throat, causing hoarseness, cough and sore throat, are possibilities with inhaled corticosteroids. If you experience these effects, try washing your mouth with water and/or cleaning the teeth after using the inhaler. Your doctor may prescribe an antifungal for you to use as a gargle immediately after using the inhaler. Alternatively, your doctor may prescribe a large plastic device called a spacer, which will help more of the drug to be deposited in the lungs and less in the mouth and throat.

Warnings: None

Interactions: None

Beclomethasone

Available preparations: Inhalers, various dry powder devices
Brand names: AeroBec, Asmabec, Becodisks, Becotide, Becloforte
Combination preparations: Ventide (beclomethasone, salbutamol)

Budesonide

Available preparations: Inhalers, Turbohaler, nebuliser solution
Brand names: Pulmicort

Fluticasone

Available preparations: Inhaler, various dry powder devices, nebules
Brand names: Flixotide

CROMONES

There are two drugs of the type called cromones – cromoglycate and nedocromil. Cromones are antiallergic drugs and, like corticosteroids, they have a role as 'preventers' in asthma. They are used by inhalation to reduce the frequency and severity of asthma attacks. However, they do not relieve the symptoms of an asthma attack once it has started. Cromones are used more often in children than in adults, because children – particularly those over the age of 4 years – seem to respond better. They also work well in preventing exercise-induced asthma in children. These drugs appear to work by reducing the production of inflammatory chemicals that are produced in the body and are involved in allergic reactions.

How to use: Use the medicine exactly as prescribed by the doctor. The important thing with these medicines is to use them regularly and not just when your asthma is worse – remember that they will not relieve symptoms of asthma at all. If you miss a dose, take it as soon as you remember. However, if it is almost time for your next dose, skip the missed dose. Do not take double the dose. Do not stop taking the medicine without asking your doctor because this may cause your underlying condition to get worse.

Side effects: These are very safe drugs with virtually no side effects. Coughing and throat irritation may occur due to inhaling the powder. Rinsing your mouth out with water may help.

Precautions, warnings, interactions: None

Cromoglycate

Available preparations: Inhalers and various dry powder devices
Brand names: Cromogen, Intal
Combination preparations: Aerocrom (cromoglycate, salbutamol)

Nedocromil

Available preparations: Inhaler
Brand names: Tilade

LEUKOTRIENE RECEPTOR ANTAGONISTS

These are recently introduced drugs for the treatment of asthma. Leukotrienes are one type of the many inflammatory chemicals involved in asthma, and leukotriene receptor antagonist drugs work by blocking the effects of these chemicals. This in turn helps to dampen down the inflammation.

These drugs are normally used in conjunction with adrenoceptor stimulants and corticosteroids, in other words when these latter drugs have failed to provide adequate relief and a further drug is needed. They are given by mouth to help reduce the severity and frequency of asthma attacks and cannot be used to give rapid relief from an asthma attack.

How to use: Use the medicine exactly as prescribed by the doctor. If you miss a dose, take it as soon as you remember. However, if it is almost time for your next dose, skip the missed dose. Do not take double the dose. Do not stop taking the medicine without asking your doctor because this may cause your underlying condition to get worse.

Precautions: Tell your doctor if you are pregnant, planning to become pregnant or are breastfeeding.

Side effects: Stomach pain and headache are the most likely. Diarrhoea and dizziness may also occur.

Warnings and interactions: Nothing specific, but these are very new drugs, so discuss any symptoms with your doctor or pharmacist. Tell your doctor or pharmacist if you are taking any other medication.

Montelukast

Available preparations: Tablets
Brand names: Singulair

Zafirlukast

Available preparations: Tablets
Brand names: Accolate

DORNASE ALPHA

General information: Dornase alpha is a version of a human enzyme produced by genetic engineering. A relatively new medicine, it is used to remove excessive mucus in the chests of people with cystic fibrosis. It is administered by nebuliser.

Side effects: Irritation of the throat, voice changes and chest pain are the most likely side effects.

Precautions, warnings, interactions: No special instructions, but this is a specialist medicine so be sure to ask your doctor about anything that you do not fully understand.

Available preparations: Nebuliser solution
Brand names: Pulmozyme

COUGH MIXTURES

Very few preparations for cough are now available on NHS prescription, although a huge number are available over the counter. All cough medicines contain one or more of the following groups of drugs:

Cough suppressants (antitussives) – these act by reducing the activity of the cough centre in the brain. Most are opiate derivatives (eg Codeine Linctus, Pholcodine Linctus) – that is, the same drugs as those used in controlling severe pain (see page 62), albeit in lower doses.

Expectorants – these act by promoting the removal of mucus from the airways (eg Ammonia and Ipecacuanha Mixture)

Demulcents – these act by soothing dry irritating coughs (eg Simple Linctus)

DECONGESTANTS

Pseudoephedrine

General information: Pseudoephedrine is a decongestant used for the relief of nasal congestion, including nasal rhinitis.

How to use: Take as prescribed. You can stop using the medicine when you feel better.
Precautions: Tell your doctor if you have or have had heart disease, thyroid disease, diabetes or high blood pressure.
Side effects: Restlessness and insomnia may occur but side effects are generally rare. 'Rebound' congestion may occur.
Interactions: Pseudoephedrine interacts with several other medicines, notably some of those used in heart conditions and high blood pressure, and also with certain antidepressants.
Available preparations: Tablets, liquid
Brand names: Sudafed. A large number of products are available over the counter.

INHALATIONS

Inhalations (eg Friar's Balsam and Menthol and Eucalyptus) include mixtures of various oils that vaporise when mixed with hot water. They are used for the relief of congestion in the nose and respiratory tract. They are used by diluting specific quantities (in the order of one teaspoonful of the inhalation to a pint of hot water, but always check individual details on the packaging), and inhaling the consequent vapour. Note: never use boiling water because of the risk of scalding.

Bones, Joints and Muscles

BONES AND JOINTS, together with the tendons, ligaments and muscles, make up the musculoskeletal system, which gives support and shape to the body and makes movement possible. The skeleton, consisting of 206 individual bones, provides strength, stability and a framework for muscles to work against in producing movement. Bones also serve to protect delicate internal organs, such as the brain, heart and lungs.

Bone is not static, but a constantly changing tissue. The size of individual bones increases until the skeleton reaches its full adult size, but even after that bone tissue is continuously broken down and remade. Bone metabolism is controlled by various hormones and is influenced by calcium, vitamin D and the amount of exercise. Although bones come in different shapes, all have basically the same structure: a soft central core, consisting of the bone marrow, and a hard outer part made up of proteins such as collagen and a substance known as hydroxyapatite. Composed mainly of calcium and other minerals, hydroxyapatite is responsible for storing most of the body's calcium and for the strength of the bones.

A joint is the place where two bones meet, and which allows us to twist, turn and bend our bodies. The direction and degree of movement available is dependent on the type of joint. Some joints do not move at all, whereas others, such as the ball and socket joints found in the hips and shoulders, allow a considerable amount of free movement between the bones. Hinge joints, found in the knee and wrist, allow for bending and straightening only.

In a joint, the end of the bones are covered in a soft but tough tissue called cartilage. This acts as a 'shock absorber' and prevents the bones from grinding against each other. Joints also have a lining, known as the synovial membrane. Cells in this membrane produce a clear fluid, called the synovial fluid, which helps to reduce friction and ease movement. Other components of the joints include the ligaments, which surround joints and hold the bones together, and tendons – tough bands of tissue that attach each end of a muscle to a bone.

What can go wrong

Disorders of the musculoskeletal system are responsible for a great deal of pain and physical disability. Injuries to bones, joints and muscles, including pulled muscles, strained or torn ligaments, inflamed tendons, dislocated joints and broken bones, are very common and occur at all ages. Although such injuries can be extremely painful at the time, they usually heal completely without complications.

Joints can also become inflamed, and if this condition persists it is known as arthritis. This causes swelling, pain and stiffness, with symptoms ranging in severity from mild aches to severe pain and joint deformity. Osteoarthritis, the most common type of arthritis, is a condition in which the cartilage covering the bones becomes thin and rough, and may eventually erode away completely. The joint is stiff and painful; there may be bony enlargement and deformity and sometimes swelling and inflammation of the joint.

Rheumatoid arthritis is a disease of the synovial membrane, the lining of individual joints. Something triggers off the body's immune system, and this causes the synovial membrane in the joints to become very inflamed. The cartilage is eaten away and this results in red, puffy, painful joints. Unlike osteoarthritis, which rarely occurs before the age of 50, rheumatoid arthritis can start at any age from childhood, but often starts between the ages of 30 and 40.

Gout, another common joint disease, is caused by an excess of the substance called uric acid in the blood. Uric acid, a breakdown product of nucleic acid, is relatively insoluble; it tends to crystallise out in a joint which then becomes red, swollen and extremely painful. Joints commonly affected include the joint at the base of the big toe, knee, wrist, ankle, hand or foot. The first attack usually lasts a few days and some people never have another attack. However, second attacks can occur – usually between six months and two years after the first attack. More common in men than women, gout is associated with obesity, a high protein diet, high alcohol intake, diabetes, raised blood fats, high blood pressure and coronary artery disease. There is often a family history and some medicines, especially thiazide diuretics, may trigger attacks.

Other conditions which affect the joints include **ankylosing spondylitis** – which affects the spine and pelvic joints and causes severe stiffness – and **juvenile rheumatoid arthritis** (Still's disease), a form of arthritis which affects children.

Various disorders can affect the bones. **Osteoporosis** is caused by a reduction in the strength and density of the bone and leads to an increased risk of fracture. Largely a disease of old age, it is more common in women than men, because women start with thinner bones and they tend to lose bone density after the menopause when levels of oestrogen drop. The risk of osteoporosis can be reduced by maintaining an adequate calcium intake throughout life and taking plenty of exercise. Hormone replacement therapy (HRT) may help to reduce the risk of osteoporosis (see page 183). Calcium and Vitamin D supplements may also help.

Osteomalacia is another bone disorder. Known as rickets when it occurs in children osteomalacia is a condition in which the bones become soft and there is a risk of bone deformity and fracture. The commonest cause of osteomalacia is lack of vitamin D. This vitamin is needed to build up the calcium and other minerals – which are what give bones their strength – in the bone. Children are more obviously affected as their bones are growing. Vitamin D deficiency can be caused by insufficient exposure of the skin to sunlight and to poor dietary intake of the vitamin. People with dark skins living in northern Britain are particularly susceptible to osteomalacia, as are people with disorders of malabsorption (eg coeliac disease) in which absorption of vitamin D is reduced. Premature babies and young children are also vulnerable.

Paget's disease is a relatively rare, chronic disorder of the skeleton in which areas of bone grow abnormally and become thicker and soft. Usually it produces no symptoms, but pain and stiffness may develop gradually. There may be bone deformity and fractures.

Common conditions and drugs used to treat them

Arthritis (treatment) – non-steroidal anti-inflammatory drugs (NSAIDs – eg ibuprofen and diclofenac); corticosteroids

Arthritis (suppression of the disease process) – gold, penicillamine, chloroquine, azathioprine, cyclosporin, methotrexate, sulphasalazine

Gout – NSAIDs, colchicine, allopurinol, probenecid, sulphinpyrazone

Myasthenia gravis – neostigmine, edrophonium

Muscle spasticity – baclofen, dantrolene

Osteoporosis – hormone replacement therapy (see page 183), calcium, vitamin D, bisphosphonates

Osteomalacia and rickets – vitamin D

Paget's disease – Calcitonin, bisphosphonates

NON-STEROIDAL ANTI-INFLAMMATORY DRUGS (NSAIDs)

NSAIDs are used to relieve pain in arthritis, other musculoskeletal disorders, including gout, and period pain. The NSAID ibuprofen is available over the counter and is suitable for pain relief in headache, period pain, toothache, joint pain etc.

There are more than 20 NSAIDs currently available, and there is little to choose between them in terms of pain relief and anti-inflammatory activity. However, some people may find that one drug works when another does not. Your doctor may try several NSAIDs before finding which one works best for you.

How they work: NSAIDs work by inhibiting an enzyme that is involved in the production of inflammatory substances called prostaglandins. Prostaglandins are natural body chemicals which trigger pain and inflammation. NSAIDS do not cure arthritis, but they do help the sufferer to move about without so much pain and stiffness.

How to use: Take the medicine exactly as prescribed by the doctor. If you miss a dose, take it as soon as you remember. However, if it is almost time for your next dose, skip the missed dose. Do not take double the dose. When prescribed for short term pain relief, the drug can be stopped at any time when you feel better. However, if prescribed for long term treatment of arthritis, check with your doctor before stopping the drug.

Precautions: Tell your doctor if you are pregnant, planning to become pregnant or are breastfeeding, or if you have or have had liver or kidney problems, heart problems, peptic ulcer or other gastrointestinal problems, porphyria, asthma, or allergy to aspirin.

Side effects: The most common side effects with NSAIDs are gastrointestinal and include nausea, diarrhoea, abdominal pain, indigestion and occasionally gastrointestinal bleeding. They can also cause peptic ulcer, being responsible for about 20 per cent of cases. Other side effects include allergic reactions such as rash, wheezing and breathing difficulties. Headache, dizziness, ringing in the ears, fluid retention and swelling, and sensitivity of the skin to sunlight may also occur. NSAIDs differ in their risk of producing side effects. Ibuprofen is associated with the lowest risk and azapropazone with the highest risk. Naproxen, diclofenac, indomethacin, ketoprofen and piroxicam are associated with intermediate risk.

Warnings: Avoid excessive alcohol while taking these drugs because it may increase the risk of gastrointestinal side effects. Avoid salt substitutes containing potassium while taking NSAIDs.

Interactions: NSAIDS interact with a wide range of other drugs to increase the risk of gastrointestinal bleeding and other side effects. These include aspirin, oral anticoagulants, cyclosporin and lithium. NSAIDs may reduce the beneficial effects of diuretics and drugs used to lower blood pressure, especially ACE inhibitors, and may enhance the effects of anticonvulsants and some drugs used in diabetes.

Aceclofenac

Available preparations: Tablets
Brand names: Preservex

Acemetacin

General information: Dizziness may be a particular problem with this drug. Take care with driving until you know how the drug affects you.

Available preparations: Capsules
Brand names: Emflex

Azapropazone

General information: This drug is associated with a particularly high risk of side effects. Its use is restricted to rheumatoid arthritis, ankylosing spondylitis (another form of arthritis) and acute gout, and only after other NSAIDs have been tried and found ineffective. Avoid direct exposure to sunlight while taking this drug, or use a sunblock preparation.

Available preparations: Tablets, capsules
Brand names: Rheumox

Diclofenac

Available preparations: Tablets, dispersible tablets, suppositories, injection, gel for external use

Brand names: Voltarol, Voltarol Emulgel; modified-release: Diclomax SR, Diclomax Retard, Motifene, Voltarol SR, Voltarol Retard.

Combination preparations: Arthrotec (diclofenac and misoprostol, an anti-ulcer drug). This preparation is used to prevent peptic ulcers in patients who need an NSAID.

Diflunisal

Available preparations: Tablets

Brand names: Dolobid

Etodolac

Available preparations: Tablets, capsules

Brand names: Lodine; modified-release: Lodine SR

Fenbufen

Available preparations: Tablets, capsules

Brand names: Lederfen

Fenoprofen

Available preparations: Tablets

Brand names: Fenopron

Flurbiprofen

Available preparations: Tablets, suppositories

Brand names: Froben; modified-release: Froben SR

Ibuprofen

Available preparations: Tablets, modified-release tablets and capsules, granules, liquid. Gel, cream, mousse and spray for external use

Brand names: Brufen, Ibugel, Ibumousse, Ibuspray, Proflex; modified-release: Brufen Retard, Fenbid. A large number of products containing ibuprofen are on sale over the counter.

Combination preparations: Codafen Continus (ibuprofen and codeine)

Indomethacin

General information: Dizziness is a particular risk with this drug. Take care with driving and other similar tasks until you know how the drug affects you. In addition to the precautions (see page 147), make sure that your doctor knows if you have epilepsy or Parkinson's disease.

Available preparations: Capsules, modified-release tablets and capsules, liquid, suppositories
Brand names: None

Ketoprofen

Available preparations: Capsules, modified-release capsules, suppositories, injection, gel for external use
Brand names: Orudis, Oruvail, Powergel; modified-release: Oruvail

Mefenamic acid

Available preparations: Tablets, capsules, liquid
Brand names: None

Meloxicam

General information: Meloxicam is said to act more selectively on the joint and less in the stomach; it may therefore cause less stomach upset.

Available preparations: Tablets, suppositories
Brand names: Mobic

Nabumetone

Available preparations: Tablets, suspension
Brand names: Relifex

Naproxen

Available preparations: Tablets, modified-release tablets, liquid, suppositories, injection
Brand names: Naprosyn, Nycopren, Synflex; modified-release: Naprosyn SR
Combination preparations: Condrotec and Napratec (both naproxen and misoprostol – an anti-ulcer drug). These preparations are used to prevent peptic ulcers in patients who need an NSAID.

Phenylbutazone

General information: This drug is restricted for use in alkylosing spondylitis (a form of arthritis) only after other NSAIDs have failed to work. It is prescribed under hospital supervision and can cause many side effects. In addition to the precautions (see page 147), make sure your doctor knows if you have thyroid disease.

Available preparations: Tablets
Brand names: Butacote

Piroxicam

Available preparations: Tablets, dispersible tablets, capsules, suppositories, injection, gel for external use
Brand names: Feldene

Sulindac

Available preparations: Tablets
Brand names: Clinoril

Tenoxicam

Available preparations: Tablets, injection
Brand names: Mobiflex

Tiaprofenic acid

General information: This drug has been associated with severe cystitis. You should not take it if you have a urinary tract disorder. If you experience urinary frequency, urgency, pain on urination or blood in the urine, stop taking the drug immediately.

Available preparations: Tablets, modified-release capsules
Brand names: Surgam; modified-release: Surgam SA

TOPICAL NSAIDs

NSAIDs are also available in the form of creams, gels and sprays, both on prescription and over the counter, for the relief of muscular aches and pains. If used in large amounts, they may be absorbed into the blood. The same precautions (particularly concerning asthma) apply to topical preparations. Below you will a find a list of the products available on prescription, together with their main ingredients.

Algesal: A cream containing a salicylate (related to aspirin)
Balmosa: A cream containing a salicylate (related to aspirin)
Difflam: A cream containing benzydamine (NSAID)
Feldene: A gel containing piroxicam (NSAID)
Ibugel: A gel containing ibuprofen (NSAID)
Ibumousse: A mousse containing ibuprofen (NSAID)
Ibuspray: A spray containing ibuprofen (NSAID)
Intralgin: A gel containing a salicylate (related to aspirin)
Movelat: A gel or cream containing salicylic acid (related to aspirin)
Oruvail: A gel containing ketoprofen (NSAID)
Powergel: A gel containing ketoprofen (NSAID)
Proflex: A cream containing ibuprofen (NSAID)
Transvasin: A cream or spray containing a salicylate (related to aspirin)
Traxam: A gel or foam containing felbinac (NSAID)
Voltarol Emulgel: a gel containing diclofenac (NSAID)

CORTICOSTEROIDS

Corticosteroids have an anti-inflammatory effect and have many uses including asthma (see page 140) and inflammatory bowel disorders (see page 124). They are also used in arthritic conditions when other drugs (eg NSAIDs) have failed to work. They relieve pain, reduce inflammation, increase mobility and reduce deformity of the joint. Prednisolone is the most commonly used corticosteroid for arthritis and is given by mouth.

Local corticosteroid injections

Some corticosteroids are given by injection for arthritis, tennis elbow, tendivitus and other musculoskeletal conditions. They are given locally into the joint by your doctor or nurse and the dose may be repeated on a few occasions, depending on the product used and the response achieved.

Dexamethasone

Brand names: Decadron

Hydrocortisone

Brand names: Hydrocortistab

Methylprednisolone

Brand names: Depomedrone, Depomedrone with Lidocaine (dexamethasone and lignocaine)

Prednisolone

Deltastab

Triamcinolone

Adcortyl, Kenalog, Lederspan

DISEASE-MODIFYING ANTIRHEUMATIC DRUGS

Certain drugs, such as chloroquine, gold, penicillamine and sulphasalazine, are thought to modify the disease processes that cause rheumatoid arthritis. They can reduce pain, swelling and stiffness. Unlike NSAIDs, they do not have an immediate effect and they may take from four to six months to produce a full beneficial effect. All these drugs tend to have a high incidence of side effects and you will require regular monitoring (eg blood tests) during treatment. These drugs are generally not started immediately when rheumatoid arthritis is first diagnosed. This is because the disease is somewhat unpredictable and your doctor will usually wait for a few months to see how it progresses.

How to use: Take the medicine exactly as prescribed by the doctor. If you miss a dose, take it as soon as you remember. However, if it is almost time for your next dose, skip the missed dose. Do not take double the dose. Do not stop taking the medicine without checking with your doctor because symptoms may recur.

Gold

General information: Gold is used in rheumatoid arthritis. It may be given by injection in the form of sodium aurothiomalate or by mouth in the form of auranofin. Treatment may continue indefinitely provided a beneficial response is achieved and the side effects not too troublesome

How to use: As disease-modifying antirheumatic drugs (see above).
Precautions: Make sure your doctor knows if you are pregnant, planning to become pregnant or are breastfeeding, or you have long term liver or kidney problems, blood disorders, eczema or other skin conditions.
Side effects: Side effects can be serious and unpleasant. Tell your doctor immediately if you experience itching skin or rash, metallic taste, fever, sore throat or tongue, mouth ulcers, bleeding gums, bruising, diarrhoea or menstrual disturbances.
Warnings: No problems with alcohol. You will be asked to attend for regular blood tests. Keep your appointments.
Interactions: None
Available preparations: Tablets, injection
Brand names: Myocrisin, Ridaura

Hydroxychloroquine

General information: Hydroxychloroquine is used in rheumatoid arthritis. It is a similar drug to the anti-malarial chloroquine, and both are effective as disease-modifying drugs in rheumatoid arthritis.

How to use: As disease-modifying antirheumatic drugs (see above).
Precautions: Make sure your doctor knows if you are pregnant, planning to become pregnant or are breastfeeding, or you have long term liver or kidney problems, epilepsy or other neurological conditions, glucose 6-phosphate deficiency (G6PD) or porphyria. Hydroxychloroquine is very toxic in overdose, so adhere strictly to quantities prescribed.
Side effects: Nausea, diarrhoea, abdominal pain, headache, rashes and skin reactions, blurred vision. Tell your doctor immediately if you experience any visual changes.
Warnings: No problems with alcohol. You will be asked to attend for regular eye tests. Keep your appointments.
Interactions: Hydroxychloroquine interacts with few other drugs. Check with your doctor or pharmacist before taking any other medicine.
Available preparations: Tablets
Brand names: Plaquenil

Penicillamine

General information: Penicillamine is used in the treatment of rheumatoid arthritis. It is also used as a chelating (binding) agent in cases of metal poisoning to eliminate copper or lead from the body. Penicillamine is used in Wilson's disease, a rare disorder in which excess copper is deposited in the liver and brain, and in a certain type of urinary stone.

How to use: As disease-modifying antirheumatic drugs (see page 152).
Precautions: Make sure your doctor knows if you are pregnant, planning to become pregnant or are breastfeeding, or you have long term liver or kidney problems. In addition tell your doctor if you are allergic to penicillin. Some people who are allergic to penicillin are also allergic to penicillamine.
Side effects: Side effects are common and include: nausea, loss of appetite, taste loss, fever, rash and itching and blood in the urine. Tell your doctor immediately if you experience sore throat, mouth ulcers, bruising, fever, lethargy and tiredness or rash.
Warnings: No problems with alcohol. You will be asked to attend for regular blood tests. Keep your appointments.
Interactions: Penicillamine reduces the absorption of minerals (eg iron and zinc) and vice versa. Do not take any supplements containing minerals. Check with your doctor or pharmacist before taking any other medicine.
Available preparations: Tablets
Brand names: Distamine, Pendramine

Other disease-modifying antirheumatic drugs include azathioprine (see page 308), chloroquine (see page 276), cyclosporin (see page 308), methotrexate (see page 299) and sulphasalazine (see page 125).

DRUGS USED FOR THE TREATMENT OF GOUT

Two approaches are used in the drug treatment of gout. First, drugs are used in the short term to control the symptoms of pain and inflammation in acute attacks of gout. Non steroidal anti-inflammatory drugs (NSAIDs), such as diclofenac, indomethacin, ketoprofen, naproxen, piroxicam or sulindac, are commonly used. Colchicine is an alternative to the NSAIDs – in people who are allergic to NSAIDs – but it is more toxic, especially in high doses.

The other approach is to try to control the disease and prevent the recurrence of gout attacks. Drugs such as allopurinol, probenecid and sulphinpyrazone are used for this purpose. They are given indefinitely and work by controlling the production of uric acid crystals – the cause of gout – in the joints, which they do by reducing the level of uric acid in the blood. Initially, they may increase the frequency of gout attacks and they should never be started during an acute attack of gout. Often an NSAID is given for the first six weeks of treatment to prevent any acute attacks.

How to use: Take the medicine exactly as prescribed by the doctor. If you miss a dose, take it as soon as you remember. However, if it is almost time for your next dose, skip the missed dose. Do not take double the dose. If the drug is taken for short term relief of gout, you can stop the drug when the symptoms disappear. However, if the drug is prescribed for long term prevention of attacks, do not stop taking the medicine without checking with your doctor.

Allopurinol

General information: Allopurinol is used in the long term prevention of gout. It is not for the treatment of acute attacks.

How to use: As drugs for gout (see page 153).
Precautions: Make sure your doctor knows if you are pregnant, planning to become pregnant or are breastfeeding, or if you have or have had liver or kidney problems. Your doctor may suggest occasional blood tests to monitor the effectiveness of treatment and adjust the dose if appropriate.
Side effects: Side effects are uncommon, but the following may occur: rash and other allergic reactions and nausea. Less common effects include headache, dizziness, drowsiness, visual and taste disturbances and hair loss.
Warnings: Avoid alcohol because it may increase the adverse effects of this drug.
Interactions: Allopurinol interacts with a few drugs, the most important of which are the anticancer drugs mercaptopurine and azathioprine.
Available preparations: Tablets
Brand names: Zyloric

Colchicine

General information: Colchicine has been in use for more than 200 years, and although it has been superseded by newer drugs, it is effective in treating acute attacks of gout. It is sometimes used in the first few months of treatment with other drugs (eg allopurinol, probenecid) used to prevent gout attacks, because these drugs may in the initial stages of treatment increase the frequency of gout attacks.

How to use: As drugs for gout (see page 153).
Precautions: Make sure your doctor knows if you are pregnant, planning to become pregnant or are breastfeeding, or if you have or have had liver or kidney problems, heart problems or gastrointestinal disease (eg peptic ulcer, inflammatory bowel disease).
Side effects: The most common side effects are nausea, vomiting, abdominal pain, diarrhoea and rash. Numbness and tingling, hair loss and bleeding or bruising may occur. Tell your doctor immediately if you experience any of these effects.
Warnings: Avoid excessive alcohol as this may increase the adverse effects of the drug.
Interactions: Cochicine and cyclosporin interact to increase the risk of adverse effects on the kidney.
Available preparations: Tablets
Brand names: None

Probenecid

General information: Probenecid is used in the long term prevention of gout. It is not for the treatment of acute attacks. It is sometimes used to enhance the effects of penicillin and cephalosporin antibiotics.

How to use: As drugs for gout (see page 153). It is important to maintain a high fluid intake (ie at least 2 litres a day).
Precautions: Make sure your doctor knows if you are pregnant, planning to become pregnant or are breastfeeding, or if you have kidney problems, peptic ulcer or porphyria. Your doctor will arrange blood tests to monitor levels of uric acid in the blood and adjust the dose, if appropriate.
Side effects: Side effects are uncommon, but the following may occur: nausea, vomiting, headache, flushing, dizziness, sore gums, hair loss, fever. Tell your doctor if you experience any of these effects.
Warnings: Avoid excessive alcohol because it may increase the adverse effects of this drug.
Interactions: Probenecid interacts with many drugs. Check with your doctor or pharmacist before taking any other medicines.
Available preparations: Tablets
Brand names: Benemid

Sulphinpyrazone

General information: Sulphinpyrazone is used in the long term prevention of gout. It is not for the treatment of acute attacks.

How to use: As drugs for gout (see page 153).
Precautions: Make sure your doctor knows if you are pregnant, planning to become pregnant or are breastfeeding, or if you have or have had heart, liver or kidney problems. Your doctor will arrange blood tests to monitor levels of uric acid in the blood and adjust the dose, if appropriate.
Side effects: Side effects are uncommon, but the following may occur: rash and other allergic reactions, nausea, fluid retention. Less common effects include gastrointestinal bleeding and jaundice.
Warnings: Avoid alcohol because it may increase the adverse effects of this drug.
Interactions: Sulphinpyrazone interacts with a few drugs, the most important of which are the anticancer drugs mercaptopurine and azathioprine.
Available preparations: Tablets
Brand names: Anturan

DRUGS USED IN MYASTHENIA GRAVIS

Myasthenia gravis is a serious and rare disease resulting in muscle weakness. It is an auto-immune disorder in which the body produces a type of antibody. This antibody attaches itself to a receptor on the muscle and blocks transmission of nerve impulses from the nerve to the muscle. Drugs are used to enhance the nerve impulses and so improve muscle strength, but they do not cure the disease.

Note: If you suffer from myasthenia gravis, you will be very sensitive to many drugs. Always tell your doctor if you have this condition.

How to use: Take the medicine exactly as prescribed by the doctor. If you miss a dose, take it as soon as you remember. However, if it is almost time for your next dose, skip the missed dose. Do not take double the dose. Do not stop taking the medicine without checking with your doctor because symptoms may recur.

Precautions: Make sure your doctor knows if you are pregnant, planning to become pregnant or are breastfeeding, or if you have difficulty in passing urine or other kidney problems, intestinal obstruction, asthma, heart problems, epilepsy, Parkinson's disease, peptic ulcer.

Side effects: The most common side effects are: nausea, vomiting, increased salivation and abdominal cramps. Tell your doctor immediately if you experience any side effects, because they may be a sign of overdosage.

Warnings: None

Interactions: These drugs interact with several others. Check with your doctor or pharmacist before taking any other medicine.

Distigmine

Available preparations: Tablets
Brand names: Ubretid

Neostigmine

Available preparations: Tablets, injection
Brand names: None

Pyridostigmine

Available preparations: Tablets
Brand names: Mestinon

MUSCLE RELAXANTS

Muscle relaxants are used for the relief of chronic muscle spasm, rigidity, and cramping caused by disorders such as multiple sclerosis and spinal cord injury. They are also used in cases of spasticity caused by stroke, cerebral palsy or brain injury. They are not for spasm associated with minor injury. Most of these drugs, except dantrolene, act on the central nervous system, probably by increasing the activity of the neurotransmitter known as GABA (gamma-amino butyric acid). In addition to the drugs listed below, diazepam is also used for this purpose (see page 28).

How to use: Take the medicine exactly as prescribed by the doctor. If you miss a dose, take it as soon as you remember. However, if it is almost time for your next dose, skip the missed dose. Do not take double the dose. Do not stop taking the medicine without checking with your doctor because symptoms may recur.

Baclofen

How to use: As muscle relaxants (see page 156).
Precautions: Tell your doctor if you are pregnant, planning to become pregnant or are breastfeeding, or if you have or have had peptic ulcer, psychiatric illness, epilepsy, liver or kidney problems or breathing problems.
Side effects: The most common side effects are drowsiness, and nausea. Dizziness, confusion, headache, insomnia, muscle pain and weakness and mental disturbances may also occur.
Warnings: Avoid alcohol because it may increase the sedative effects of the drug. Take care with driving and other similar activities until you know how the drug affects you.
Interactions: Baclofen interacts with several other drugs including some used for heart conditions and those with a sedative action.
Available preparations: Tablets, liquid, injection
Brand names: Lioresal

Carisoprodol

How to use: As muscle relaxants (see page 156). In particular, do not stop taking these tablets suddenly.
Precautions: Tell your doctor if you are pregnant, planning to become pregnant or are breastfeeding, or you have or have had lung disease or breathing problems, liver or kidney problems or porphyria.
Side effects: Drowsiness is very common. Light-headedness, confusion, forgetfulness, headache, dizziness, blurred vision, rashes, low blood pressure, dry mouth or mouth watering, difficulty in passing urine, changes in libido and digestive disorders may occur, but these tend to be quite rare.
Warnings: Avoid alcohol with this drug. Take care with driving or other similar activities until you know how you react to this drug.
Interactions: Carisoprodol interacts with other drugs that act on the central nervous system, including drugs used for anxiety, depression and insomnia, to increase the sedative effect.
Available preparations: Tablets
Brand names: Carisoma

Dantrolene

How to use: As muscle relaxants (see page 156).
Precautions: Tell your doctor if you are pregnant, planning to become pregnant or are breastfeeding, or if you have or have had liver, heart or breathing problems. You will be asked to attend for regular liver function tests while taking this drug.

Side effects: Common side effects include drowsiness, dizziness, fatigue, weakness, muscle weakness, diarrhoea, loss of appetite, nausea, headache and rash.

Warnings: Avoid alcohol because it may increase the sedative effects of the drug. Take care with driving and other similar activities until you know how the drug affects you.

Interactions: Dantrolene interacts with several other drugs, including some used for heart conditions and those with a sedative action.

Available preparations: Capsules, injection

Brand names: Dantrium

Methocarbamol

How to use: As muscle relaxants (see page 156).

Precautions: Tell your doctor if you are pregnant, planning to become pregnant or are breastfeeding, or if you have or have had liver or kidney problems, epilepsy or myasthenia gravis.

Side effects: Common side effects include drowsiness, dizziness, restlessness, anxiety, confusion, nausea and allergic rash.

Warnings: Avoid alcohol because it may increase the sedative effects of the drug. Take care with driving and other similar activities until you know how the drug affects you.

Interactions: Methocarbamol interacts with several other drugs, including some used for heart conditions and those with a sedative action.

Available preparations: Tablets, injection

Brand names: Robaxin

Tizanadine

How to use: As muscle relaxants (see page 156).

Precautions: Tell your doctor if you are pregnant or breastfeeding, or if you have or have had liver or kidney problems.

Side effects: Common side effects include drowsiness, fatigue, dizziness, dry mouth, nausea and other gastrointestinal disturbances.

Warnings: Avoid alcohol because it may increase the sedative effects of the drug. Take care with driving and other similar activities until you know how the drug affects you.

Interactions: Tizanadine interacts with several other drugs including some used for heart conditions and those with a sedative action.

Available preparations: Tablets

Brand names: Zanaflex

DRUGS USED IN BONE DISORDERS

The bones can be affected by various disorders, including osteoporosis, osteomalacia and Paget's disease. Hormone replacement therapy (HRT – see page 183) has an important role in diminishing bone loss after the menopause and hence reducing the risk of osteoporosis. Calcium and vitamin D (see pages 313 and 316) may also have an important role.

This section covers drugs which are used in Paget's disease of the bone (see page 146) and similar conditions where there is a high level of calcium in the blood. Some of these drugs (eg alendronic acid, etidronate) are also used to treat osteoporosis and some (eg pamidronate, sodium clodronate) are used in bone cancer.

How to use: Take the medicine exactly as prescribed by the doctor. If you miss a dose, take it as soon as you remember. However, if it is almost time for your next dose, skip the missed dose. Do not take double the dose. Do not stop taking the medicine without checking with your doctor because symptoms may recur.

Alendronic acid

General information: Alendronic acid is a drug belonging to the bisphosphonate group. It is used in the treatment of postmenopausal osteoporosis. It works by reducing the activity of the bone cells and helps to reduce bone loss.

How to use: As drugs used in bone disorders (see above). In addition, swallow tablets whole with a full glass of water on an empty stomach at least 30 minutes before breakfast and any other oral medication. You must stay upright for at least 30 minutes. Do not take tablets at bedtime or before rising.
Precautions: Tell your doctor if you are pregnant, planning to become pregnant or are breastfeeding, or if you have or have had kidney problems or abnormalities of the oesophagus.
Side effects: The most common side effects are oesophagitis and ulceration of the oesophagus, abdominal pain and distension, diarrhoea, constipation, flatulence, bone pain, headache and rash. Tell your doctor immediately if you experience difficulty or pain on swallowing or heartburn.
Warnings: None
Interactions: Absorption of this drug is reduced by antacids and iron. If you are taking any of these products, leave a gap of two hours before or after to minimise effects on absorption.
Available preparations: Tablets
Brand names: Fosfamax

Calcitonin

General information: Calcitonin is a hormone produced by the thyroid gland which helps to control loss of calcium from the bones. It causes calcium to move from the blood to bones. Used in Paget's disease, it reduces blood calcium by transferring the mineral into the bones, thus helping to stop abnormal bone formation and prevent the spread of the disease. There are two forms of the drug – one derived from the pig's thyroid and synthetic salmon calcitonin (salcatonin). Synthetic human salcatonin is becoming available.

How to use: As drugs used in bone disorders (see above).

Precautions: Tell your doctor if you are pregnant, planning to become pregnant or are breastfeeding.
Side effects: Side effects are common and include nausea, vomiting, flushing, tingling of hands and unpleasant taste.
Warnings: None
Interactions: None
Available preparations: Injection
Brand names: Calcitare, Calsynar, Micalcic

Etidronate

General information: Etidronate is a drug belonging to the bisphosphonate group. It is used in the treatment of Paget's disease and in postmenopausal osteoporosis. It works by reducing the activity of the bone cells and helps to reduce bone loss.

How to use: As drugs used in bone disorders (see page 159). In addition, avoid food for at least 2 hours before and after taking the tablets (particularly calcium-containing foods such as milk and cheese).
Precautions: Tell your doctor if you are pregnant, planning to become pregnant or are breastfeeding, or if you have kidney problems.
Side effects: The most common side effects are diarrhoea, constipation, abdominal pain and nausea. Bone pain and skin itching may also occur.
Warnings: None
Interactions: Absorption of this drug is reduced by antacids and iron. If you are taking any of these products, leave a gap of two hours before or after to minimise effects on absorption.
Available preparations: Tablets
Brand names: Didronel
Combination preparation: Didronel PMO (etidronate with calcium). This preparation is specifically for treatment of postmenopausal osteoporosis.

Pamidronate

General information: Pamidronate is a drug belonging to the bisphosphonate group. It is used in the treatment of Paget's disease and in bone cancer. It works by reducing the activity of the bone cells and helps to reduce bone loss.

How to use: As drugs used in bone disorders (see page 159).
Precautions: Tell your doctor if you are pregnant, planning to become pregnant or are breastfeeding, or if you have kidney problems, heart problems or if you have had thyroid surgery.
Side effects: The most common side effects are fever, flu-like symptoms, bone pain, nausea, vomiting and headache. Loss of appetite, abdominal pain, muscle cramps, diarrhoea, constipation, dyspepsia, confusion, agitation, dizziness, insomnia and rash may also occur.
Warnings: Take care with driving until you know how the drug affects you.
Interactions: Absorption of this drug is reduced by antacids and iron. If you are tak-

ing any of these products, leave a gap of two hours before or after to minimise effects on absorption.
Available preparations: Injection
Brand names: Aredia

Sodium clodronate

General information: Sodium clodronate is a drug belonging to the bisphosphonate group and used in the treatment of bone cancer. It works by reducing the activity of the bone cells and helps to reduce bone loss.

How to use: As drugs used in bone disorders (see page 159). Avoid food, particularly calcium-containing food (eg milk) for one hour before and after taking the medicine.
Precautions: Tell your doctor if you are pregnant or breastfeeding, or if you have or have had kidney problems.
Side effects: The most common side effects are nausea, diarrhoea and skin reactions.
Warnings: None
Interactions: Absorption of this drug is reduced by antacids and iron. If you are taking any of these products, leave a gap of two hours before or after to minimise effects on absorption.
Available preparations: Tablets, capsules, injection
Brand names: Bonefos, Loron

Tiludronic acid

General information: Tiludronic acid is a drug belonging to the bisphosphonate group. It is used in Paget's disease. It works by reducing the activity of the bone cells and helps to reduce bone loss.

How to use: As drugs used in bone disorders (see page 159). Avoid food, particularly calcium-containing food (eg milk) for two hours before and after taking the medicine.
Precautions: Tell your doctor if you are pregnant, planning to become pregnant or are breastfeeding, or if you have or have had kidney problems.
Side effects: The most common side effects are nausea, diarrhoea and stomach pain. Skin reactions, dizziness and headache may also occur.
Warnings: None
Interactions: Absorption of this drug is reduced by antacids and iron. If you are taking any of these products, leave a gap of two hours before or after to minimise effects on absorption.
Available preparations: Tablets
Brand names: Skelid

The Endocrine System

THE ENDOCRINE SYSTEM consists of a group of organs, more commonly known as glands, whose main function is to produce and secrete hormones directly into the bloodstream. Hormones act as chemical messengers to co-ordinate activities in various parts of the body. They ebb and flow through the bloodstream, providing the glands with precisely the information they need. Hormones have a wide range of fundamental functions, such as growth, repair and metabolism, for sexual development and function, and for governing the processes of reproduction, (see the reproductive system, page 177). The release of hormones into the bloodstream also helps us to cope with intense emotional experiences, for example fear, stress and sudden trauma.

The major glands of the endocrine system are the pituitary gland, the hypothalamus, the thyroid gland, the parathyroid glands, the pancreas, the adrenal glands, the testes and the ovaries. Each gland produces and secretes one or more hormones.

The pituitary gland is often known as the master gland because it co-ordinates so many of the activities of the other glands. It releases a whole host of hormones into the bloodstream, some of which have direct effects, while others control the rate at which other endocrine glands release their hormones. It secretes growth hormone, and hormones controlling the activity of the thyroid, adrenal glands and reproductive glands. It also helps to control water levels in the body by producing the substance known as anti-diuretic hormone (ADH). The hypothalamus gland is connected to the pituitary gland. It secretes several hormones, some of which trigger the release of pituitary hormones and some of which suppress them.

The thyroid gland secretes the hormones thyroxine and tri-iodothyronine. These play a part in regulating growth and metabolism.

The parathyroid glands are four small glands which lie behind the thyroid gland. They secrete two hormones – parathyroid hormone and calcitonin – which, working with vitamin D in the bone and kidneys, help to maintain blood levels of calcium at an appropriate level.

The pancreas has important functions in digestion, but it also acts as an endocrine gland. It produces insulin and glucagon which work together to maintain blood glucose at the appropriate level.

The two adrenal glands are situated just above each kidney and are composed of two distinct parts. The first part is the outer zone, which produces three types of steroid hormones: the sex hormones; the glucocorticoid hormones, commonly known as steroids (eg cortisol – a stress hormone); and mineralocorticoids, such as aldosterone, which help to control blood pressure and the body's salt balance. The second part is the core of the gland, which produces adrenaline and noradrenaline. Adrenaline is often known as the body's 'fight and flight hormone' because it is produced in response to stimuli such as fear, excitement or shock.

The ovaries and testes are targets for various hormones from the pituitary gland and they also produce their own hormones. As well as releasing eggs, the ovaries produce the female sex hormones oestrogen and progesterone. The testicles manufacture the male sex hormones, including testosterone, and also produce sperm.

What can go wrong

Hormones are vital for our health. When endocrine glands malfunction, hormone levels can become abnormally high or low, disrupting body functions. Because the pituitary gland controls the whole endocrine system, disturbances in the activities of endocrine glands are sometimes caused by problems with the pituitary gland.

Common examples of illnesses involving the endocrine system include diabetes, of which there are two main types. Type I diabetes (often known as insulin-dependent diabetes) usually starts in young people, but it can occur at any age and is caused by a severe lack of insulin. Type II diabetes (often known as non-insulin-dependent diabetes) occurs either when there is insufficient insulin or when the body cannot use what insulin is produced properly. It commonly develops in middle-aged people, especially in those who are overweight.

When there is not enough insulin, the level of glucose in the blood rises too high. Indeed, blood glucose may rise so high that the kidneys cannot hold it back and glucose spills over into the urine. This is why, if a doctor suspects a person has diabetes, a urine sample is tested for glucose. High blood glucose levels have several implications. First, the glucose in the urine makes it difficult for the kidney to concentrate the urine. This results in frequent urination and thirst, both of which are typical symptoms of diabetes. Second, glucose which stays in the blood does not get into the cells, and the tissues are therefore starved of their principal fuel and energy, resulting in feelings of lethargy and tiredness. The cells then switch to using other sources of energy – mainly fat. When fat is used, chemicals called ketoacids are produced which can cause nausea, vomiting and excessive accumulation of acid in the blood. The body responds to this by overbreathing to reduce the amount of acid in the blood. The loss of glucose in the urine and the excessive fat breakdown result in weight loss.

Diabetic patients tend to develop longer term complications too, such as blindness, infections, damage to the nerve endings, kidney disease and cardiovascular disease, including high blood pressure. As a result of poor circulation, patients may also develop foot and leg problems including ulcers. The risk of these complications can be substantially reduced by controlling the blood glucose level tightly. This involves careful attention to diet, and normally the use of drugs and/or insulin.

Disorders of the thyroid gland are caused by an excess or a deficiency of thyroid hormones. They lead to conditions such as hyperthyroidism, hypothyroidism and goitre (an enlarged thyroid gland). Hyperthyroidism causes restlessness, anxiety, weight loss, diarrhoea and slight tremor. Common consequences of hypothyroidism are slowness and lethargy, weight gain, deafness, constipation, feeling cold, dry skin and hair, joint pains and menstrual problems.

Disturbances in the function of the adrenal glands can lead to a number of disorders. Underactive adrenal glands, for example, often result in Addison's disease, a condition in which there is a failure to make adequate amounts of glucocorticoid and mineralocorticoid hormones. Conditions caused by overproduction of the adrenal hormones vary, depending on which hormones are affected. Overproduction of testosterone and other male sex hormones can lead to virilisation – the development of exaggerated masculine characteristics in either men or women. Overproduction of steroid hormones can result in Cushing's syndrome, a condition which is often characterised by a large, round 'moon' face. Excessive production of aldosterone, which is much rarer, can lead to high blood pressure, salt retention, and also low levels of potassium in the blood which in turn can cause weakness, tingling and muscle spasms.

Because the pituitary gland controls the activity of the whole endocrine system, problems with its function can cause disorders affecting any endocrine gland. For example the adrenal glands, thyroid and reproductive glands will cease to function properly if the pituitary fails to produce sufficient amounts of the appropriate hormones. However, the pituitary gland also produces hormones with their own direct effects, and failure in the production of any of these can also cause problems. Failure in the production of growth hormone, for example, results in stunted growth, and the inability to produce adequate amounts of anti-diuretic hormone (ADH) leads to excessive excretion of urine and the condition known as diabetes insipidus.

Drugs used to treat all these conditions aim either to replace deficient hormones (eg insulin) or to reduce hormone levels when they are excessive.

Common conditions and drugs used to treat them

Diabetes – insulin, oral antidiabetic drugs (oral hypoglycaemics)

Hypothyroidism (myxoedema) – thyroid hormones (eg thyroxine)

Hyperthyroidism – antithyroid drugs (eg carbimazole)

Adrenal insufficiency (eg Addison's disease) – glucorticoids (eg hydrocortisone) and mineralocorticoids (eg fludrocortisone)

Diabetes insipidus – desmopressin, vasopressin.

INSULIN

Insulin is the hormone produced by the pancreas. When the production of natural insulin is inadequate – as happens in diabetes – the hormone can be replaced by giving insulin injections. However, natural insulin secretion fluctuates throughout the day in response to blood glucose levels, and this means that artificial insulin doses have to be calculated very carefully to try to match these fluctuations as much as possible and respond to the person's individual needs.

Insulin is used in both types of diabetes (Type I and Type II), but is most commonly needed by patients with Type I diabetes. There are four types of insulin which vary in their speed of onset of action, total duration of action and time to reach maximum effect. Short acting insulin starts to work within 30 minutes to one hour, with a maximum effect at two to four hours and a duration of action of eight hours. Intermediate acting insulin starts to work after 30 minutes to three hours, with a maximum effect at 2–16 hours and a duration of 24 hours. Long acting insulin starts to work after 2–6 hours, producing a peak effect at 8–24 hours and with a duration of action of 36 hours. Biphasic insulins are ready-made mixtures of short and intermediate acting insulins in one bottle. The short acting insulin starts to work very quickly and the intermediate acting insulin prolongs the effect for 24 hours, thus providing the best of both worlds in one preparation.

Most patients use insulin twice a day. This normally involves giving a mixture of a short and an intermediate acting insulin before breakfast and again before the evening meal. However, multiple regimens are becoming increasingly popular, with the aim of controlling blood glucose levels even more precisely. This may involve, for example, giving short acting insulin before meals and intermediate or long acting insulin at bedtime.

Insulin has to be given by injection; it is destroyed in the stomach and cannot therefore be given by mouth. It is normally injected just under the skin (subcutaneously) into the upper arms, abdomen, thighs or buttocks. Reactions at the injection site – albeit rare - can to some extent be prevented by rotating the location used.

Nowadays, insulin is often administered using injection devices known as 'pens', which contain the insulin in a cartridge. This is easy for the patient to change and meters the right dose, so that the patient does not have to measure anything. However, conventional needles and syringes are still used by some patients. Insulin was traditionally obtained from the pancreas of animals (eg beef and pork insulin), but nowadays about 85 per cent of insulin is manufactured to resemble human insulin very closely, using genetic engineering techniques.

How to use: Use exactly as prescribed. Do not stop using insulin without asking your doctor. This can lead to very serious consequences, including coma. If you miss a dose, the appropriate course of action will be determined by the type of insulin you are using, but in general you should not double up. Simply carry on with your usual regime at the correct time. Check with your doctor. In addition to using insulin, you should also follow any dietary advice you have been given by your doctor or dietitian. Remember to monitor your blood glucose levels regularly, using the equipment and instructions you have been given. If you are unsure about any aspects of your insulin prescription or glucose monitoring, check with your doctor or pharmacist. Do not stop using insulin if you are ill as your body's need for insulin is greater during illness. If you have persistent vomiting, check with your doctor.

Precautions: Tell your doctor if you have kidney disease and if you have ever had an allergic reaction to any type of insulin. If you are pregnant or breastfeeding, your insulin dose may be adjusted and you will be carefully monitored, but it is essential to continue using your insulin.

Side effects: Irritation and dimpling of the skin at the injection site may occur and can to some extent be prevented by rotation of the injection site. Allergic reactions, including rash and shortness of breath, may occur, but are rare.

Interactions: Many medicines (eg some antibiotics) can reduce blood sugar levels, while others (eg beta-blockers) can mask the signs of low blood sugar. Some cough and cold mixtures also contain ingredients which can upset diabetic control. Check with your doctor or pharmacist before taking any other medicines.

Warnings: Symptoms such as sweating, weakness, dizziness and confusion indicate low blood sugar. You should always carry a diabetes warning card with you so that appropriate treatment can be given should these symptoms develop. It is also advisable to carry a source of rapidly available sugar, for example glucose sweets. Alcohol need not be avoided entirely, but is best consumed in moderate amounts only (eg one glass of wine a day) and always with meals. Finally, there are many brands of insulin. Always check that the one you receive on each occasion is exactly what you are expecting.

Biphasic isophane insulin

General information: Biphasic isophane insulin is an intermediate acting insulin.

Available preparations: Conventional injections and various pen devices
Brand names: Animal insulins: Hypurin Porcine Biphasic Isophane 30/70 Mix, Pork Mixtard 30; Human insulins: Human Mixtard, Humulin M

Insulin lispro

General information: Insulin lispro is a relatively new, short acting insulin manufactured by genetic engineering.

Available preparations: An injection pen device
Brand names: Humalog

Insulin zinc suspension

General information: Insulin zinc suspension is a long acting insulin.

Available preparations: Conventional injections and pen devices
Brand names: Animal insulins: Hypurin Bovine Lente, Lentard MC; Human insulins: Human Monotard, Human Ultratard, Humulin Lente, Humulin Zinc

Isophane insulin

General information: Isophane insulin is an intermediate acting insulin.

Available preparations: Conventional injections and pen devices
Brand names: Animal insulins: Hypurin Bovine Isophane, Hypurin Porcine Isophane, Pork Insulatard; Human insulins: Human insulatard ge, Humulin I

Soluble insulin

General information: Soluble insulin is one of the oldest forms of insulin. It is a short acting insulin.

Available preparations: Conventional injection and various pen devices
Brand names: Animal insulins: Hypurin Bovine Neutral, Hypurin Porcine Neutral, Pork Velosulin; Human insulins: Human Actrapid, Humulin S

ORAL ANTIDIABETIC DRUGS

Oral antidiabetic drugs, often called oral hypoglycaemics, are used in the treatment of diabetes. They are given mainly in Type II diabetes, which normally develops in middle age.

How they work: Oral antidiabetic drugs work by reducing blood glucose levels, but they achieve this in different ways. Most stimulate the pancreas to increase its production of insulin, but one drug – metformin – works by stimulating the body cells to take up excess glucose from the blood. Another drug – acarbose – works by delaying the digestion of carbohydrate, which reduces the increase in blood glucose that normally occurs after eating a meal.

How to use: Take the medicine exactly as prescribed by the doctor. If you miss a dose, take it before your next meal. Do not take double the dose. Do not stop taking the medicine without asking your doctor because this may cause your underlying condition to get worse. If you are vomiting or not eating, do not continue with the treatment but ask your doctor for advice.

Precautions: Tell your doctor if you are pregnant, planning to become pregnant or are breastfeeding (although these drugs are not normally used in women of this age group), or if you have liver or kidney disease.

Side effects: These are generally mild and infrequent and include nausea, vomiting, diarrhoea, headache and allergic reactions including rash. Most of these drugs (with the exception of metformin and acarbose) can cause weight gain, so attention to diet is very important.

Warnings: Symptoms such as sweating, weakness, dizziness and confusion indicate low blood sugar. You should always carry a diabetes warning card with you so that appropriate treatment can be given should such symptoms develop. It is also advisable to carry glucose sweets. Alcohol need not be avoided entirely, but is best consumed in only moderate amounts (eg one glass of wine a day) and always with meals.

Interactions: Many medicines (eg some antibiotics) can reduce blood sugar levels, while others (eg beta-blockers) can mask the signs of low blood sugar. Some cough and cold mixtures also contain ingredients which can upset diabetic control. Check with your doctor or pharmacist before taking any other medicines.

Acarbose

General information: Acarbose is used in diabetes which is inadequately controlled by diet and other oral antidiabetic drugs.

Precautions, warnings, interactions: As oral antidiabetics (see above). In addition,

tell your doctor if you have any gastrointestinal disorder or obstruction.
Side effects: Diarrhoea, abdominal pain and flatulence may occur.
Available preparations: Tablets
Brand names: Glucobay

Chlorpropamide

General information: Chlorpropamide is used in diabetes. Alcohol should be avoided with this drug as it causes flushing.

Available preparations: Tablets
Brand names: None

Glibenclamide

General information: Glibenclamide is used in diabetes.

Available preparations: Tablets
Brand names: Daonil, Semi-Daonil, Euglucon

Gliclazide

General information: Gliclazide is used in diabetes, particularly in the elderly.

Available preparations: Tablets
Brand names: Diamicron

Gliquidone

General information: Gliquidone is used in diabetes.

Available preparations: Tablets
Brand names: Glurenorm

Guar gum

General information: Guar gum is used in diabetes which is inadequately controlled by diet and other oral antidiabetic drugs.

Precautions, warnings, interactions: As oral antidiabetics (see page 167). In addition, tell your doctor if you have any gastrointestinal disorder or obstruction. Take this preparation with plenty of water.
Side effects: Diarrhoea, abdominal pain and flatulence may occur.
Available preparations: Granules
Brand names: Guarem

Metformin

General information: Metformin is used in diabetes which is inadequately controlled by diet and antidiabetic drugs, for example glibenclamide and gliclazide. It is particularly useful in overweight patients, and has a lower risk of causing low blood sugar than the other antidiabetic drugs.

Precautions, side effects, warnings, interactions: As oral antidiabetics (see page 167). In addition, tell your doctor if you have heart failure or kidney disease.
Available preparations: Tablets
Brand names: Glucophage

Repaglinide

General information: Repaglinide is used in diabetes, either or its own or in combination with metformin.

Available preparations: Tablets
Brand names: NovoNorm

Tolazamide

General information: Tolazamide is used in diabetes.

Available preparations: Tablets
Brand names: Tolanase

Tolbutamide

General information: Tolbutamide is used in diabetes, especially in the elderly.

Available preparations: Tablets
Brand names: Rastinon

Hypoglycaemia

Good diabetes control depends on maintaining an appropriate amount of insulin in the blood in relation to the amount of sugar. Sometimes, however, there may be too much insulin in proportion to the amount of glucose in the blood and your blood sugar level may fall. This condition is known as hypoglycaemia, or a 'hypo'; it usually occurs because you have missed a meal or snack or taken unexpected exercise.

Hypoglycaemia is easy to recognise. Its symptoms include trembling, sweating, faintness, headache, unsteadiness, blurred vision, irritability, palpitations, confusion and difficulty in concentration. If you suffer a 'hypo', stop what you are doing immediately and take two lumps of sugar, three glucose tablets, a glass of milk, a glass of Lucozade or other sparkling glucose drink, or a non-diet version of Ribena or Coca-Cola. Within a few minutes the symptoms should have disappeared, but if not take another couple of glucose tablets. Occasionally you may lose consciousness due to hypoglycaemia, but when the blood sugar drops this low, your body responds by making glucose and you will always recover. You may on very rare occasions have a convulsion, but this is a reaction to the low blood sugar and does not mean that you have developed epilepsy.

Always carry some form of sugar with you that you can easily swallow should these symptoms occur. In addition, always carry an identification card to say that you are diabetic and always make sure that people round you – for example, at work, school or home – know exactly what to do if you become hypoglycaemic.

There is also an injection known as glucagon, which causes the blood sugar level in the body to rise. It is available on prescription and friends, family and colleagues can be trained to give you this injection. You may feel a bit sick or actually vomit after this injection, but you will soon feel better.

THYROID HORMONES

Thyroid hormones (thyroxine and liothyronine) are used to replace natural thyroid hormones when the thyroid gland is underactive and production of the hormones is deficient. Low levels of natural thyroid hormones (hypothyroidism) cause different conditions depending on the age of the patient. In adults, hypothyroidism causes slowing of mental activity, lethargy, slow heart rate, weight gain, dry skin, puffy face and eyelids, hair loss and sensitivity to cold. In children, the condition may be similar, but including failure of growth and stunting and delayed puberty in adolescence. However, untreated hypothyroidism in infants leads to permanent neurological and intellectual damage as well as stunting (cretinism). In most parts of the UK babies are screened for this in the first week of life and early treatment restores normal development.

How to use: Take the medicine exactly as prescribed by the doctor. If you miss a dose, take it as soon as you remember. Do not take double the dose. Do not stop taking the medicine without asking your doctor because this may cause your underlying condition to get worse.

Precautions: Tell your doctor if you are pregnant, planning to become pregnant or are breastfeeding, or if you have a heart condition, high blood pressure or any other disorder of the endocrine system (eg diabetes, adrenal insufficiency). None of these conditions is a contraindication to treatment, but may affect the dose. You will be asked to attend for regular blood tests to monitor the dose.

Side effects: Side effects are rare unless the dose is excessive in which case the following may occur: chest pains, palpitations, muscle cramps, diarrhoea, vomiting, restlessness, agitation, insomnia, headache, flushing, sweating and excessive weight loss. Tell your doctor if you experience any of these side effects.

Warnings: None

Interactions: Thyroid hormones interact with several drugs, of which oral anticoagulants (eg warfarin) are the most important.

Thyroxine

General information: Thyroxine is a thyroid hormone used in hypothyroidism.

Available preparations: Tablets
Brand names: None

Liothyronine sodium

General information: Liothyronine sodium is similar to thyroxine, but it works faster. It can therefore be used (by injection) in severe cases of hypothyroidism when a rapid response is needed.

Available preparations: Tablets, injection
Brand names: Tertroxin

ANTITHYROID DRUGS

Antithyroid drugs are used in cases of overactive thyroid gland (hyperthyroidism or thyrotoxicosis). They can be used for long term treatment, or short term while the patient is waiting for surgery to remove part of the thyroid gland. There are two antithyroid drugs – carbimazole and propylthiouracil – of which carbimazole is the more commonly used. Both work primarily by interfering with the production of thyroid hormones.

Radioactive iodine is also used for hyperthyroidism, especially where antithyroid drugs fail to work properly. Ordinary iodine solution may also be given for 10–14 days before surgery to help control of the condition, but is not used for long term treatment. Other drugs used in hyperthyroidism include the beta-blockers, particularly propranolol (see page 86). These drugs do not alter thyroid function, but they do reduce some of the symptoms of the condition (eg agitation, restlessness and fast heart beat).

How to use: Take the medicine exactly as prescribed by the doctor. If you miss a dose, take it as soon as you remember. Do not take double the dose. Do not stop taking the medicine without asking your doctor because this may cause your underlying condition to get worse.

Precautions: Tell your doctor if you are pregnant, planning to become pregnant or are breastfeeding, or if you have or have had liver or kidney problems.

Side effects: Nausea, headache, joint pain and hair loss may occur. Tell your doctor immediately if you develop a sore throat, mouth ulcers, bruising or fever, or if any other illness develops.

Warnings: None

Interactions: None

Carbimazole

Available preparations: Tablets
Brand names: Neo-Mercazole

Propylthiouracil

Available preparations: Tablets
Brand names: None

CORTICOSTEROIDS

Corticosteroids, often known as steroids for short, have a variety of uses. They may be used to replace natural steroid hormones (mineralocorticoids and glucocorticoids) produced by the adrenal glands in disorders such as Addison's disease. However, they are used more commonly in a variety of allergic and inflammatory conditions, for example asthma (see page 140), inflammatory bowel disease (see page 124) and arthritis (see page 151). They are also used in some cancers (see page 308) and systemic lupus erythematus. Creams and ointments containing steroids are used in inflammatory skin conditions such as eczema (see page 205) and steroids are included in certain drops to treat inflammatory conditions of the eye (see page 226) and ear (see page 235). They work by reducing inflammation and suppress allergic reactions and immune system activity.

This section lists all the corticosteroids used systemically – that is, by mouth or injection – together with precautions for use, side effects, warnings and interactions.

How to use: Take the medicine exactly as prescribed by the doctor. If you miss a dose, take it as soon as you remember. Do not take double the dose. Do not stop taking the medicine without asking your doctor because this may cause your underlying condition to get worse. If your doctor thinks it advisable to stop taking the medicine s/he may recommend that you reduce your dose gradually.

Precautions: Tell your doctor if you are pregnant, planning to become pregnant or are breastfeeding, or if you have an infection, a history of tuberculosis, heart problems, high blood pressure, liver or kidney problems, diabetes, osteoporosis, glaucoma, epilepsy, peptic ulcer or an underactive thyroid gland.

Side effects: Corticosteroids are powerful drugs, particularly when given by mouth or injection in high doses over long periods of time. In these circumstances, they can cause serious side effects such as high blood pressure, fluid retention, muscle weakness, thinning of the skin and delay in wound healing, reduced ability to fight infection, increased hair growth on the face, chest and stomach, osteoporosis, indigestion and peptic ulcer, mood changes and mental disturbances, diabetes, weight gain and acne.

However, when used topically, that is in the form of inhalers, creams, ointments, eye, ear and nose preparations, steroids are unlikely to cause severe side effects.

Interactions: Corticosteroids interact with several other drugs including some antibiotics, anticonvulsants and cyclosporin. Always check with your doctor or pharmacist before taking any other medication.

Warnings: Avoid excessive alcohol intake because it may increase the risk of adverse effects from these drugs. You will be given a steroid treatment card by your pharmacist who dispenses your medicine. Always carry this with you. Steroids increase susceptibility to infection, including common infections such as chickenpox. Seek medical advice immediately if you have been in contact with people with infections or if an infection develops. In addition, steroids often dampen down the body's own reaction to infection and trauma, and this reaction may persist for some months after steroids have been stopped. If you have been on steroids and become ill or need an operation, you should tell the doctor that you have had steroids recently. If you are on steroids, you may need to increase the dose during an acute illness. Always check with your doctor.

Betamethasone

Available preparations: Tablets, injection
Brand names: Betnelan, Betnesol

Cortisone

Available preparations: Tablets
Brand names: Cortisyl

Deflazacort

Available preparations: Tablets
Brand names: Calcort

Dexamethasone

Available preparations: Tablets, injection
Brand names: Decadron, Decadron Shock-Pak

Fludrocortisone

Available preparations: Tablets
Brand names: Florinef

Hydrocortisone

Available preparations: Tablets, injection
Brand names: Efcortesol, Hydrocortone, Solu-Cortef

Methyprednisolone

Available preparations: Injection
Brand names: Medrone, Solu-Medrone

Prednisolone

Available preparations: Tablets
Brand names: Precortisyl Forte, Prednesol

Prednisone

Available preparations: Tablets
Brand names: None

Triamcinolone

Available preparations: Injection
Brand names: Kenalog

ANTI-ADRENAL DRUGS

Two drugs are available which are used occasionally to treat conditions such as Cushing's syndrome, in which there is excessive secretion of corticosteroids from the adrenal glands. These drugs are supervised by specialists in hospital.

How to use: Take the medicine exactly as prescribed by the doctor. If you miss a dose, take it as soon as you remember. Do not take double the dose. Do not stop taking the medicine without asking your doctor because this may cause your underlying condition to get worse.

Metyrapone

General information: Metyrapone is used to treat Cushing's syndrome and also in the diagnosis of a type of Cushing's syndrome (as a test of pituitary function).

Precautions: Tell your doctor if you are pregnant, planning to become pregnant or are breastfeeding.
Side effects: Nausea, vomiting, dizziness, headache and drowsiness may occur.
Warnings, interactions: None
Available preparations: Capsules
Brand names: Metopirone

Trilostane

General information: Trilostane is used to treat overactivity of the adrenal glands.

Precautions: Tell your doctor if you are pregnant, planning to become pregnant or are breastfeeding.
Side effects: Flushing, tingling, swelling of the mouth, runny nose, nausea, vomiting, diarrhoea and rash may occur.
Warnings, interactions: None
Available preparations: Capsules
Brand names: Modrenal

ANABOLIC STEROIDS

When people think of steroids it is usually the anabolic steroids – rather than the corticosteroids – that they are thinking of. Anabolic steroids are synthetic derivatives of male sex hormones, but with rather different properties. They promote tissue growth by increasing protein manufacture. They are little used in medicine, but are sometimes used illegally by athletes to improve performance in sports events. In the past they were used in osteoporosis, but newer drugs have now superseded them.

How to use: Use exactly as prescribed.

Precautions: Tell your doctor if you are pregnant, planning to become pregnant or are breastfeeding, or you have prostate cancer, breast cancer (men only), high blood pressure, diabetes or epilepsy.

Side effects: Acne, increased hair growth, menstrual disturbances and a range of other side effects may occur.

Warnings: None

Interactions: Anabolic steroids enhance the effects of oral anticoagulants.

Nandrolone

General information: Nandrolone is an anabolic steroid used in a specific type of anaemia (aplastic anaemia). It can also be used in osteoporosis, but is now very rarely prescribed for this purpose.

Available preparations: Injection
Brand names: Deca-Durabolin

Stanozolol

General information: Stanozolol is an anabolic steroid used in hereditary angio-edema (a serious allergic disorder) and Behcet's disease.

Available preparations: Tablets
Brand names: Stromba

ANTI-DIURETIC HORMONE

Anti-diuretic hormone is a hormone produced by the pituitary gland. It helps to regulate the amount of water in the body by reducing, as its name suggests, the volume of urine lost. If the pituitary gland fails to produce ADH, the person develops the condition known as diabetes insipidus in which very large amounts of urine are lost. This condition, like the more well-known form of diabetes, diabetes mellitus, is treated by replacing the missing hormone. In diabetes insipidus, the hormone ADH, also known as vasopressin, is given. Similar drugs, such as desmopressin and lypressin, are also used; most forms are broken down in the intestine, so must be given by injection or nasal spray. All work by reducing the volume of urine output.

How to use: Take the medicine exactly as prescribed by the doctor. If you miss a dose, take it as soon as you remember. Do not take double the dose. Do not stop taking the medicine without asking your doctor because this may cause your underlying condition to get worse.

Precautions: Tell your doctor if you are pregnant, planning to become pregnant or are breastfeeding, or if you have problems with the liver, kidney, heart or circulation.

Side effects: Nausea, stomach pain and headache may occur.

Warnings: None

Interactions: None

Desmopressin

General information: Desmopressin is similar to anti-diuretic hormone (ADH) and is used in the treatment of diabetes insipidus. It is also used to boost blood clotting in some patients with haemophilia, for bedwetting and testing kidney function.

Available preparations: Tablets, nasal spray, injection
Brand names: DDAVP, Desmotabs, Desmospray

Lypressin

General information: Lypressin is similar to anti-diuretic hormone (ADH) and is used in the treatment of diabetes insipidus.

Available preparations: Nasal spray
Brand names: Syntopressin

Terlipressin

General information: Terlipressin is used to treat bleeding from the oesophagus

Available preparations: Injection
Brand names: Glypressin

Vasopressin

General information: Vasopressin is anti-diuretic hormone (ADH) itself. It is used in diabetes insipidus and to treat bleeding from the oesophagus.

Available preparations: Injection
Brand names: Pitressin

GROWTH HORMONE

Somatropin

General information: Somatropin is growth hormone produced using genetic engineering. It is used in the treatment of growth hormone deficiency.

Precautions: Tell your doctor if you are pregnant or breastfeeding, or if you have diabetes.
Side effects: Headache, visual problems, nausea and vomiting may occur.
Available preparations: Injection
Brand names: Genotropin, Humatrope, Norditropin, Saizen, Zomacton

The Reproductive System

THE REPRODUCTIVE SYSTEM in the male consists of the penis, scrotum and testes (testicles) together with other structures such as the prostate gland, the seminal vesicles, the vas deferens and the urethra. The overall function of the male reproductive system is to produce sperm and deliver sperm to the vagina. Sperm is made in the testes and stored in the seminal vesicles. During sexual intercourse the sperm is transported along with fluid called semen through the vas deferens and the erect penis.

The male reproductive system is controlled by one main hormone – testosterone – which is produced in the testes. The secretion of testosterone is itself controlled by a hormone from the pituitary gland (see page 162), called luteinising hormone (LH). LH is itself also controlled by gonadotrophin-releasing hormone from the hypothalamus – both the pituitary gland and the hypothalamus being situated in the brain. The synthetic form of this hormone, gonadorelin, is used as a drug. Testosterone is responsible for the development of the male genitals and the secondary sexual characteristics such as the deepening of the voice, growth of facial and pubic hair and strengthening of the muscles. Sperm production in the testis is stimulated by a second hormone secreted by the pituitary gland called follicle-stimulating hormone (FSH).

In the female, the reproductive system consists of the vulva (the external female genitalia), the vagina, the uterus (womb), the fallopian tubes and the ovaries. The function of the female reproductive system is to produce eggs, receive sperm from the male, protect and feed the unborn child and finally to give birth.

The female sex hormones are the oestrogens and progestogens, and their secretion is controlled by two hormones from the pituitary gland: follicle-stimulating hormone (FSH) and luteinising hormone (LH), which are themselves also controlled by hormones from the hypothalamus. A complex interaction of these hormones regulates the menstrual cycle and allows an egg to be released from the ovaries once a month, which if fertilized implants itself into the uterus. If the egg is not fertilised, the uterine lining is shed and the woman experiences vaginal bleeding or menstruation. Menstruation begins on average around the age of 11–12 years and continues until the time of the menopause, which generally occurs around the age of 50. Each menstrual cycle is normally about 28 days, but this can vary enormously between individuals and even within one individual.

What can go wrong

Reproductive function can be disrupted by various hormonal disturbances. These can sometimes lead to infertility and drugs may be used to restore the balance and to stimulate normal reproductive function. In addition, women may suffer from various menstrual disorders, such as painful periods and endometriosis – problems which do not necessarily affect fertility, but may be painful or uncomfortable.

The menopause is associated with a range of symptoms such as hot flushes, mood changes, headaches and sleeplessness – symptoms which may be caused by falling oestrogen levels that occur at this time in a woman's life, and which are sometimes helped by hormone replacement therapy (HRT). Moreover, post-menopausal women are at increasing risk of developing conditions such as osteoporosis and coronary heart disease, and HRT may sometimes be prescribed for several years beyond the menopause to help reduce the risk of these conditions.

Common conditions and drugs used to treat them

Contraception – hormonal contraceptives (eg oral contraceptives)

Menopause – hormone replacement therapy

Menstrual disorders such as painful periods and endometriosis – progestogens, danazol, gestrinone

Infertility – various hormonal preparations

Male sex hormone deficiency – testosterone

HORMONAL CONTRACEPTIVES

There are several methods of contraception, including condoms, diaphragms, intra-uterine devices (coils), natural family planning, sterilisation and hormonal contraceptives. Only hormonal contraceptives will be covered in this section.

Hormonal contraceptives, which first became popular in the 1960s, are the most reliable way of preventing conception, but they are not suitable for all women because of the side effects they can cause. Of the three main types of hormonal contraceptives – combined oral contraceptives, progestogen-only pills and progestogen implants and injections – the combined oral contraceptive pill is the most widely used.

Combined oral contraceptives

All combined oral contraceptives contain two main ingredients – a synthetic oestrogen and a synthetic progestogen. Ethinyloestradiol is the most common oestrogen used, although mestranol, which is converted to ethinyloestradiol in the body, is used occasionally. A range of progestogens are used, of which norethisterone and levonorgestrel are the most common.

Most combined oral contraceptives contain an oestrogen and a progestogen in a fixed amount in each tablet. Available in monthly calendar packs which normally contain 21 tablets, they are known as monophasic pills and are taken once a day for 21 days followed by seven pill-free days during which a form of withdrawal bleeding (ie not a normal period) occurs. However, a few products contain 28 tablets in a monthly pack. Known as ED (every day) preparations, they contain 21 tablets with hormones, and seven tablets with inactive ingredients ('dummy tablets'). One tablet is taken each day throughout the whole month and bleeding takes place during the time when the seven hormone-free tablets are taken.

Some combined oral contraceptives are formulated into what is known as phased pills. Each month's calendar pack contains 21 tablets, but not all of these tablets contain the same proportions of oestrogen to progestogen. Each pack contains two (biphasic) or three (triphasic) different strengths of tablet, indicated by different colours. Thus, there may be seven white tablets all of one strength and 14 pink tablets all of a different strength. The aim of these preparations is to try to provide a hormonal balance that more closely resembles that of the natural menstrual cycle.

How they work: Combined oral contraceptives disrupt the body's normal hormonal control of ovulation, implantation and fertilisation. The oestrogens and progestogens in combined oral contraceptives add to the body's natural supply of sex hormones, and mimic the hormone levels in pregnancy, when ovulation temporarily ceases. The extra oestrogen suppresses FSH and LH secretion by the pituitary gland and hence stops ovulation, which will only take place on instruction by the pituitary gland. The progestogen acts on the cervix (at the top of the vagina) to produce a sticky mucous plug, which helps to prevent sperm from entering.

How to use: Take exactly as prescribed. If you forget a pill take it as soon as you remember, followed by the next one at your normal time. If you are 12 or more hours late with any pill, especially the first in the packet, the pill may not work. As soon as you remember, continue normal pill taking. However, you will not be protected for the next seven days, so if you have sex, use another method, such as a condom. If these seven days run beyond the end of your packet, start the next packet at once when you have finished the present packet. Do not leave a gap between the packets. This may mean that you have no bleeding until the end of two packets, but this does no harm. If you are using ED (every day) tablets, miss out the seven inactive pills. If you are not sure which these are, check with your doctor. Always be careful if you change from one make of pill to another. Ask your doctor for instructions regarding exactly what day you should start the new pill and whether you need to take additional contraceptive precautions for a period of time.

Diarrhoea and vomiting can also interfere with the pill. If you have an episode of either diarrhoea or vomiting, use additional contraceptive precautions during the illness and for seven days after. If the illness occurs during the last seven days, start the next packet immediately you have finished the current pack. Do not leave a gap between packets. If you are using ED tablets, miss out the seven inactive pills.

Precautions: Tell your doctor if you are pregnant, planning to become pregnant or are breastfeeding, or if you have any heart or circulatory condition, high blood pressure, migraine, liver problems, jaundice porphyria, gallstones, severe depression, inflammatory bowel disease (eg Crohn's disease), diabetes, varicose veins or if you smoke. You should be seen by your doctor at least once every 6 months for blood pressure and weight checks. Your doctor may decide not to prescribe the combined oral contraceptive for you if you are obese, a heavy smoker or over 35 years of age.

Side effects: Nausea, vomiting, headache, breast tenderness, changes in body weight, changes in libido and depression may occur. However, use of the pill is associated with various advantages for health – reduced menstrual bleeding, less iron-deficiency anaemia, reduction in pre-menstrual tension and painful periods, and reduced risk of endometrial and ovarian cancer and inflammatory disease of the pelvis.

Warnings: Tell your doctor at once if you experience chest pain, breathlessness, severe pain in the stomach, severe pain in the calf of one leg, severe, prolonged headache (particularly if associated with visual disturbances), fainting, weakness or numbness affecting one side or part of your body. This is because the combined contraceptive pill can cause deep-vein thrombosis. If you need to have any surgery, tell your doctor that you are taking the pill. You will need to stop the pill four weeks before any major surgery.

Interactions: The effectiveness of combined oral contraceptives may be affected by several drugs, including some antibiotics, carbamazepine, griseofulvin, phentyoin, phenobarbitone, primidone, rifabutin, rifampicin and topiramate. You will need to take additional contraceptive precautions while taking these drugs. Ask your doctor or pharmacist to advise you.

Brand names
ORDINARY (MONOPHASIC) PILLS
Brevinor (ethinyloestradiol, norethisterone)
Cilest (ethinyloestradiol, norgestimate)
Eugynon 30 (ethinyloestradiol, levonorgestrel)
Femodene (ethinyloestradiol, gestodene)
Femodene ED (ethinyloestradiol, gestodene)
Loestrin 20 (ethinyloestradiol, norethisterone)
Loestrin 30 (ethinyloestradiol, norethisterone)
Marvelon (ethinyloestradiol, desogestrel)
Mercilon (ethinyloestradiol, desogestrel)
Microgynon 30 (ethinyloestradiol, levonorgestrel)
Microgynon 30 ED (ethinyloestradiol, levonorgestrel)
Minulet (ethinyloestradiol, gestodene)
Norimin (ethinyloestradiol, norethisterone)
Norinyl-1 (mestranol, norethisterone)
Ovran (ethinyloestradiol, levonorgestrel)
Ovran 30 (ethinyloestradiol, levonorgestrel)
Ovranette (ethinyloestradiol, levonorgestrel)
Ovysmen (ethinyloestradiol, norethisterone)

PHASED PILLS
BiNovum (ethinyloestradiol, norethisterone)
Logynon (ethinyloestradiol, levonorgestrel)
Logynon ED (ethinyloestradiol, levonorgestrel)
Synphase (ethinyloestradiol, norethisterone)

Triadene (ethinyloestradiol, gestodene)
Tri-Minulet (ethinyloestradiol, gestodene)
Trinordiol (ethinyloestradiol, levonorgestrel)
TriNovum (ethinyloestradiol, norethisterone)

PROGESTOGEN-ONLY CONTRACEPTIVES

Progestogen-only contraceptives, sometimes called the 'mini-pill', contain one type of female hormone only – a progestogen. Unlike the combined oral contraceptives, they contain no oestrogen and are sometimes suitable for women in whom oestrogens are inappropriate. This may include those who have a history of thrombosis, a heart condition, high blood pressure, diabetes or migraine, as well as those who are heavy smokers or are over the age of 35. However, progestogen-only pills are not quite so effective at preventing contraception as the combined pill, and menstrual irregularities are more common. If the method fails, the risks of a tubal or ectopic pregnancy (when the fertilised egg implants in the fallopian tube rather than the womb) are greater than with the combined pill or a barrier method like a condom.

Progestogen-only contraceptives are also available in the form of an injection. In general, these are more effective than the progestogen-only pills, with a failure rate slightly less than the combined pill. There is also a progestogen-containing coil, which releases progestogen locally. This is useful in women who are either intolerant of the side effects of oral contraceptives or who require control of heavy menstrual bleeding as well as contraception.

Common progestogens in these contraceptives include ethynodiol, norethisterone, norgestrel and levonorgestrel.

How they work: Progestogen-only pills work by causing the cervix to produce a thick mucus which prevents the penetration of sperm. They also affect the lining of the womb, making it less hospitable for implantation of a fertilised egg. Unlike the combined pill, progestogen-only pills do not prevent ovulation, and this is what makes them less reliable as contraceptives.

How to use: Take exactly as prescribed and at exactly the same time every day. If you miss a pill take it as soon as you remember and carry on with the next pill at the right time. If the pill was more than 3 hours overdue, you are not protected. Continue with your pills as normal, but use an additional method of contraception (eg condoms) for the next seven days. If you have an episode of diarrhoea or vomiting, use additional contraceptive precautions during the illness and for seven days after.

Precautions: Tell your doctor if you are pregnant or planning to become pregnant, or if you have heart disease, migraine, liver disease, porphyria or inflammatory bowel conditions (eg Crohn's disease). It is safe to breastfeed with these preparations.

Side effects: Irregular bleeding is more likely with progestogen-only pills than combined pills, but is not usually heavy. Nausea, headache, dizziness, vomiting, depression, breast discomfort, weight changes, disturbance of appetite and change in libido may occur.

Warnings: None

Interactions: The effectiveness of progestogen–only pills may be affected by several drugs, including carbamazepine, griseofulvin, phenytoin, phenobarbitone, primidone, rifabutin, rifampicin and topiramate. You will need to take additional contraceptive precautions while taking these drugs. Ask your doctor or pharmacist to advise you.

Available preparations: Tablets, implant, injection, intra–uterine system

Brand names:
TABLETS
Femulen (ethynodiol)
Micronor (norethisterone)
Microval (levonorgestrel)
Neogest (norgestrel, levonorgestrel)
Norgeston (levonorgestrel)
Noriday (norethisterone)

INJECTIONS
Depo–Provera (medroxyprogesterone)
Noristerat (norethisterone)

INTRA–UTERINE SYSTEM
Mirena (levonorgestrel)

EMERGENCY CONTRACEPTION

Emergency hormonal contraception (the 'morning–after' pill) is available for use after unprotected sexual intercourse.

How to use: Take exactly as prescribed. This involves taking the first dose within 72 hours of unprotected sexual intercourse, although the method probably works better if the tablets are taken within the first 24 hours. Take two tablets followed by two more tablets after a further 12 hours. If you vomit within the first two hours of taking either dose of tablets, call your doctor immediately. You need to use a barrier method of contraception (eg a condom) until your next period.

Side effects: Nausea, headache, dizziness, breast discomfort, menstrual irregularities.

Precautions: Tell your doctor if you have migraine at the time you ask for the tablets, and if you have a history of thrombosis.

Warnings: Your next period may be early or late. Contact your doctor immediately if you have any lower abdominal pain, heavy bleeding or persistent spotting or blood–stained discharge.

Interactions: The effectiveness of these pills may be affected by several drugs, including carbamazepine, griseofulvin, phenytoin, phenobarbitone, primidone, rifabutin, rifampicin and topiramate. Tell your doctor if you are taking any other medication.

Available preparations: Tablets

Brand names: Schering PC4

HORMONE REPLACEMENT THERAPY (HRT)

Hormone replacement therapy is used to replace the female sex hormones – oestrogens and progesterone – whose levels fall dramatically at the time of the menopause. Loss of these hormones often causes several symptoms such as hot flushes, emotional instability and dryness of the hair, skin and vagina, as well as increased risk of heart disease and osteoporosis. By replacing these lost hormones, HRT may help to reduce both menopausal symptoms and the risk of heart disease and osteoporosis after the menopause.

Most HRT preparations contain a combination of an oestrogen with a progestogen. In this respect they are similar to combined oral contraceptives, but the dose of the hormones is lower. Various oestrogens are used, the most common of which are oestradiol and conjugated oestrogens. Progestogen used include norethisterone, levonorgestrel, norgestrel, medroxyprogesterone acetate and dydrogesterone.

Some HRT preparations contain oestrogens on their own without any progestogen. However, these preparations are suitable only for women who have had a hysterectomy. This is because oestrogens increase the risk of cancer of the womb (endometrial cancer). Progestogens oppose the effects of oestrogens and thus reduce the risk of endometrial cancer. Women with a uterus should therefore always use HRT that contains both types of hormones. For women who have had a hysterectomy, however, there is no risk of endometrial cancer so an oestrogen on its own can be used.

How to use: Use exactly as prescribed, following the instructions on the package carefully. If you are prescribed patches, apply them to clean, dry, unbroken areas of skin below the waistband. Do not apply them near the breasts or under the waistband. Apply to a different site each time you change the patch. If a patch falls off in the bath, wait for the skin to dry before applying a new one.

Precautions: Tell your doctor if you are pregnant, planning to become pregnant or are breastfeeding, or if you have liver disease, any history of breast disease, porphyria, uterine fibroids, endometriosis, gall bladder disease or a history of thrombosis.

Side effects: Nausea, vomiting, abdominal cramps, breast tenderness, weight changes, fluid retention, changes in libido, headache, dizziness and migraine may occur. There is an increased risk of breast cancer with HRT, but this is very small, particularly in those who use HRT for five years or less.

If you have not had a hysterectomy, you will still experience a regular monthly bleed while using most HRT preparations. Although some products are now available which avoid this, these products are not suitable until after 12 months following the last menstrual period.

Warnings: HRT does not provide contraception.

Interactions: Interactions are unlikely.

Available preparations: There are four different types of HRT preparations:

• **Tablets:** These are normally in calendar packs.

• **Skin patches:** These release the hormones slowly through the skin and generally have to be changed every three or four days, although some patches can now be left on continuously for seven days. Some packs contain patches and tablets, with the patches containing the oestrogen and the tablets the progestogen.

• **Implants:** These contain oestrogen only and are inserted under the skin where they release the hormone over a period of months. They may be used in women who have had a hysterectomy and thus do not need to take a progestogen. Women who have a uterus will need to take a progestogen as well.

• **Gel:** This contains oestrogen only and is applied to the skin, from where it is absorbed into the blood.

Brand names:
OESTROGENS ONLY
Climaval (oestradiol) – tablets
Dermestril (oestradiol) – patches
Elleste-Solo (oestradiol) – tablets
Elleste-Solo MX (oestradiol) – patches
Estraderm MX (oestradiol) – patches
Estraderm TTS (oestradiol) – patches
Evorel (oestradiol) – patches
Fematrix (oestradiol) – patches
FemSeven (oestradiol) – patches
Harmogen (oestriol) – tablets
Hormonin (oestradiol, oestriol, oestrone) – tablets
Menorest (oestradiol) – patches
Oestradiol Implants (oestradiol) – implant
Oestrogel (oestradiol) – gel
Ovestin (oestriol) – tablets
Premarin (conjugated oestrogens) – tablets
Progynova (oestradiol) – tablets
Progynova TS (oestradiol) – tablets
Sandrena (oestradiol) – gel
Zumenon (oestradiol) – tablets

OESTROGENS AND PROGESTOGENS
Climagest (oestradiol, norethisterone) – tablets
Climesse (oestradiol, norethisterone) – tablets
Cyclo-Progynova (oestradiol, levonorgestrel) – tablets
Elleste-Duet (oestradiol, norethisterone) – tablets
Estracombi (oestradiol patches, norethisterone tablets)
Estrapak 50 (oestradiol patches, norethisterone tablets)

Evorel Conti (oestradiol, norethisterone) – patches
Evorel Pak (oestradiol patches, norethisterone tablets)
Evorel Sequi (oestradiol and oestradiol/norethisterone) – patches
Femapak (oestradiol patches, dydrogesterone tablets)
Femoston (oestradiol, dydrogesterone) – tablets
Improvera (estropipate, medroxyprogesterone acetate) – tablets
Kliofem (oestradiol, norethisterone) – tablets
Kliovance (oestradiol, norethisterone) – tablets
Menophase (mestranol, norethisterone) – tablets
Nuvelle (oestradiol, levonorgestrel) – tablets
Nuvelle TS (oestradiol, oestradiol/levonorgestrel) – patches
Premique (conjugated oestrogens, medroxyprogesterone acetate) – tablets
Prempak-C (conjugated oestrogen, norgestrel) – tablets
Tridestra (oestradiol, medroxyprogesterone acetate) – tablets
Trisequens (oestradiol, norethisterone) – tablets

Tibolone

General information: Tibolone is a synthetic drug and not a hormone as such. However, it has oestrogenic and progestogenic activity. It is used for menopausal hot flushes and for prevention of osteoporosis. Most women do not have bleeds while taking this drug.

How to use: Take exactly as prescribed. If you forget a dose, take it as soon as you remember. Do not stop taking without asking your doctor.
Precautions: Tell your doctor if you are pregnant, planning to become pregnant or breastfeeding, or if you have heart disease, a history of thrombosis, liver or kidney disease, epilepsy, migraine or diabetes. This medicine is not suitable if you have had a menstrual period within the last 12 months.
Side effects: Weight changes, ankle swelling, dizziness, skin rash, headache and abdominal pain may occur.
Warnings: Tibolone is not a contraceptive.
Interactions: Tibolone interacts with few drugs. Check with your doctor or pharmacist before taking any other medicines.
Available preparations: Tablets
Brand names: Livial

Raloxifene

General information: Raloxifene is a new drug which is not itself a hormone. It binds to oestrogen receptors in the bone without stimulating oestrogen receptors in the womb or breast. It is used in the prevention of fractures in postmenopausal women at risk of osteoporosis. Its effects on blood fats are broadly beneficial.

How to use: Take exactly as prescribed. If you miss a dose, take it as soon as you remember. Do not stop taking the medicine without checking with your doctor.
Precautions: Tell your doctor if you are still having menstrual periods. This medi-

cine should not be used in women who could become pregnant. Tell your doctor if you have a history of thrombosis or liver or kidney problems.

Side effects: This is a new drug, but side effects reported so far include fluid retention and leg cramps. Tell your doctor immediately if you develop any pain in the chest or the calf of the leg, or if you have any uterine bleeding.

Warnings: None

Interactions: Raloxifene interacts with warfarin and cholestyramine.

Available preparations: Tablets

Brand names: Evista

TOPICAL HRT

Lack of oestrogen at the time of the menopause may cause vaginal dryness and soreness. Oestrogens may be applied locally in the form of creams or pessaries to the vagina to help these symptoms. They are generally prescribed on a short term basis only.

Brand names:
Estring (oestradiol) – vaginal ring
Ortho-Dienoestrol (dienoestrol) – cream
Ortho-Gynest (oestriol) – cream and pessaries
Ovestin (oestriol) – cream
Premarin (conjugated oestrogens) – cream
Tampovagan (stilboestrol) – pessaries
Vagifem (oestradiol) – vaginal tablets

PROGESTOGENS

Progestogens are one of the female sex hormones (oestrogens are the other). Medically, their most well-known uses are in oral contraceptives (see page 178) and hormone replacement therapy (see page 183). However, they are also used on their own to treat various menstrual disorders such as amenorrhoea (absence of periods), painful periods (dysmenorrhoea), pre-menstrual syndrome and endometriosis. Endometriosis is a condition in which tissue from the lining of the uterus occurs outside of the uterus (womb). This causes extremely painful periods, and bleeding outside of periods themselves.

How they work: Progestogens work in menstrual disorders by influencing the pattern of hormonal changes that is causing the problem.

How to use: Take exactly as prescribed. If you miss a dose, take as soon as you remember. Do not stop taking the medicine without checking with your doctor because it may make the underlying condition worse.

Precautions: Tell your doctor if you are pregnant, planning to become pregnant or are breastfeeding, or if you have or have had liver, kidney, heart or circulatory disease or porphyria.

Side effects: Acne, itchy skin, fluid retention, weight changes, breast discomfort, irregular menstruation, changes in sexual function and mood changes may occur.

Warnings: None

Interactions: Several medicines reduce the effectiveness of these drugs. Check with your doctor or pharmacist before taking any other medicines.

Dydrogesterone

Available preparations: Tablets
Brand names: Duphaston; Duphaston HRT (this product is used in combination with oestrogens for HRT)

Hydroxyprogesterone

Available preparations: Injection
Brand names: Proluton Depot (this product is used for habitual miscarriage only)

Medroxyprogesterone

Available preparations: Tablets
Brand names: Provera

Norethisterone

Available preparations: Tablets
Brand names: Primulot N, Utovlan, Micronor HRT (this product is used in combination with oestrogens for HRT)

Progesterone

Available preparations: Vaginal gel, pessaries, injection
Brand names:
Crinone gel: This product is used in combination with oestrogens for HRT and also in some cases of infertility treatment
Cyclogest pessaries: This product is used for pre-menstrual syndrome and post-natal depression
Gestone: This product is used for abnormal uterine bleeding and habitual abortion

TOPICAL PREPARATIONS FOR VAGINAL INFECTIONS

Creams and pessaries containing various anti-infective drugs are used to treat vaginal and vulval infections. Most of them contain an anti-fungal drug (eg clotrimazole, econazole, miconazole, nystatin) because the most common vaginal infection is fungal, ie thrush. Some of these products are available over the counter and a tablet containing fluconazole (brand name: Diflucan – see page 265) is also available over the counter for the treatment of thrush. Other ingredients (eg povidone-iodine, clindamycin, metronidazole) are used to treat non-specific or mixed bacterial infections or a protozoal infection called trichomonas vaginitis.

Warning: Some of these products may damage condoms and diaphragms. Contraceptive protection may be reduced.

Brand names (with ingredients in brackets):
Aci-Jel – vaginal jelly (acetic acid)
Betadine – vaginal cleansing kit, vaginal gel, pessaries (povidone–iodine)
Canesten – cream, vaginal cream, pessaries, combination pack containing pessaries and cream (clotrimazole)
Dalacin – cream (clindamycin)
Ecostatin – cream, pessaries, twin pack containing pessaries and cream (ecostatin)
Femeron – cream, pessary (miconazole)
Gyno-Daktarin – intravaginal cream, pessaries, combination pack containing pessaries and cream, vaginal capsule (miconazole)
Gyno-Pevaryl – cream, pessaries, combination packs containing pessaries and cream (econazole)
Lomexin – pessaries (fenticonazole)
Masnoderm – cream (clotrimazole)
Nizoral – cream (ketoconazole)
Nystan – gel, vaginal cream, pessaries (nystatin)
Pevaryl – cream (econazole)
Sultrin – cream (sulphathiazole)
Travogyn – vaginal tablets (isoconazole)
Zidoval – vaginal gel (metronidazole)

MALE SEX HORMONES

The main male sex hormone is testosterone. Medically, male sex hormones (testosterone and the synthetic drug mesterolone) are used in men with sex hormone deficiency. However, this is a fairly rare condition. These drugs will restore secondary sexual characteristics such as the need to shave or libido, but they do not restore fertility (ie sperm production) – in fact they tend to depress it.

How to use: Take exactly as prescribed. If you miss a dose, take as soon as you remember. Do not stop taking the medicine without checking with your doctor because it may make the underlying condition worse.

Precautions: Tell your doctor if you have had any type of cancer, liver, heart or kidney disease, epilepsy or migraine.

Side effects: Headache, depression, nausea, jaundice, prostate abnormalities and a range of changes in libido may occur.

Warnings: None

Interactions: Male sex hormones interact with few drugs. Check with your doctor or pharmacist before taking any other medicines.

Mesterolone

Available preparations: Tablets
Brand names: Pro-Viron

Testosterone

Available preparations: Capsules, skin patch, implant, injection
Brand names: Andropatch, Primosten Depot, Restandol, Sustanon, Virormone.

ANTAGONISTS OF MALE SEX HORMONES

Cyproterone acetate

General information: Cyproterone acetate inhibits the production of sperm and is used in severe hypersexuality and sexual deviation in men. Fully informed consent is recommended before this drug is prescribed for this purpose. Cyproterone is also prescribed for prostate cancer. In women, it is used to overcome relatively high levels of androgens in conditions such as polycystic ovaries, hirsutism (excessive facial and body hair) or severe acne. In these cases it is combined with ethinyloestradiol and is another form of oral contraceptive.

How to use: Take exactly as prescribed.
Precautions: Tell your doctor if you have liver disease, diabetes, sickle cell anaemia, severe depression or a history of thrombosis. Note: these precautions do not apply if you are being treated for prostate cancer.
Side effects: Tiredness, weight changes, less oily skin, breast swelling, change in hair growth. There are also some adverse effects on blood fats. **Interactions:** None reported.
Warnings: None
Interactions: None reported
Available preparations: Tablets
Brand names: Androcur, Cyprostat, Dianette (the brand name for the preparation containing cyproterone acetate and ethinyloestradiol, suitable for use in women)

Finasteride

General information: Finasteride inhibits an enzyme in the body responsible for producing a very active form of testosterone. It leads to a reduction in prostate size and improves urinary flow rate. It is used in men with an enlarged prostate gland (benign hypertrophic hyperplasia: BPH).

How to use: Take exactly as prescribed. If you miss a dose, take it as soon as you remember. Do not stop taking the medicine without checking with your doctor.
Precautions: Your doctor may wish to do a blood test before starting finasteride. The blood test is to measure prostate specific antigen (PSA) which is raised in prostate cancer.
Side effects: Impotence, decreased sexual function, breast tenderness and enlargement, allergic reactions (eg lip swelling and rash)

Warnings: Use condoms as the drug is secreted in the semen, particularly if your partner is pregnant.
Interactions: None
Available preparations: Tablets
Brand names: Proscar

MISCELLANEOUS DRUGS FOR DISORDERS OF THE REPRODUCTIVE SYSTEM

Bromocriptine

General information: Bromocriptine is used in some types of female infertility, benign breast pain, some menstrual disorders and tumours of the pituitary gland. It can also be used to suppress lactation in women who do not want to breast feed, although it is rarely used for this purpose nowadays. It is also used in Parkinson's disease (see page 54).

How it works: Bromocriptine inhibits the secretion of the hormone prolactin from the pituitary gland by binding directly to inhibitory dopamine receptors in the gland. Some reproductive disorders are associated with high prolactin production and bromocriptine can be helpful in these conditions. Its direct action on dopamine receptors accounts for its beneficial action in Parkinson's disease.
How to use: Take exactly as prescribed. If you miss a dose, take it as soon as you remember. Do not stop taking the medicine without asking your doctor.
Precautions: Tell your doctor if you are pregnant or planning to become pregnant, or if you have heart or circulatory problems, a stomach ulcer, or a history of severe mental illness.
Side effects: Nausea, vomiting, constipation and other gastrointestinal disturbances, headache, dizziness and drowsiness may occur.
Warnings: Avoid excessive alcohol because it may increase the adverse effects of this medicine. Take care with driving and other similar activities until you know how this drug affects you.
Interactions: Domperidone, metoclopramide and antipsychotic drugs may reduce the effects of bromocriptine. Medicines containing sympathomimetics also interact with bromocriptine. Several over-the-counter medicines (eg remedies for coughs, colds and flu, including nose drops) contain sympathomimetics, so always check with your pharmacist or doctor before taking any other medication.
Available preparations: Tablets, capsules
Brand names: Parlodel

Buserelin

General information: Buserelin is a similar substance to the hormone gonadorelin, which is produced by the hypothalamus. Although single doses of this drug stimulate FSH and LH production, continuous use of buserelin results in reduced secretion of FSH and LH, and consequently reduced secretion of the sex hormones by the ovaries and testes. In women, it is used to treat endometriosis (a painful condition in which uterine tissue occurs outside the uterus), to shrink fibroids before surgery and may also be given to prepare the ovaries prior to *in vitro* fertilisation. In men, it is used to treat prostate cancer, when it is combined with cyproterone (an anti-androgen) to overcome the initial stimulation phase.

How to use: Use exactly as prescribed.
Precautions: Tell your doctor if you are pregnant, planning to become pregnant or are breastfeeding (although this is very unlikely to be the case if you have a condition for which this drug is used).
Side effects: In women, there may be menopausal-like symptoms (eg hot flushes, increasing sweating, vaginal dryness), breakthrough bleeding, breast tenderness and breast milk production. In men and women there may be nausea, vomiting, diarrhoea, constipation, anxiety, concentration and memory disturbances, dizziness, drowsiness, palpitations, dry skin, back and limb pain.
Warnings: Women should make sure that they do not become pregnant while using this drug. Use a non-hormonal method of contraception.
Interactions: Avoid the use of nasal decongestants before and for at least 30 minutes after treatment with this drug.
Available preparations: Nasal spray, injection
Brand names: Suprecur

Cabergoline

General information: Cabergoline is a similar drug to bromocriptine (see above).

Available preparations: Tablets
Brand names: Dostinex

Chorionic gonadotrophin

General information: Chorionic gonadotrophin is a hormone which is secreted by the placenta. It stimulates the ovaries and testes to produce sex hormones. It is obtained from the urine of pregnant women and used to treat infertility in women and occasionally to treat male sex hormone deficiencies.

Precautions: Tell your doctor if you have heart or kidney problems, asthma, epilepsy or migraine.
Side effects: Headache, tiredness and mood changes may occur. Breast swelling and fluid retention may occur in men.
Available preparations: Injection
Brand names: Choragon, Pregnyl, Profasi

Clomiphene

General information: Clomiphene is used in the treatment of female infertility. It stimulates ovulation by increasing the secretion of hormones from the pituitary gland.

How to use: Take exactly as prescribed. If you miss a dose take as soon as you remember. Stopping the drug will reduce your chances of conception.
Precautions: Tell your doctor if you have liver problems.
Side effects: Hot flushes, abdominal discomfort, breast tenderness, headache, insomnia, dizziness and rashes may occur. Tell your doctor immediately if you experience any visual disturbances. There is a risk of ovarian hyperstimulation with this drug, which can lead to multiple births and ectopic pregnancies.
Interactions: None reported
Warnings: This drug should not be used for longer than six menstrual cycles.
Available preparations: Tablets
Brand names: Clomid, Serophene

Danazol

General information: Danazol is a synthetic steroid hormone that inhibits certain pituitary hormones. It has a range of effects on sex hormone production and is used in the treatment of endometriosis (a painful condition in which uterine tissue occurs outside the uterus), menstrual disorders such as menorrhagia, breast tenderness (in women) and breast swelling (in men).

How to use: Take exactly as prescribed. If you miss a dose take it as soon as you remember. Do not stop taking the medicine without checking with your doctor.
Precautions: Tell your doctor if you are pregnant, planning to become pregnant or are breastfeeding, or if you have liver, heart or kidney problems or porphyria.
Side effects: Nausea, dizziness, skin reactions, acne, mood changes, weight changes, menstrual irregularities and a range of other side effects.
Warnings: None
Interactions: Danazol interacts with anticoagulants, anticonvulsants and cyclosporin.
Available preparations: Capsules
Brand names: Danol

Follitropin

General information: Follitropin is a follicle-stimulating hormone produced by the pituitary gland which stimulates the ovaries and testes to produce sex hormones. It is used to treat infertility in women and occasionally to treat male sex hormone deficiencies. This drug is used under specialist supervision only.

Warnings: If used for infertility, it can result in multiple pregnancies.
Available preparations: Injection
Brand names: Puregon

Gestrinone

General information: Gestrinone is similar to danazol and is used in endometriosis.

Precautions: Tell your doctor if you are pregnant or breastfeeding, or have heart, kidney or liver disease.
Side effects: Acne, fluid retention, unusual hair growth, voice changes.
Available preparations: Capsules
Brand names: Dimetriose

Gonadorelin

General information: Gonadorelin is a synthetic version of gonadotrophin-releasing hormone, a hypothalamic hormone, which acts on the pituitary gland to release various other hormones (eg FSH, LH). As a drug it is used in infertility.

Side effects: Side effects are rare, but nausea, headache, abdominal pain, increased menstrual bleeding and allergic reactions may occur.
Available preparations: Injection
Brand names: Fertiral

Goserelin

General information: Goserelin is similar to buserelin (see page 190). It is used in endometriosis, and in prostate and breast cancer.

Available preparations: Implant
Brand names: Zoladex

Human menopausal gonadotrophins

General information: Human menopausal gonadotrophins are extracted from the urine of postmenopausal women. They contain the hormones follicle-stimulating hormone and luteinising hormone, which stimulate the ovaries and testes to secrete sex hormones. It is used as a drug to treat female infertility.

Warnings: This drug can result in multiple pregnancies.
Available preparations: Injection
Brand names: Humegon, Menogon, Normegon, Pergonal.

Leuprorelin

General information: Leuprorelin is similar to buserelin (see page 190). It is used in endometriosis and in prostate cancer.

Available preparations: Injection
Brand names: Prostap

Nafarelin

General information: Nafarelin is similar to buserelin (see page 190). It is used in endometriosis and to prepare the ovaries before *in vitro* fertilisation.

Available preparations: Nasal spray
Brand names: Synarel

Quinagolide

General information: Quinagolide is a newly introduced drug and is similar to bromocriptine (see page 190).

Available preparations: Tablets
Brand names: Dostinex

Triptorelin

General information: Triptorelin is similar to buserelin (see page 190). It is used in endometriosis and in prostate cancer.

Available preparations: Injection
Brand names: De-capeptyl

Urofollitrophin

General information: Urofollitrophin is extracted from the urine of postmenopausal women. It contains the hormone follicle-stimulating hormone which stimulates the ovaries and the testes to secrete sex hormones. It is used in female infertility.

Warnings: This drug may result in multiple pregnancies.
Available preparations: Injection
Brand names: Metrodin High Purity, Orgafol

DRUGS FOR IMPOTENCE

Alprostadil

General information: Alprostadil is a prostaglandin. It is used to treat erectile dysfunction in men.

How to use: This drug is given by injection into the penis. The first dose will be given by a medically trained person. S/he will then train you to use the injection yourself.
Precautions: Tell your doctor if you have ever had a tendency to prolonged erection. This can occur in conditions such as leukaemia, other forms of cancer and sickle cell anaemia.

Side effects: Pain may be felt in the penis, and local reactions such as rash, swelling, haemorrhage and inflammation may occur at the injection site.
Warnings: Tell your doctor if you have an erection lasting 4 hours or longer.
MUSE only (see brand names below): Use condoms if your partner is pregnant.
Interactions: None
Available preparations: Injection, urethral application
Brand names: Injections: Caverject, Viridal; Topical: MUSE is a pellet of alprostadil (urethral application) placed in the urethra. It produces an erection in about 5 minutes.

Sildenafil

How to use: Sildenafil is taken in tablet form and the prescribed dose should be taken one hour before sexual activity.
Precautions: Tell your doctor if you have any serious heart condition, particularly angina, low blood pressure, peptic ulcer or liver disorder.
Side effects: Headache, flushing, dizziness, indigestion, nasal congestion and visual changes (eg blurred vision, change in colour and light perception) may occur.
Warnings: None
Interactions: Some antibiotics and cimetidine may interact with sildenafil. This drug must not be taken by anyone on nitrates. Check with your doctor or pharmacist before taking any other medicine.
Available preparations: Tablets
Brand names: Viagra

Thymoxamine

How to use: This drug is given by injection into the penis. The first dose will be given by a medically trained person. S/he will then train you to use the injection yourself.
Precautions: Tell your doctor if you have ever had a tendency to prolonged erection. This can occur in conditions such as leukaemia, other forms of cancer and sickle cell anaemia. Tell your doctor if you have a heart condition or low blood pressure.
Side effects: Pain may be felt in the penis, and local reactions such as haemorrhage may occur at the injection site. Tiredness, drowsiness, nausea, dizziness, headache, flushing, dry mouth, sinus congestion and runny nose may occur.
Warnings: Tell your doctor immediately if you have an erection lasting three hours or longer.
Interactions: None reported
Available preparations: Injection
Brand names: Erecnos

The Urinary System

THE MAIN FUNCTION of the urinary system is to remove waste products from the blood and eliminate them in the urine. Blood flows from the general circulation into the kidneys. The kidneys filter metabolic waste products and produce the liquid known as urine. Normally, a person has two kidneys. Each kidney has a tube, called a ureter, which drains urine from the kidney into the bladder. The bladder, which is expandable, gradually increases in size to accommodate the increasing volume of urine. When the bladder is full, nerve signals are sent to the brain conveying the need to urinate. From the bladder urine passes through the urethra, which leaves the body either through the penis in males or the vulva in females.

What can go wrong

Apart from infection, the most common urinary problems are due to poor bladder function. Urine can be released involuntarily (urinary incontinence) and with increased frequency (urgency) or it may be retained in the bladder (urinary retention). Prostate problems, particularly an enlarged prostate gland, commonly cause difficulties in passing urine in older men.

Infection can occur anywhere in the urinary tract, but most commonly in the bladder (cystitis). Women are more prone to this than men because the distance from the urethra to the bladder is shorter in women, making it easier for infection to get to the bladder.

Common conditions and drugs used to treat them

Infections – antibiotics (see page 246)

Benign prostatic hyperplasia (BPH) – alpha-blockers (eg doxazosin, prazosin)

Urinary retention – parasympathomimetics (eg bethanecol)

Urinary incontinence – flavoxate, oxybutinin

ALPHA-BLOCKERS

Drugs such as doxazosin and prazosin belong to the group of drugs known as alpha-blockers. Some of these drugs are used in the treatment of high blood pressure (see page 90). However, they are also used in benign prostatic hyperplasia (BPH). They work by relaxing the muscle in the tubes in the urinary tract, which helps to improve the flow of urine and reduce any symptoms of obstruction.

Use, precautions, side effects, warnings, interactions: As alpha-blockers (see page 90). Dizziness, due to the drop in blood pressure, is a particularly common side-effect, and patients already on blood pressure tablets may need a reduction in dosage. It is best to take the first dose of any of these drugs at bedtime and to lie down in case dizziness develops.

This section contains a list of alpha-blockers used in BPH.

Alfuzosin

Available preparations: Tablets, modified-release tablets
Brand names: Xatral, Xatral SR

Doxazosin

Available preparations: Tablets
Brand names: Cardura

Indoramin

Available preparations: Tablets
Brand names: Doralese

Prazosin

Available preparations: Tablets
Brand names: Hypovase

Tamsulosin

Available preparations: Capsules
Brand names: Flomax MR

Terazosin

Available preparations: Tablets
Brand names: Hytrin BPH

PARASYMPATHOMIMETICS

Bethanecol, carbachol and distigmine belong to the group of drugs known as parasympathomimetics. These drugs are licensed to treat urinary retention, particularly after surgery, although they are now used much less frequently than they were 20 years ago. They work by increasing the contraction of the muscle in the urinary tract and help to improve the flow of urine.

How to use: Take exactly as prescribed. If you miss a dose, take it as soon as you remember. Do not stop the drug without checking with your doctor.

Precautions: Tell your doctor if you are pregnant, planning to become pregnant or are breastfeeding, or if you have any obstruction in the gastrointestinal tract, asthma, a heart or thyroid condition, epilepsy, Parkinson's disease or a peptic ulcer.

Side effects: Nausea, sweating, vomiting, blurred vision and slow heart rate may occur, particularly in elderly people.

Warnings: None

Interactions: These drugs interact with a number of other drugs, including beta-blockers and anti-arrhythmics. Check with your doctor or pharmacist before taking any other medication.

Bethanecol

Available preparations: Tablets
Brand names: Myotonine

Carbachol

Available preparations: Tablets, injection
Brand names: None

Distigmine

Available preparations: Tablets
Brand names: Ubretid

DRUGS FOR URINARY INCONTINENCE

Urinary urgency and frequency in adults can be treated with several drugs. They all have an antispasmodic action and work basically by improving the capacity of the bladder to hold urine. In addition to the drugs listed below, propantheline (see page 117) is also used occasionally for this condition. The tricyclic antidepressants (see page 32) are also used in low doses for night-time frequency, particularly in children.

How to use: Take exactly as prescribed. If you miss a dose, take it as soon as you remember. Do not stop taking the medicine without checking with your doctor.

Precautions: Tell your doctor if you are pregnant, planning to become pregnant or are breastfeeding, or if you have glaucoma, any type of gastrointestinal disease, liver or kidney disease, heart disease or an overactive thyroid gland.

Side effects: These drugs may cause dry mouth, blurred vision, nausea, constipation and facial flushing.

Warnings: Alcohol is not a problem. Take care with driving and other similar activities until you know how you react to the medicine.

Interactions: Several other drugs may interact with these to increase the risk of adverse effects. Check with your doctor or pharmacist before taking any other medication.

Flavoxate

Available preparations: Tablets
Brand names: Urispas 200

Oxybutinin

Available preparations: Tablets, liquid
Brand names: Cystrin, Ditropan

Propiverine

Available preparations: Tablets
Brand names: Detrunorm

Tolterodine

Available preparations: Tablets
Brand names: Detrusitol

The Skin

THE SKIN IS THE BODY'S largest organ. It forms a waterproof and flexible covering around the body tissue and protects the delicate internal organs. However, the skin is also an active organ system which regulates body temperature, senses various stimuli – both pleasant and painful – and provides a shield from the harmful effects of the sun, as well as acting as a barrier to infection.

There are two layers within the skin – the epidermis and dermis – and both of these perform specific tasks. The top layer, the epidermis, is very thin – actually thinner over most of the body than clingfilm. The surface of the epidermis contains keratin, formed from the remains of dead cells that are constantly shed to dislodge bacteria and other micro-organisms. At the bottom of the epidermis are the melanocytes, the cells that produce the skin's pigment, melanin, and also a layer of cells that divides and replenishes the cells which are lost.

Below the epidermis lies the dermis, which acts as the skin's support layer. It contains pain and touch receptors and many of the other important structures of the skin. When body temperature rises, the nerves cause the blood vessels in the skin to widen, allowing blood to flow to the surface of the skin from where heat is lost. Sweat glands produce sweat which evaporates from the skin and helps the cooling process. Other structures in the skin include the sebaceous glands, which produce oil to help keep the skin moist and protected against bacteria. At the base of the hair follicle is a tiny muscle. This contracts during periods of heat loss or emotional arousal, causing the hair to stand on end and goose pimples to appear.

Below the dermis lies a layer of fat, the third layer of the skin. This helps to insulate the body from heat and cold.

What can go wrong

Anything that goes wrong with the skin's function or appearance can have important consequences for physical and mental health. The skin tends to change considerably throughout a person's lifetime. Thinning and wrinkling of the skin, for example, are a natural consequence of age, but can be accelerated by exposure to sunlight. Damaged skin tends to heal more slowly in older than in young people.

Dermatitis (eczema) is one of the most common skin conditions. Characterised by red, itchy, scaly skin, it can be caused by irritants such as detergents and chemicals, and is common in nurses, hairdressers or anyone who spends a lot of time with his or her hands in detergent. There are several different types. Contact eczema occurs when people develop an allergic reaction to a chemical, often after repeated exposure, for example to substances in cosmetics or to nickel in jewellery and buckles. Atopic eczema is common in babies and children, often starting in the first year of life. It often occurs with asthma and hayfever, particularly if there is a family history of these conditions. The skin is sensitive to irritants and sometimes woollen clothes. Infection may aggravate the condition and diet is sometimes a trigger. Another form of dermatitis is seborrhoeic dermatitis – an itching, scaly condition caused by a reaction to a common yeast which occurs on the face or the scalp. On the scalp, seborrhoeic dermatitis is known more commonly as dandruff (in adults) or cradle cap (in children).

Psoriasis is a skin condition in which thickening of the epidermis takes place. Featuring patches of salmon pink dry skin covered by silvery scales, psoriasis is caused by rapid cell turnover in the epidermis, leaving heaps of dead skin on the surface. It can start at any age, but commonly begins in the late teens and early 20s. The scalp, knees, elbows and knuckles are the areas most often affected, and itching is a common symptom.

Acne is a common skin complaint, especially in adolescents, and it tends to occur more in boys than girls. Because of the hormonal changes in the teenage years, the oil-producing sebaceous glands often become very active. They produce large amounts of sebum which can block the sebaceous glands, leading to blackheads. The blackheads may rupture, with a resulting release of sebum into the dermis, where it is acted on by bacteria in the skin, creating consequent inflammation and pustules.

Like any other part of the body, the skin can become infected with bacteria, fungi and viruses. Impetigo is a common bacterial infection of the skin, while frequently encountered fungal infections include athlete's foot and ringworm. Cold sores and shingles are among the most common viral infections. Warts and veruccas, caused by various types of wart virus, are also infections of the skin. The skin can also be affected by parasitic insects such as lice and mites, including the itch mite which causes scabies.

Common conditions and medicines used to treat them

Dermatitis (eczema) – moisturising and barrier creams, corticosteroids, tar preparations, evening primrose oil (gamolenic acid)

Psoriasis – creams and ointments containing coal tar, salicylic acid, dithranol or calcipotriol (a vitamin D derivative). Severe cases may require oral treatment with acitrecin (a vitamin A derivative) or the immunosuppressants cyclosporin or methotrexate

Acne – creams and ointments, oral antibiotics, hormones or retinoids (vitamin A derivatives)

Warts, veruccas and calluses – various paints and ointments containing ingredients such as salicylic acid, podophyllum, formaldehyde or glutaraldehyde

Skin infections – topical or oral antimicrobials

Lice and scabies – lotions and shampoos containing various ingredients such as malathion, permethrin or phenothrin

EMOLLIENTS (MOISTURISERS)

Emollients are used to soothe, smooth and moisturise the skin. Consisting of a mixture of waxes, paraffins and other moisturisers, they work either by preventing water loss from the skin or by improving the binding of water to it. The effects last only a short time, and emollients need to be applied very frequently even after the condition has improved. Emollients are used in the treatment of all dry skin conditions and eczema, and to some extent in psoriasis. They are available in the form of creams which are light, non greasy and able to disappear into the skin when applied; more greasy preparations are also available for dry skin conditions. Emollients can be added to the bath or used in the shower, and are especially useful for atopic eczema. Some may also be used as soap substitutes. The particular emollient prescribed will depend on the severity and site of the condition being treated and, to some extent, on the individual's preference.

Some emollients contain ingredients which may occasionally cause sensitisation. Tell your doctor immediately if your skin condition gets worse or you develop a rash.

This section contains a list of emollient preparations with their main ingredients. Use them exactly as prescribed.

NON-BRANDED PREPARATIONS

Aqueous cream: contains wax, white soft paraffin and liquid paraffin in a light, non-greasy cream formulation, often used as a soap substitute

Emulsifying ointment: contains wax, white soft paraffin and liquid paraffin in a greasy formulation

Hydrous ointment: contains wool alcohols and various paraffins in a greasy formulation

White soft paraffin (white petroleum jelly) and yellow soft paraffin (yellow petroleum jelly); both often used as diluents in ointments containing active ingredients

Zinc cream: contains zinc oxide and peanut oil in a cream formulation

Zinc ointment: contains zinc oxide with various fats and paraffins in a greasy ointment formulation

Zinc and castor oil ointment: contains zinc oxide, castor oil, peanut oil and beeswax in a greasy ointment formulation

BRANDED PRODUCTS

Alcoderm: A cream containing liquid paraffin and other emollient ingredients; additives include hydroxybenzoates (parabens) and isopropyl palmitate

Alpha Keri Bath: A bath oil containing liquid paraffin and lanolin

Aquadrate: A cream containing urea (a hydrating agent that binds water in the skin)

Aveeno: Available as a cream, bath oil or bath additive, containing oatmeal in an emollient base

Balneum: A bath oil containing soya oil

Balneum Plus: A cream containing urea (a hydrating agent that binds water in the skin); also available as a bath additive containing soya oil with other emollients

Calmurid: A cream containing urea (a hydrating agent – binds water to the skin)

Dermamist: A spray containing white soft paraffin and other emollient ingredients

Dermol 500: A lotion containing liquid paraffin with antiseptics

Diprobase: Available as a cream or ointment containing liquid paraffin and other emollients

Diprobath: A bath additive containing liquid paraffin in an oily liquid

E45: A cream containing various paraffins and hypoallergenic lanolin; also available as a wash cream containing zinc oxide in an emollient base, and as a bath oil containing cetyl dimethicone in an emollient base.

Emmolate: A bath oil containing wool alcohols and liquid paraffin

Emulsiderm: A bath additive containing liquid paraffin in an oily liquid with benzalkonium

Epaderm: A cream containing various paraffins and wax

Eucerin: A cream containing urea (a hydrating agent – binds water to the skin)

Hewletts Cream: A cream containing zinc oxide, peanut oil and lanolin in an emollient base

Humiderm: A cream containing pyrrolidone carboxylic acid in an emollient base

Hydromol: A cream containing various paraffins and peanut oil; also available as a bath additive containing liquid paraffin in an oily liquid

Kamillosan: An ointment containing chamomile extracts in an emollient base

Keri: A lotion containing various oils

LactiCare: A lotion containing lactic acid and pyrrolidine carboxylic acid

Lipobase: A cream containing various fats

Morhulin: An ointment containing cod liver oil and zinc oxide in an emollient base

Neutrogena Dermatological Cream: A cream containing glycerol in an emollient base

Nutraplus: A cream containing urea (a hydrating agent that binds water to the skin)

Oilatum: Available as a cream, bath additive and shower gel, containing various oils and paraffins

Oilatum Plus: A bath additive containing light liquid paraffin, benzalkonium and triclosan

Sudocrem: A cream containing zinc oxide, benzyl alcohol, benzyl benzoate, and lanolin

Ultrabase: A cream containing various paraffins

Unguentum Merck: A cream containing various paraffins

Vaseline Dermacare: Available as a cream or lotion containing dimethicone with various paraffins in an emollient base; the lotion contains lanolin

BARRIER PREPARATIONS

Barrier preparations are used for napkin rash, urinary rash and various pressure sores, including bed sores. They contain substances that repel water such as dimethicone.

Brand names:

Conotrane: A barrier cream containing dimethicone

Drapolone: A barrier cream containing various fats and paraffins with an antiseptic

Metanium: A barrier cream containing titanium salts with dimethicone and paraffin

Siopel: A barrier cream containing dimethicone, an antiseptic and peanut oil

Sprilon: A barrier preparation in spray form containing dimethicone, zinc oxide with various fats and paraffins

Vasogen: A barrier cream containing dimethicone, calamine and zinc oxide

ANTI-ITCH PREPARATIONS

Itching skin (pruritus) may be caused by sensitivity to drugs or to internal disease or skin disease (eg eczema). Adequate treatment of eczema with emollients and steroids often helps the irritation. Probably the two most widely prescribed types of preparation for itching are those containing calamine (eg calamine cream and calamine lotion) or crotamiton (see below). Crotamiton cream is often used after treatment of scabies.

A wide range of creams and ointments containing local anaesthetics (to numb pain and itching) and antihistamines (to soothe itching) is available over the counter, but these products are very rarely prescribed. They should not be used to treat eczema and never applied for longer than 3 days. They are generally best avoided in young children.

Brand names:

Eurax: A cream containing crotamiton; also available as a lotion

TOPICAL CORTICOSTEROIDS

Corticosteroids are used topically in the form of creams and ointments for inflammatory skin conditions, such as eczema and other allergic rashes, nappy rash and psoriasis. Creams are generally best for moist lesions and ointments for dry, thickened lesions; both forms work by preventing the production of inflammatory chemicals in the skin.

Steroids come in various potencies including mild (eg hydrocortisone), moderate (eg clobetasone), potent (eg betamethasone) and very potent (eg clobetasol). They may be combined with antimicrobial ingredients to treat infected eczema, or with urea or salicylic acid to increase the penetration of corticosteroid to the skin.

How to use: Use exactly as prescribed. (Be particularly careful with children.) This usually involves applying the preparation sparingly once or twice a day. Do not apply in large amounts or more frequently than prescribed. The stronger the steroid, the more care is required. As a guide, the following quantities are suitable for an adult for twice daily application for one week: face and neck, or the scalp, or both hands, or the groin and genitals – 15 to 30g; both arms – 30 to 60g; both legs or the trunk – 100g.

Side effects: The risk of side effects depends on the strength of the steroid and the length of time for which it is used. Steroids are potent drugs and can be absorbed through the skin (particularly from the face, genitals and raw areas); they should always be applied sparingly. Local side effects on the skin include: thinning of the skin (which is to some extent reversible), increased hair growth, acne, mild loss of skin pigment, inflammatory rash on the face or near the mouth, stretch marks and exacerbation of any untreated skin infection.

Warnings: Do not use these preparations in acne, scabies or leg ulcers. If you develop a skin infection, check with your doctor before continuing to use the preparation. Do not use on the face without consulting a doctor. In general, potent and very potent steroids are not suitable for use on babies under the age of one year.

Aclometasone (a moderately potent corticosteroid)

Available preparations: Cream, ointment
Brand names: Modrasone

Beclomethasone (a potent corticosteroid)

Available preparations: Cream, ointment
Brand names: Propaderm

Betamethasone (a moderately potent to potent corticosteroid)

Available preparations: Cream, ointment, lotion, scalp application
Brand names: Betacap, Betnovate, Betnovate RD, Bettamousse, Diprosone
Combination preparations: Betnovate C (betamethasone with the antimicrobial,

clioquinol); Betnovate N (betamethasone with the antibiotic, neomycin); Diprosalic (betamethasone with salicyclic acid); Fucibet (betamethasone with the antibiotic, fusidic acid); Lotriderm (betamethasone with the antifungal clotrimazole)

Clobetasol (a very potent corticosteroid)

Available preparations: Cream, ointment, scalp application
Brand names: Dermovate
Combination preparations: Dermovate NN (clobetasol with the antimicrobials, nystatin and neomycin)

Clobetasone (a moderately potent corticosteroid)

Available preparations: Cream, ointment
Brand names: Eumovate
Combination preparations: Trimovate (clobetasone with the antimicrobials, oxytetracycline and nystatin)

Desoxymethasone (a moderately potent corticosteroid)

Available preparations: Cream, lotion
Brand names: Stiedex

Diflucortolone (a potent corticosteroid)

Available preparations: Cream, oily cream, ointment
Brand names: Nerisone, Nerisone Forte

Fluocinolone (a potent corticosteroid)

Available preparations: Cream, gel, ointment
Brand names: Synalar, Synalar 1 in 4 Dilution, Synalar 1 in 10 Dilution
Combination preparations: Synalar C (fluocinolone with the antimicrobial, clioquinol); Synalar N (fluocinolone with the antibiotic, neomycin)

Fluocinonide (a potent corticosteroid)

Available preparations: Cream, ointment, scalp application
Brand names: Metosyn

Fluocortolone (a moderately potent corticosteroid)

Available preparations: Cream, ointment
Brand names: Ultralanum Plain

Flurandrenolone (a moderately potent corticosteroid)

Available preparations: Cream, ointment, tape
Brand names: Haelan

Fluticasone (a potent corticosteroid)

Available preparations: Cream, ointment
Brand names: Cutivate

Halcinonide (a very potent corticosteroid)

Available preparations: Cream
Brand names: Halciderm Topical

Hydrocortisone (a mild corticosteroid)

Available preparations: creams, gels and ointments
Brand names: Cobadex, Dioderm, Efcortelan, Hydrocortisyl, Mildison.
Combination preparations: Alphaderm (hydrocortisone and the moisturising ingredient, urea); Alphosyl HC (hydrocortisone with coal tar); Calmurid HC (hydrocortisone, lactic acid and urea, a moisturising ingredient); Canesten HC (hydrocortisone with the antifungal clotrimazole); Daktacort (hydrocortisone with the antifungal miconazole); Econacort (hydrocortisone with the antifungal econazole); Eurax Hydrocortisone (hydrocortisone with the anti-itch ingredient, crotamiton); Fucidin H (hydrocortisone with the antibiotic, fusidic acid); Gregoderm (hydrocortisone with the antimicrobials, neomycin, nystatin and polymixin B); Nystaform HC (hydrocortisone with the antifungal nystatin and the antimicrobial chlorhexidine); Quinocort (hydrocortisone with the antimicrobial, potassium hydroxyquinoline sulphate); Tarcortin (hydrocortisone with coal tar); Terra-Cortril (hydrocortisone with the antibiotic oxytetracycline); Terra-Cortril Nystatin (hydrocortisone with the antifungal nystatin and the antibiotic oxytetracycline); Timodine (hydrocortisone with dimethicone and the antimicrobial, benzalkonium chloride); Vioform Hydrocortisone (hydrocortisone with the antimicrobial clioquinol)

Hydrocortisone butyrate (a potent corticosteroid)

Available preparations: Cream, ointment, scalp lotion
Brand names: Locoid, Locoid Crelo
Combination preparations: Locoid C (hydrocortisone butyrate with the antimicrobial chlorquinaldol)

Mometasone (a potent corticosteroid)

Available preparations: Cream, ointment, scalp application
Brand names: Elocon

Triamcinolone (a potent corticosteroid)

Available preparations: Cream, ointment
Brand names: Adcortyl
Combination preparations: Adcortyl with Graneodin (triamcinolone with the antibiotics, gramicidin and neomycin); Aureocort (triamcinolone with the antibiotic, chlortetracycline); Nystadermal (triamcinolone with the antifungal, nystatin); Pevaryl TC (triamcinolone with the antifungal, econazole); Tri-Adcortyl (triamcinolone with the antimicrobials, gramicidin, neomycin and nystatin)

PREPARATIONS FOR ECZEMA AND PSORIASIS

Both eczema and psoriasis may be treated with emollients (see page 202) and/or topical corticosteroids (see page 205). However, various other topical and oral preparations are used in some cases. Below is a list of these drugs with preparations available on prescription. Drugs used for psoriasis and not covered in this section include cyclosporin (see page 308) and methotrexate (see page 299).

Acitretin

General information: Acitretin is a synthetic retinoid (a derivative of vitamin A) given by mouth for severe psoriasis. It is prescribed by or under the supervision of consultant dermatologists only and is available mainly in hospitals.

How to use: Take exactly as prescribed.
Precautions: Tell your doctor if you are pregnant, plan to become pregnant or are breastfeeding, or if you have liver or kidney problems. You will be asked to attend for various tests to monitor your liver function and blood lipids. Avoid excessive exposure to sunlight and sunlamps.
Side effects: The main side effects are dryness and irritation of the skin and eyes, although a range of other side effects has been reported. Tell your consultant if you experience any unusual effects.
Warnings: Avoid pregnancy for at least one month before, during and two years after treatment. This is because there is a risk of damage to the foetus. Use adequate contraceptive protection. Do not donate blood for at least a year after stopping the drug.
Interactions: Avoid taking vitamin A while you are on this drug. Also avoid tetracyclines. Check with your consultant before taking any other medication.
Available preparations: Capsules
Brand names: Neotigason

Calcipotriol

General information: Calcipotriol is a derivative of vitamin D which is widely used as a topical preparation for certain types of psoriasis. It reduces overproduction of cells in the epidermis.

How to use: Apply exactly as prescribed and use no more than instructed. Avoid getting the preparation on the face or other areas of the body away from the site of the skin condition. Wash your hands immediately after you have applied it.

Precautions: Tell your doctor if you are pregnant and if you have any disorders of calcium metabolism.

Side effects: The preparations may cause local irritation of the skin and dermatitis.

Available preparations: Cream, ointment, scalp solution

Brand names: Dovonex

Coal tar

General information: Coal tar has anti-inflammatory and anti-scaling properties. Preparations containing this ingredient have been used for many years, but its use has now largely been superseded by newer preparations. It is used in psoriasis and occasionally in chronic atopic eczema.

How to use: Apply exactly as prescribed. Avoid getting the preparation on the eyes and broken or inflamed skin.

Side effects: Coal tar may irritate the skin.

Warnings: Coal tar stains skin, hair and clothes.

Available preparations: Calamine and Coal Tar Ointment, Coal Tar and Salicylic Acid Ointment, Coal Tar Paste, Zinc and Coal Tar Paste, Coal Tar Solution. (Coal tar is also contained in several shampoos which are used in scaly scalp conditions, including eczema, psoriasis and dandruff.)

Brand names: Alphosyl (cream and lotion); Alphosyl 2 in 1 (shampoo); Balneum with Tar (bath oil); Baltar (shampoo); Capasal (shampoo); Carbo-Dome (cream); Clinitar (cream and shampoo); Cocois (scalp ointment); Exorex (lotion); Gelcosal (gel); Gelcotar (gel and shampoo); Ionil T (shampoo); Pentrax (shampoo); Polytar Liquid, Polytar AF and Polytar Plus (shampoos); Polytar Emollient (bath additive); Pragmatar (cream); Psoriderm (cream, bath additive and shampoo), Psorigel (gel); T/Gel (shampoo)

Dithranol

General information: Dithranol is very effective in the treatment of psoriasis.

How to use: Apply exactly as prescribed. Avoid getting the preparation on the eyes and broken or inflamed skin. Use very carefully because dithranol can cause quite severe skin irritation. Wash your hands after applying it. Your doctor will probably prescribe a low strength preparation to start, to see how you react to it, and then change to a higher strength preparation after about a week. The strength will be gradually increased until a preparation is found that produces a beneficial effect without causing irritation.

Side effects: Dithranol may cause burning and irritation of the skin.

Warnings: Dithranol stains skin, hair and clothes.

Available preparations: Dithranol Ointment, Dithranol Paste

Brand names: Dithrocream (cream); Micanol (cream), Psorin (ointment and scalp gel)

Gamolenic Acid (evening primrose oil)

General information: Gamolenic acid is the main ingredient in evening primrose oil. It is available on prescription for eczema, and also breast pain. It is thought to produce an anti-inflammatory effect by altering the balance of various inflammatory chemicals in the body.

Precautions: Tell your doctor if you have a history of epilepsy.
Side effects: Side effects are uncommon, but nausea, indigestion, headache and allergic rash may occur.
Available preparations: Capsules
Brand names: Epogam

Lithium succinate

General information: Lithium succinate is a relatively new agent, used to treat seborrhoeic dermatitis.

Available preparations: Ointment
Brand names: Efalith

Salicylic acid

General information: Salicylic acid is related to aspirin and preparations have been in use for many years for all skin conditions such as psoriasis where there is scaling. It works by increasing the rate of loss of surface scales.

How to use: Apply as prescribed. Avoid broken or inflamed skin.
Side effects: Salicylic acid may cause skin irritation and dry skin.
Available preparations: Salicylic Acid Ointment, Zinc and Salicylic Acid Paste; also available in combination preparations with steroids (eg Capasal shampoo)
Brand names: Meted (shampoo – for scaly scalp disorders, including psoriasis and dandruff)

Selenium sulphide

General information: Selenium sulphide is antimicrobial and is contained in shampoos which are used for dandruff.

How to use: Apply as directed. Avoid using 48 hours before or after applying hair colouring or waving products.
Available preparations: Shampoo
Brand names: Lenium, Selsun

Tacalcitol

General information: Tacalcitol is a newly introduced vitamin D derivative which is used for plaque psoriasis. It works by reducing the production of surface skin cells.

How to use: Apply exactly as prescribed and use no more than instructed. Avoid getting the preparation on the face or other areas of the body away from the site of the skin condition. Wash your hands immediately after you have applied it.
Precautions: Tell your doctor if you are pregnant.
Side effects: Local irritation of the skin.
Available preparations: Ointment
Brand names: Curatoderm

Tazarotene

General information: Tazarotene is a synthetic retinoid (vitamin A derivative) used topically for the treatment of mild to moderate plaque psoriasis. It reduces inflammation and the rate of formation of skin surface cells.

Precautions: Tell your doctor if you are pregnant, planning to become pregnant or are breastfeeding.
Side effects: Skin irritation, burning, and dermatitis may occur.
Warnings: Avoid in pregnancy. Use adequate contraceptive protection.
Available preparations: Gel
Brand names: Zorac

PREPARATIONS FOR ACNE

Mild acne may be helped by regular washing with acne soaps to remove grease. There are also various preparations – both topical in the form of creams, ointments and gels, and also for oral use. Topical treatments include those containing benzoyl peroxide, salicylic acid and antibiotics (eg erythromycin, clindamycin, tetracycline). All these treatments work basically by unblocking the oil-producing sebaceous ducts and improving the flow of sebum. Oral medicines include antibiotics (eg oxytetracycline, erythromycin and minocycline), which help reduce inflammation in the skin, and also hormones (eg cyproterone acetate – see page 189) which reduce sebum production. Synthetic retinoids (vitamin A derivatives) are used both orally and topically in acne. These dramatically reduce sebum production as well as keratin production at the hair follicle, lowering the grease content of the skin.

Adapalene

General information: Adapalene is a synthetic retinoid (vitamin A derivative). It is used topically for mild to moderate acne.

Precautions: Tell your doctor if you are pregnant, plan to become pregnant or are breastfeeding.
Side effects: Skin irritation may occur.
Warnings: Avoid pregnancy. Use an adequate method of contraception.
Available preparations: Gel
Brand names: Differin

Azelaic acid

General information: Azelaic acid has an antibacterial effect and is used in mild to moderate acne. Improvement usually occurs after one month of treatment, but five or six months may be needed to resolve the condition entirely.

Precautions: Tell your doctor if you are pregnant or breastfeeding.
Side effects: Skin irritation may occur and occasionally the skin may become sensitive to sunlight.
Available preparations: Cream
Brand names: Skinoren

Antibiotics

General information: Various antibiotics (eg erythromycin, clindamycin, tetracycline) are used topically in the treatment of mild to moderate acne. They are quite effective, but resistance of bacteria to these preparations is a problem.

Available preparations: Gel, lotion
Brand names: Dalacin T (clindamycin), Eryacne (erythromycin), Stiemycin (erythromycin), Topicycline (tetracycline), Zineryt (erythromycin)

Benzoyl peroxide

General information: Benzoyl peroxide has an antibacterial effect and is used in acne. It should be used daily for a prolonged period to produce an improvement.

Precautions: Avoid getting the product in the eyes and mouth.
Side effects: Skin irritation and dryness, especially during the first two weeks of treatment. Use of a bland moisturiser will help. Benzoyl peroxide may bleach fabrics, so keep away from clothing.
Available preparations: Creams, gels, lotions
Brand names: Acnecide, Nericur, PanOxyl
Combination preparations: Acnidazil (benzoyl peroxide with the antifungal miconazole); Benzamycin (benzoyl peroxide with the antibiotic, erythromycin); Quinoderm (benzoyl peroxide with the antimicrobial, potassium hydroxyquinoline sulphate)

Corticosteroids

General information: One topical corticosteroid preparation is available for acne, but it is now used very rarely.

Available preparations: Lotion
Brand names: Actinac (hydrocortisone with the antibiotic chloramphenicol and other ingredients)

Isotretinoin

General information: Isotretinoin is a synthetic retinoid (vitamin A derivative). It is used topically or orally for severe acne that has not responded to other treatments. When used orally, it is prescribed under the supervision of a consultant dermatologist.

Precautions: Avoid pregnancy. Use an adequate method of contraception. Minimise exposure to sunlight. Oral preparation only: avoid pregnancy for one month before, during and for one month after treatment. Use an adequate method of contraception. Avoid giving blood during treatment or for one month after. You may be asked to attend for blood tests before and during treatment.
Side effects: Skin irritation and dryness may occur, together with a range of side effects from the oral preparation. Discuss with your consultant.
Available preparations: Capsules, gel
Brand names: Isotrex, Roaccutane
Combination preparation: Isotrexin (isotretinoin with the antibiotic, erythromycin)

Nicotinamide

General information: Nicotinamide is a vitamin B3 derivative which has anti-inflammatory properties. It is used in acne.

Precautions: Avoid getting the product in the eyes, nose and mouth.
Side effects: Skin irritation and dryness, especially during the first two weeks of treatment. Use of a bland moisturiser will help.
Available preparations: Gel
Brand names: Papulex

Tretinoin

General information: Tretinoin is a synthetic retinoid (vitamin A derivative). It is used topically for mild to moderate acne.

Precautions: Avoid pregnancy. Use an adequate method of contraception.
Side effects: Skin irritation may occur.
Available preparations: Cream, gel, lotion
Brand names: Retin-A

MISCELLANEOUS PREPARATIONS

General information: Various abrasive agents, salicylic acid and sulphur are used in preparations for acne, but these products are rarely prescribed.

Brand names: Acnisal (contains salicyclic acid); Brasivol (contains aluminium oxide, an abrasive agent); Eskamel (contains sulphur and resorcinol); Ionax Scrub (contains polyethylene granules, an abrasive agent with an antiseptic)

WART AND CALLUS REMOVERS

Preparations for warts work by destroying cells that are infected by wart viruses. Preparations containing formaldehyde, glutaraldehyde and salicylic acid have a physical action and cause destruction of the keratin layer in the skin of the wart and surrounding tissue. This is a slow process; you must be prepared to be patient and to spend time paring down the wart, applying the preparation carefully over several weeks. One preparation contains podophyllin, an ingredient that destroys wart cells chemically by disrupting cell division.

Formaldehyde

How to use: Apply as prescribed. Always protect the surrounding skin and avoid broken skin. Do not put on the face, anus, or genitals.
Available preparations: Gel, lotion
Brand names: Veracur

Glutaraldehyde

How to use: Apply as prescribed. Always protect the surrounding skin and avoid broken skin. Do not put on the face, anus, or genitals.
Available preparations: Lotion
Brand names: Glutarol

Podophyllum

General information: Podophyllum is used for genital warts only.

How to use: Use exactly as prescribed. Check with your doctor or pharmacist if you do not understand the instructions. Avoid normal skin, open wounds and the face.
Precautions: Tell your doctor if you are pregnant, planning to become pregnant or are breastfeeding. This preparation must not be used in pregnancy.
Side effects: Podophyllum can cause considerable irritation at the site of application and can cause severe toxicity if applied in excessive amounts.
Available preparations: Cream, liquid
Brand names: Condyline, Warticon

Salicylic acid

How to use: Apply as prescribed. Always protect the surrounding skin and avoid broken skin. Do not put on the face, anus, or genitals.
Precautions: Tell your doctor if you have diabetes.
Available preparations: Paints, gels, ointments
Brand names: Cuplex, Duofilm, Occlusal, Salactol, Salactac, Verrugon.
Combination preparation: Posalfilin (contains salicylic acid and podophyllum resin)

ANTI-INFECTIVE SKIN PREPARATIONS

There are a large number of anti-infective preparations available for direct application to the skin. They contain antibiotics (eg framycetin, fusidic acid), antifungals (eg clotrimazole), antivirals (eg acyclovir) and antiseptics (eg chlorhexidine, cetrimide, iodine, hexachlorophane). Doctors rarely prescribe topical antibiotics these days, mainly because of the risk that resistance to the bacteria will occur. In addition, bacterial skin infections are normally best treated systemically with a medicine taken by mouth.

Topical antibiotics should not be confused with antiseptics. Antiseptics are used fairly frequently – for skin cleansing and disinfection, and also for swabbing wounds and burns. They are useful for helping to prevent infection and are also regularly used by doctors and nurses for disinfecting their hands before operations and diagnostic procedures.

This section contains a list of the anti-infective drugs used in topical products for skin infection, together with the available products.

How to use: Apply as prescribed.

Precautions: Tell your doctor if you are pregnant, planning to become pregnant or breastfeeding.

Side effects: All these preparations may cause skin irritation.

Warnings: Avoid getting the preparations in your eyes.

Aciclovir

General information: Aciclovir is an antiviral drug used topically to treat viral infections caused by herpes, such as cold sores and genital herpes.

Available preparations: Cream
Brand names: Zovirax

Amorolfine

General information: Amorolfine is an antifungal drug which is used topically for fungal skin infections, including those of the nails.

Available preparations: Cream, nail lacquer
Brand names: Loceryl

Benzoic acid

General information: Benzoic acid is an antifungal which is used topically to treat the fungal infection known as ringworm (ointment only).

Available preparations: Ointment
Brand names: None
Combination preparations: Aserbine cream and solution (benzoic acid, malic acid, propylene glycol, salicylic acid) – for wound cleaning

Benzoyl peroxide

General information: Benzoyl peroxide is an antifungal which is used topically to treat fungal infections, particularly athlete's foot.

Available preparations: Cream
Brand names: Quinoped

Chlorhexidine

General information: Chlorhexidine is a disinfectant for general skin cleansing, including swabbing of wounds and burns.

Available preparations: Cleansing solution, dusting powder, cream
Brand names: Chlorhexidine 0.05%, CX Antiseptic Dusting Powder, Hibiscrub, Hibisol, Hibitane 5% Concentrate, Hibitane Obstetric, pHiso-Med, Sterexidine, Steripod Chlorhexidine, Unisept.
Combination preparations: Hibicet Hospital Concentrate (chlorhexidine, cetrimide); Steripod Chlorhexidine/Cetrimide, Tisept (chlorhexidine, cetrimide); Travsept 100 (chlorhexidine, cetrimide)

Chlortetracycline

General information: Chlortetracycline is an antibiotic and can be used topically for bacterial skin infections.

Available preparations: Ointment
Brand names: Aureomycin

Clotrimazole

General information: Clotrimazole is an antifungal drug which is used topically for fungal skin infections.

Available preparations: Cream, liquid, spray, dusting powder
Brand names: Canesten, Masnoderm

Econazole

General information: Econazole is an antifungal drug which is used topically for fungal skin infections.

Available preparations: Cream, lotion
Brand names: Ecostatin, Pevaryl

Framycetin

General information: Framycetin is an antibiotic and can be used topically for bacterial skin infections.

Available preparations: Ointment
Brand names: Soframycin

Fusidic acid

General information: Fusidic acid is an antibiotic and can be used topically for bacterial skin infections.

Available preparations: Cream, gel, ointment
Brand names: Fucidin

Hexachlorophane

General information: Hexachlorophane is used as a pre-operative scrub (cream only) and for the prevention of staphylococcal skin infections (powder only).

Available preparations: Cream, dusting powder
Brand names: Ster-Zac, DC Skin Cleanser, Ster-Zac Powder

Hydrogen peroxide

General information: Hydrogen peroxide is used for skin disinfection, especially for cleaning and deodorising wounds, pressure sores and ulcers.

Available preparations: Cream, solution
Brand names: Hioxyl

Idoxuridine

General information: Idoxuridine is available for topical use in viral infections caused by herpes, such as cold sores and chickenpox. However, it has now been superseded by newer preparations and is now rarely prescribed.

Available preparations: Liquid
Brand names: Herpid

Iodine

General information: Iodine is used in skin disinfection.

Precautions: In addition to the precautions on page 215, do not use any product containing iodine if you have a thyroid problem or if you take lithium.
Available preparations: Paints, solutions, sprays, dry powder spray.
Brand names: Betadine, Savlon Dry Powder

Ketoconazole

General information: Ketoconazole is an antifungal drug which is used topically for fungal skin infections. It is available in the form of a shampoo for seborrhoeic dermatitis and dandruff.

Available preparations: Cream, shampoo
Brand names: Nizoral

Metronidazole

General information: Metronidazole is an antibiotic and can be used topically for acne rosacea (an inflammatory condition of the face) and skin tumours.

Available preparations: Cream, gel
Brand names: Ababact, Metrogel, Metrotop, Noritate, Rozex

Miconazole

General information: Miconazole is an antifungal drug which is used topically for fungal skin infections.

Available preparations: Cream, dusting powder, spray powder
Brand names: Daktarin

Mupirocin

General information: Mupirocin is an antibiotic and can be used topically for bacterial skin infections.

Available preparations: Nasal ointment
Brand names: Bactroban

Neomycin

General information: Neomycin is an antibiotic and can be used topically for bacterial skin infections.

Available preparations: Cream, ointment, dusting powder
Brand names: Cicatrin, Graneodin

Nystatin

General information: Nystatin is an antifungal drug which is used topically for fungal skin infections.

Available preparations: Cream, gel, ointment
Brand names: Nystaform, Nystan, Tinaderm-H

Penciclovir

General information: Penciclovir is an antiviral drug used topically to treat viral infections caused by herpes, such as cold sores and genital herpes.

Available preparations: Cream
Brand names: Vectavir

Polmyxins

General information: Polmyxins are antibiotics and can be used topically for bacterial skin infections.

Available preparations: Ointment, powder
Brand names: Colomycin, Polyfax

Potassium permanganate

General information: Potassium permanganate is used for cleaning the skin and deodorising wounds and exuding eczema. It must be diluted with water before use.

Available preparations: Solution, tablets (for making into a solution)
Brand names: Permitabs

Salicylic acid

General information: Salicylic acid has antifungal properties and can be used for fungal skin infections, particularly ringworm.

Available preparations: Paint
Brand names: Phytex

Sodium chloride

General information: Sodium chloride is used for general cleaning of skin and wounds.

Available preparations: Solution for external use
Brand names: Irriclens, Normasol, Sterac Sodium Chloride, Steripod Sodium Chloride

Sulconazole

General information: Sulconazole is an antifungal drug which is used topically for fungal skin infections.

Available preparations: Cream
Brand names: Exelderm

Terbinafine

General information: Terbinafine is an antifungal drug which is used topically for fungal skin infections.

Available preparations: Cream
Brand names: Lamisil

Tioconazole

General information: Tioconazole is an antifungal drug which is used topically for fungal skin infections.

Available preparations: Nail solution
Brand names: Trosyl

Triclosan

General information: Triclosan is used for disinfection of the skin.

Available preparations: Liquid skin cleanser, hand rub and bath concentrate
Brand names: Aquasept, Manusept, Ster-Zac Bath Concentrate

Undecanoates

General information: These substances are antifungals which are used topically to treat fungal infections, particularly athlete's foot

Available preparations: Cream, paint
Brand names: Monphytol, Mycota

SCABICIDES AND LICE PREPARATIONS

Benzyl benzoate

General information: Benzyl benzoate is used in the treatment of scabies.

How to use: Apply to the whole body and wash off after 24 hours.
Precautions: Tell your doctor if you are pregnant or are breastfeeding.
Side effects: Skin irritation may occur.
Warnings: Avoid contact with eyes, nose and mouth and broken skin.
Available preparations: Liquid for external use
Brand names: None

Carbaryl

General information: Carbaryl is used in the treatment of head and crab lice. It has recently been restricted to prescription-only status because research has shown that it may cause cancer.

How to use: Apply to dry hair and rub into hair and scalp and affected areas. Allow to dry. Wash off after 12 hours and comb hair.
Precautions: Tell your doctor if you are pregnant or are breastfeeding, or if you have asthma.
Side effects: Skin irritation.

Warnings: Avoid contact with eyes, nose and mouth and broken skin.
Available preparations: Lotion for external use
Brand names: Carylderm (not suitable for asthmatics); Derbac C; Suleo C (not suitable for asthmatics)

Malathion

General information: Malathion is used in the treatment of scabies, head lice and pubic lice.

How to use: For scabies, apply to the whole body and wash off after 24 hours.
For lice, apply the lotion to dry hair, scalp and affected areas. Allow to dry. Wash off and comb hair. Apply the shampoo to hair for 5 minutes, rinse, repeat, rinse again. Repeat twice at intervals of 3 days.
Precautions: Tell your doctor if you have asthma.
Side effects: Skin irritation may occur.
Warnings: Avoid contact with eyes, nose and mouth and broken skin.
Available preparations: Lotion for external use
Brand names: Derbac M (not suitable for asthmatics); Prioderm Lotion (not suitable for asthmatics; Prioderm Shampoo; Suleo M (not suitable for asthmatics)

Permethrin

General information: Permethrin is used in the treatment of scabies and head lice.

How to use: Cream rinse (for lice) – apply to clean damp hair, leave on for 10 minutes, rinse and dry. Cream (for scabies) – apply over whole body and wash off after 8–12 hours. If hands are washed within 8 hours of application, reapply the cream.
Side effects: Skin irritation may occur.
Warnings: Avoid contact with eyes, nose and mouth and broken skin.
Available preparations: Cream, cream rinse (similar to a conditioner)
Brand names: Lyclear

Phenothrin

General information: Phenothrin is used in the treatment of scabies and head lice.

How to use: Liquid: apply to dry hair, allow to dry naturally. Shampoo after 12 hours or next day. Comb while wet. Lotion: apply to dry hair, allow hair to dry naturally. Shampoo after 2 hours, comb hair while it is still wet.
Precautions: Tell your doctor if you have asthma.
Side effects: Skin irritation may occur.
Warnings: Avoid contact with eyes, nose and mouth and broken skin.
Available preparations: Liquid, lotion
Brand names: Full Marks Liquid; Full Marks Lotion (not suitable for asthmatics)

MISCLELLANEOUS SKIN PRODUCTS

Aluminium chloride

General information: Aluminium chloride is a potent antiperspirant and is used for excessive sweating affecting the armpits, hands or feet.

Precautions: Do not shave or use a hair remover within 12 hours of using the preparation. Avoid contact with eyes and mouth.
Side effects: Skin irritation may occur.
Available preparations: Solution for external use
Brand names: Anhydrol Forte, Driclor

Heparinoid

General information: Heparinoid-containing preparations are used to improve circulation in conditions such as bruising, chilblains, varicose veins and superficial thrombophlebitis, but they are very rarely prescribed.

Available preparations: Cream, gel, ointment
Brand names: Hirudoid, Lasonil

Minoxidil

General information: Minoxidil is used for male baldness. It may encourage hair growth in some adults, but if no improvement is seen after one year, its use should be discontinued. It is not available on the NHS and is not for use by women.

Precautions: Avoid contact with the skin, nose, mouth and broken skin.
Available preparations: Solution for external use
Brand name: Regaine

The Eye

THE EYE IS A COMPLEX and fascinating organ. Similar to, but more sophisticated than, a digital camera, the eye detects light and captures it as an electrical impulse on the back of the eye. It is composed of various structures which help to control the amount of light entering the eye and to focus it. Light enters the eye through the cornea, which, together with the thin transparent skin that covers it (known as the conjunctiva), helps to protect the eye. In addition, the cornea (with the lens) helps to focus light on the retina, a 'screen' at the back of the eye.

Light then passes through the pupil, which is the pinhole in the middle of the iris – the circular area which gives your eyes their colour. The iris is actually a muscle which expands and contracts to control the size of the pupil. When it is dark, the pupil dilates and the iris allows more light into the eye. In brighter conditions, the pupil reduces in size and less light is allowed in. Behind the iris is the lens, which, by changing its shape, focuses light on to the retina to form an image. The retina contains the light-sensitive cells that convert the image into electrical impulses, which are transported to the brain by the optic nerve. The brain receives these impulses and uses them to form a picture, enabling us to 'see'.

The inside of the eye (the eyeball) is divided into two compartments, each filled with fluid. The front compartment extends from the cornea to the lens and the back compartment from the back of the lens to the retina. Both compartments are filled with fluid which helps the eyeball to retain its shape. In the front compartment, this is known as aqueous humour, and in the back compartment it is known as vitreous humour.

What can go wrong

Defects in vision include short sight and long sight. In cases of short sight, the eye is too long and light from distant objects falls in front of the retina. This is corrected by using glasses with a concave lens, which bends the rays to focus correctly on the retina. In long sight, the eye ball is too short, with the result that light from distant objects falls behind the retina. Normal changes in the lens compensate for this situation in distant vision, but it means that for close work the lens cannot focus any further, causing possible eye strain. Glasses with a convex lens, again bringing the rays of light to a correct focus on the retina, are therefore prescribed for long sight. Astigmatism, a condition in which the cornea is misshapen, also affects vision, particularly in older people. As people age, the lens becomes less flexible. It is increasingly less able to change shape and thus focus on nearby objects – a condition known as presbyopia. Older people again need glasses to correct the defect for reading and close work. Surgery is also now used to correct visual defects – a practice that will become more common in the future. Cataract, a condition in which the lens turns cloudy, is also treated surgically.

Like any other part of the body, the eye is prone to infection and injury – the front of the eye, which is relatively unprotected, is particularly vulnerable. A common condition is conjunctivitis or 'red eye', in which the thin skin (conjunctiva) covering the cornea becomes inflamed, either as a result of infection or as part of an allergic reaction such as hayfever. Conjunctivitis is common and highly infectious, although it is not usually dangerous. However, infection can affect the cornea and sometimes the inside of the eye, and in these cases vision can be affected.

Glaucoma, which occurs mainly in older people, and also sometimes in those with high blood pressure, is a condition in which the pressure inside the eye is raised. Although it is painless, glaucoma leads to a progressive loss of vision, but early detection, and appropriate treatment with drugs or surgery, can prevent blindness.

There are two types of glaucoma – simple and acute. In each case drugs are used to treat the condition. The most common type is simple glaucoma, in which pressure in the eye builds up slowly and insidiously, gradually damaging the optic nerve and reducing the field of vision. If treated in the early stages, further deterioration can be prevented, although damage already suffered cannot be restored. Acute glaucoma develops suddenly and is a medical emergency. There is a sudden blockage in the flow of aqueous humour out of the eye, and pressure from excess fluid increases rapidly. The eye becomes red and painful, watering copiously, and vision is significantly reduced.

The retina itself is prone to many disorders which can cause loss of vision. Diabetes may affect the retina as well as other parts of the eye, as may high blood pressure. Degenerative conditions, for example macular degeneration, can affect vision in the elderly. Retinal detachment, a condition in which a tear in the retina enables fluid to peel it off the protective layer behind, causes sudden visual loss and is commoner in people with very short sight. Laser treatment may help to repair the damage. With any eye condition, contact lens wearers should check with a doctor.

Common conditions and drugs used to treat them

Eye infections (eg conjunctivitis) – antibacterials (eg chloramphenicol, framycetin, gentamicin)

Inflammation of the eye – corticosteroids (eg betamethasone, clobetasone)

Allergic conjunctivitis – sodium cromoglycate, antazoline

Glaucoma – adrenaline, beta-blockers (eg betaxolol, timolol), acetazolamide

DRUGS USED TO TREAT EYE INFECTIONS

Eye infections are usually treated with eye drops and eye ointments that contain antibacterial drugs. The only antiviral drug available as an eye preparation is aciclovir and this is used to treat herpes simplex infections. If the eye infection is serious, it will be treated with antibiotics given by mouth (see page 246). This section lists only those anti-infective drugs available in the form of eye drops and/or eye ointments.

How to use: Eye drops: Use as prescribed. This usually involves applying one drop at least every 2 hours, reducing frequency of application as the infection gets better. Continue using the eye drops for 24 hours after the infection is completely better. Eye drops should not be used for more than four weeks after first opening the container. See also page 17.

Eye ointments: Use as prescribed. This usually involves applying the eye ointment at night, particularly if eye drops are used during the day. However, if the eye ointment is used on its own (ie without eye drops), it should be used 3–4 times a day. See also page 18.

Side effects: Side effects of eye drops and eye ointments are usually limited to transient stinging, burning and irritation. Allergic reactions may develop to some antibacterials or preservatives in eye drops, causing burning, irritation and redness in the eye and around the eye.

Warnings: Contact lens wearers should check with their doctor before continuing to wear them.

Aciclovir

Available preparations: Eye ointment
Brand names: Zovirax

Chloramphenicol

Available preparations: Eye drops, eye ointment
Brand names: Chlormycetin, Sno Phenicol, Minims Chloramphenicol

Chlortetracycline

Available preparations: Eye ointment
Brand names: Aureomycin

Ciprofloxacin

Precautions: Tell your doctor if you are pregnant or breastfeeding.
Side effects: Burning, itching, crusting of the eye lids, corneal staining and visual disturbances may occur with these drops. The eyes may also become over-sensitive to light.
Available preparations: Eye drops
Brand names: Ciloxan

Framycetin

Available preparations: Eye drops, eye ointment
Brand names: Soframycin

Fusidic acid

Available preparations: Eye drops
Brand names: Fucithalmic

Gentamicin

Available preparations: Eye drops, eye ointment
Brand names: Cidomycin, Garamycin, Genticin, Minims Gentamicin

Neomycin

Available preparations: Eye drops, eye ointment
Brand names: Minims Neomycin Sulphate, Neosporin

Ofloxacin

Precautions: Do not use these drops for more than 10 days. Tell your doctor if you are pregnant or breastfeeding.
Side effects: The eye may become over-sensitive to light and eye irritation can occur. Nausea, headache and dizziness may occur, but these side effects are rare.
Available preparations: Eye drops
Brand names: Exocin

Polymixin B

Available preparations: Eye drops, eye ointment
Brand names: Polyfax, Polytrim

Propamidine

Available preparations: Eye drops, eye ointment
Brand names: Brolene

EYE PREPARATIONS CONTAINING CORTICOSTEROIDS

Corticosteroids are used in the treatment of many inflammatory conditions, and they are available in the form of eye drops and eye ointments. They are sometimes given along with antibiotics in one preparation. They are used after surgery to treat local inflammation of the eye.

How to use: Use corticosteroid preparations exactly as prescribed.

Side effects: These medicines can cause allergic reactions and irritation of the eye. Report any unusual reactions to your doctor.

Betamethasone

Available preparations: Eye drops, eye ointment
Brand names: Betamethasone, Vista-Methasone
Combination preparations: Betnesol N, Vista-Methasone N (both contain betamethasone and neomycin)

Clobetasone

Available preparations: Eye drops
Brand names: Cloburate

Dexamethasone

Available preparations: Eye drops, eye ointment
Brand names: Maxidex, Minims Dexamethasone
Combination preparations: Maxitrol, Sofradex (both contain dexamethasone with antibiotics)

Fluorometholone

Available preparations: Eye drops
Brand names: FML
Combination preparations: FML-Neo

Hydrocortisone

Available preparations: Eye drops, eye ointment
Brand names: None
Combination preparations: Neo-Cortef (hydrocortisone, neomycin)

Prednisolone

Available preparations: Eye drops
Brand names: Minims Prednisolone, Pred Forte, Predsol
Combination preparations: Predsol N (prednisolone, neomycin)

EYE PREPARATIONS FOR ALLERGIC CONJUNCTIVITIS

Allergic conditions, for example hayfever, often cause itchy, watery eyes and conjunctivitis. Various eye preparations are available to treat this condition. Most of them in the list below (apart from nedocromil and sodium cromoglycate) are antihistamines. In severe cases, topical steroids may be used.

Antazoline

Available preparations: Eye drops
Combination preparations: Otrivine-Antistin (antazoline with xylometazoline, a decongestant)

Azelastine

Available preparations: Eye drops
Brand names: Optilast

Levocabastine

Available preparations: Eye drops
Brand names: Livostin

Lodoxamide

Available preparations: Eye drops
Brand names: Alomide

Nedocromil

Available preparations: Eye drops
Brand names: Rapitil

Sodium cromoglycate

Available preparations: Eye drops
Brand names: None.

MEDICINES FOR GLAUCOMA

Glaucoma can be treated topically with several types of drugs – miotics (eg carbachol and pilocarpine), beta-blockers (eg betaxolol, timolol), sympathomimetics (eg adrenaline) and carbonic anhydrase inhibitors (eg dorzolamide). It can also be treated orally with acetazolamide.

How they work: Drugs used to treat glaucoma work in different ways to achieve the same effect – reduction of pressure in the eye. Miotics improve the drainage of fluid from the eye and constrict the pupil, while beta-blockers (see page 82) reduce the production of fluid in the eye, and sympathomimetics increase outflow of fluid from the eye.

How to use: Use exactly as prescribed

Acetazolamide

General information: Acetazolamide is a carbonic anhydrase inhibitor which is used systemically (by mouth or injection) to treat glaucoma.

Precautions: Tell your doctor if you are pregnant, planning to become pregnant or are breastfeeding, or if you have liver or kidney disease.
Side effects: Side effects can be troublesome with acetazolamide. They may include gastrointestinal disturbances, headache, dizziness, fatigue, irritability, depression, rash and thirst.
Interactions: Acetazolamide interacts with a few other drugs. Check with your doctor or pharmacist before taking any other medicine.
Available preparations: Tablets, injection
Brand names: Diamox, Diamox SR

Adrenaline

General information: Adrenaline is a sympathomimetic and used topically in the treatment of certain forms of glaucoma.

Precautions: Tell your doctor if you have heart problems or hypertension, or if you are taking monoamine oxidase inhibitors (MAOIs).
Side effects: These eye drops can cause severe smarting or redness of the eye.
Available preparations: Eye drops
Brand names: Eppy, Simplene

Betaxolol

General information: Betaxolol is a beta-blocker used topically in the treatment of glaucoma.

Precautions: Tell your doctor if you have heart problems or asthma, or if you are taking other medication.
Side effects: Dry or itchy eyes may develop.
Available preparations: Eye drops
Brand names: Betoptic

Brimonidine

General information: Brimonidine is a sympathomimetic and used topically in the treatment of glaucoma.

Precautions: Tell your doctor if you are pregnant or breastfeeding, or if you have heart or circulatory problems, liver or kidney problems or depression.
Available preparations: Eye drops
Brand names: Alphagan

Carbachol

General information: Carbachol is a miotic and used topically in the treatment of glaucoma.

Precautions: Tell your doctor if you have or have had any other eye problems, heart problems, high blood pressure, asthma, peptic ulcer, Parkinson's disease or urinary tract problems.
Side effects: Burning, itching and smarting of the eyes, blurred vision, headache and browache may occur.
Available preparations: Eye drops
Brand names: Isopto Carbachol

Carteolol

General information: Carteolol is a beta-blocker used topically in the treatment of glaucoma.

Precautions: Tell your doctor if you have heart problems or asthma, or if you are taking any other medication.
Side effects: Dry or itchy eyes may develop.
Available preparations: Eye drops
Brand names: Teoptic

Dipivefrine

General information: Dipivefrine is a sympathomimetic and used topically in the treatment of glaucoma.

Precautions: Tell your doctor if you have heart problems or hypertension.
Available preparations: Eye drops
Brand names: Propine

Dorzolamide

General information: Dorzolamide is a carbonic anhydrase inhibitor used topically in the treatment of glaucoma.

Precautions: Tell your doctor if you are pregnant or breastfeeding, or if you have or have had kidney or liver problems.
Side effects: Burning, stinging and itching of the eye may occur. Allergic reactions (eg rash), blurred vision, bitter taste, headache, dizziness and nausea are also possible.
Available preparations: Eye drops
Brand names: Trusopt
Combination preparations: Cosopt (dorzolamide with timolol, a beta-blocker)

Guanethidine

General information: Guanethidine is a sympathomimetic and used topically in the treatment of glaucoma.

Precautions: Tell your doctor if you have or have had heart problems or hypertension. You should have your eyes checked every 6 months because these drops may cause damage to the cornea and conjunctiva while you are taking them.
Available preparations: Eye drops
Brand names: Ganda

Latanoprost

General information: Latanoprost is a prostaglandin. It is a relatively new drug and used topically in the treatment of glaucoma.

Precautions: Tell your doctor if you are pregnant or breastfeeding, or if you have asthma.
Side effects: Eye irritation and brown pigmentation of the iris may occur, so your eye colour may change.
Available preparations: Eye drops
Brand names: Xalatan

Levobunolol

General information: Levobunolol is a beta-blocker used topically in the treatment of glaucoma.

Precautions: Tell your doctor if you have or have had heart problems or asthma, or you are taking other medication.
Side effects: Dry or itchy eyes may develop.
Available preparations: Eye drops
Brand names: Betagan

Metipranolol

General information: Metipranolol is a beta-blocker used topically in the treatment of glaucoma.

Precautions: Tell your doctor if you have or have had heart problems or asthma, or if you are taking other medication.
Side effects: Dry or itchy eyes may develop.
Available preparations: Eye drops
Brand names: Minims Metipranolol

Pilocarpine

General information: Pilocarpine is a miotic and used topically in the treatment of glaucoma.

Precautions, **Side effects:** As carbachol (see page 230).
Available preparations: Eye drops, gel, long acting inserts
Brand names: Isopto Carpine, Minims Pilocarpine Nitrate, Ocusert, Pilogel, Sno Pilo

Timolol

General information: Timolol is a beta-blocker used topically in the treatment of glaucoma.

Precautions: Tell your doctor if you have or have had heart problems or asthma, or if you are taking any other medication.
Side effects: Dry or itchy eyes may develop.
Available preparations: Eye drops
Brand names: Timoptol, Timoptol LA.

MISCELLANEOUS EYE PREPARATIONS

Acetylcysteine

General information: Acetylcysteine is used topically for tear deficiency (dry eyes).

Available preparations: Eye drops
Brand names: Ilube

Carbomers

General information: Carbomers are a group of substances used topically for tear deficiency (dry eyes).

Available preparations: Eye drops
Brand names: GelTears, Viscotears

Hydroxyethylcellulose

General information: Hydroxyethylcellulose is used topically for tear deficiency (dry eyes).

Available preparations: Eye drops
Brand names: Minims Artificial Tears

Hypromellose

General information: Hypromellose is used topically for tear deficiency (dry eyes).

Available preparations: Eye drops
Brand names: Isopto Alkaline, Isopto Plain, Moisture-eyes, Tears Naturale
Combination preparations: Isopto Frin (hypromellose with phenylephrine, a decongestant)

Liquid paraffin

General information: Liquid paraffin is used topically for dry eye conditions.

Available preparations: Eye ointment
Brand names: Lacri-Lube, Lubri-Tears

Polyvinyl alcohol

General information: Polyvinyl alcohol is used topically for tear deficiency (dry eyes).

Available preparations: Eye drops
Brand names: Hypotears, Liquifilm Tears, Sno Tears

Sodium chloride

General information: Sodium chloride is used topically to flush out the eye in cases of eye irritation.

Available preparations: Solution
Brand names: Minims Sodium Chloride

Yellow soft paraffin

General information: Soft paraffin is used topically to soften eye crusts or as a lubricant.

Available preparations: Eye ointment
Brand names: Simple Eye Ointment

Zinc sulphate

General information: Zinc sulphate is used topically as an astringent in cases of excessive tear production.

Available preparations: Eye drops
Brand names: None

The Ear, Nose and Throat

THE EARS, NOSE AND THROAT are closely related both in location and function. The ear, which is the organ of hearing and balance, consists of three parts: the outer, middle and inner ear. The outer ear (the part visible on the head) captures sound waves which pass through the middle ear to the inner ear, where they are converted into nerve impulses which then travel to the brain. The inner ear also helps to maintain balance, and its lining produces wax.

The nose is the organ of smell; it provides the main passageway for air to flow in and out of the lungs. The cells in the nose produce mucus and have hair-like projections, known as cilia. The mucus helps to trap any bacterial and other particles which are then wafted out through the nose by the cilia. In addition, the nose is responsible for warming and humidifying the incoming air before its entry to the lungs.

The throat (pharynx) is located behind the mouth and above the oesophagus (foodpipe) and trachea (windpipe). Like the nose and mouth, it is lined with mucus which helps to trap foreign particles. Below the throat is the voice box (larynx) which contains the vocal cords and is responsible for producing the sounds used in speech.

What can go wrong

Like any other parts of the body, the ears, nose and throat can become infected and/or inflamed. Allergies, particularly hayfever, can cause symptoms of itching and watering in the nose.

Mouth ulcers are open sores caused by a break in the mucous membrane that lines the mouth. Many people suffer from them and over-the-counter remedies are a popular form of treatment. However, any mouth ulcers lasting for longer than two weeks should be investigated by a doctor.

Common conditions and drugs used to treat them

Ear infections – oral antibiotics (middle and inner ear – see page 246); topical antibiotics – ear drops, ear ointments (outer ear)

Inflammatory conditions – topical corticosteroids (ear drops/ointments)

Ear wax – various oils and branded ear drops

Nasal allergy – oral antihistamines (see page 284); nasal drops and sprays containing antihistamines, corticosteroids, cromoglycate

Stuffy nose – nasal decongestants

Nasal infections – Topical antibacterial preparations

Mouth ulcers and other inflammatory conditions – various lozenges, pastilles, creams, mouthwashes containing anti-infective and anaesthetic ingredients

DRUGS TO TREAT EAR INFECTIONS

Ear infections may occur in the outer, middle or inner ear. Infection of the outer ear can be treated with anti-infective ear drops, but infections of the middle ear or inner ear are usually treated with antibiotics given by mouth (see page 246). This section lists only those anti-infective drugs available in the form of ear drops. Some antibacterials are contained in combination with corticosteroids in ear drops (see below).

How to use: Use exactly as prescribed. These medicines should not generally be used for longer than one week.

Side effects: Allergic reactions and local irritation to the ear may develop occasionally.

Chloramphenicol

Brand names: None

Clotrimazole

Brand names: Canesten

Gentamicin

Brand names: Cidomycin, Garamycin, Genticin

EAR PREPARATIONS CONTAINING CORTICOSTEROIDS

Corticosteroids, available in the form of ear drops and ear ointments, are used in the treatment of many inflammatory conditions. They are particularly useful for treating local inflammation and eczema of the outer ear.

How to use: Use the medicines exactly as prescribed.

Side effects: These medicines can cause allergic reactions and irritation of the ear.

Betamethasone

Available preparations: Ear drops
Brand names: Betnesol, Vista-Methasone
Combination preparations: Betnesol-N, Vista-Methasone N (both contain betamethasone and neomycin, an antibiotic)

Dexamethasone

Available preparations: Ear drops, ear ointment, spray
Brand names: Otomize (dexamethasone, neomycin, acetic acid); Sofradex (dexamethasone, framycetin, gramicidin)

Flumethasone

Available preparations: Ear drops
Combination preparations: Locorten Vioform (flumethasone with clioquinol, an antibacterial)

Hydrocortisone

Available preparations: Ear drops, ear ointment
Combination preparations: Gentisone HC (hydrocortisone with gentamicin, an antibiotic); Neo-Cortef (hydrocortisone with neomycin, an antibiotic); Otosporin (hydrocortisone with antibiotics)

Prednisolone

Available preparations: Ear drops
Brand names: Predsol
Combination preparations: Predsol-N (prednisolone with neomycin, an antibiotic)

Triamcinolone

Available preparations: Ear drops
Combination preparations: Audicort (triamcinolone with neomycin, an antibiotic); Tri-Adcortyl Otic (triamcinolone, gramicidin, neomycin, nystatin)

PREPARATIONS USED FOR EAR WAX

Wax is a normal body secretion which provides protection to the ear canal. It should only be removed if it causes deafness or pain. If needed, wax is removed by syringing the ears, but before this, wax can be softened using almond oil, olive oil, sodium bicarbonate ear drops or one of the proprietary ear drop preparations, such as those listed below.

Cerumol – contains chlorbutol, paradichlorobenzene, arachis (peanut) oil

Exterol – contains urea, hydrogen peroxide, glycerol

Molcer – contains docusate sodium

Otex – contains urea, hydrogen peroxide

Waxsol – contains docusate sodium

PREPARATIONS FOR NASAL ALLERGY

Allergies which affect the nose, including hayfever, can be treated with oral anti-histamines (see page 284) and also various nasal preparations. These preparations contain corticosteroids, antihistamines, cromoglycate or nedocromil.

How to use: Use the preparations exactly as prescribed.

Azelastine

General information: Azelastine is an antihistamine used topically to treat nasal symptoms of hayfever and similar allergies.

Side effects: Nasal irritation is the most common side effect. Taste disturbance may also occur.

Available preparations: Nasal spray

Brand names: Rhinolast

Beclomethasone

General information: Beclomethasone is a corticosteroid used topically to treat nasal symptoms of hayfever and similar allergies.

Side effects: Nasal side effects may include dryness, irritation of the nose and throat, and taste disturbance. Allergic reactions, including breathing problems, have also been reported.

Available preparations: Nasal spray

Brand names: Beconase

Betamethasone

General information: Betamethasone is a corticosteroid used topically to treat nasal symptoms of hayfever and similar allergies.

Side effects: Nasal side effects may include dryness, irritation of the nose and throat, and taste disturbance. Allergic reactions, including breathing problems, have also been reported.

Available preparations: Nasal drops

Brand names: Betnesol

Budesonide

General information: Budesonide is a corticosteroid used topically to treat nasal symptoms of hayfever and similar allergies.

Side effects: Nasal side effects may include dryness, irritation of the nose and throat, and taste disturbance. Allergic reactions, including breathing problems, have also been reported.

Available preparations: Nasal spray

Brand names: Rhinocort Aqua

Cromoglycate

General information: Cromoglycate is an anti-inflammatory drug used topically to treat nasal symptoms of hayfever and similar allergies.

Side effects: Nasal irritation and allergic reactions, including breathing problems, may occur.
Available preparations: Nasal spray
Brand names: Rynacrom, Vividrin
Combination preparations: Rynacrom Compound (cromoglycate with xylometazoline, a decongestant)

Dexamethasone

General information: Dexamethasone is a corticosteroid used topically to treat nasal symptoms of hayfever and similar allergies.

Side effects: Nasal side effects may include dryness, irritation of the nose and throat, and taste disturbance. Allergic reactions, including breathing problems, have also been reported.
Available preparations: Nasal spray
Combination preparations: Dexarhinaspray Duo (dexamethasone with tramazoline, an antihistamine)

Flunisolide

General information: Flunisolide is a corticosteroid used topically to treat nasal symptoms of hayfever and similar allergies.

Side effects: Nasal side effects may include dryness, irritation of the nose and throat, and taste disturbance. Allergic reactions, including breathing problems, have also been reported.
Available preparations: Nasal spray
Brand names: Syntaris

Fluticasone

General information: Fluticasone is a corticosteroid used topically to treat nasal symptoms of hayfever and similar allergies.

Side effects: Nasal side effects may include dryness, irritation of the nose and throat, and taste disturbance. Allergic reactions, including breathing problems, have also been reported.
Available preparations: Nasal spray
Brand names: Flixonase

Levocobastine

General information: Levocobastine is an antihistamine used topically to treat nasal symptoms of hayfever and similar allergies.

Side effects: Nasal irritation is the most common side effect. Headache, drowsiness and fatigue may also occur.
Available preparations: Nasal spray
Brand names: Livostin

Ipratropium

General information: Ipratropium is used to dry up runny nose associated with hayfever or non-allergic conditions.

Side effects: Nasal dryness and irritation.
Available preparations: Nasal spray
Brand names: Rinatec

Mometasone

General information: Mometasone is a corticosteroid used topically to treat nasal symptoms of hayfever and similar allergies.

Side effects: Nasal side effects may include dryness, irritation of the nose and throat, and taste disturbance. Allergic reactions, including breathing problems, have also been reported.
Available preparations: Nasal spray
Brand names: Nasonex

Nedocromil

General information: Nedocromil is an anti-inflammatory drug used topically to treat nasal symptoms of hayfever and similar allergies.

Side effects: Nasal irritation and taste disturbances may occur.
Available preparations: Nasal spray
Brand names: Tilarin

Triamcinolone

General information: Triamcinolone is a corticosteroid used topically to treat nasal symptoms of hayfever and similar allergies.

Side effects: Nasal side effects may include dryness, irritation of the nose and throat, and taste disturbance. Allergic reactions, including breathing problems, have also been reported.
Available preparations: Nasal spray
Brand names: Nasacort

NASAL DECONGESTANTS

Decongestants are available for topical nasal use to treat a blocked up and stuffy nose. They work by constricting the blood vessels in the nose which helps to dry up the mucus. They should only be used for short periods of time (up to 7 days). This is because they can cause rebound dilation of the blood vessels and hence an increase in nasal congestion.

Ephedrine

Available preparations: Nasal drops
Brand names: None

Xylometazoline

Available preparations: Nasal drops, nasal spray
Brand names: None

PREPARATIONS FOR NASAL INFECTIONS

Certain nasal drops and ointments contain antibacterial ingredients and are used occasionally to treat infection in the nose.

Bactroban nasal ointment (mupirocin)
Betnesol N nasal drops (betamethasone, neomycin)
Locabiotal nasal spray (fusafungine)
Naseptin cream (chlorhexidine)
Vista-Methasone N nasal drops (betamethasone, neomycin)

PREPARATIONS FOR MOUTH CONDITIONS

There are many remedies for mouth ulcers and inflammatory conditions of the mouth, including lozenges, mouthwashes, pastes and gels. All of them aim to soothe the pain while the ulcer heals naturally. Other preparations for use in the mouth include mouthwashes for cleaning and refreshing the mouth, antifungals for use in oral thrush and saliva replacements for people with dry mouth.

Aciclovir

General information: Aciclovir is an antiviral agent used locally to treat herpes infections of the lining of the mouth, including cold sores.

Available preparations: Cream
Brand names: Zovirax

Amphotericin

General information: Amphotericin is an antifungal used locally to treat mouth infections.

Available preparations: Lozenges, oral liquid
Brand names: Fungilin

Anaesthetics

General information: Local anaesthetics are used to numb the pain of mouth ulcers.

Available preparations: Teething gels
Brand names: Various teething gels are available (eg Anbesol, Calgel, Dentinox, Rinstead, Woodward's Ulc-Aid)

Artificial saliva

General information: Artificial saliva is used to relieve dry mouth.

Available preparations: Oral sprays, gel, lozenges
Brand names: Glandosane, Luborant, Oralbalance, Saliva Orthana, Salivace, Salivese, Salivix

Benzydamine

General information: Benzydamine is an anti-inflammatory which helps to reduce the discomfort of mouth ulcers and other similar inflammatory conditions.

Available preparations: Oral rinse, spray
Brand names: Difflam

Carbenoxolone

General information: Carbenoxolone is an anti-inflammatory which helps to reduce the discomfort of mouth ulcers and other similar conditions where inflammation is causing pain.

Available preparations: Mouthwash
Brand names: Bioplex

Carmellose

General information: Carmellose is used to protect mouth ulcers while they heal naturally.

Available preparations: Oral paste, oral powder
Brand names: Orabase, Orahesive,

Cetylpyridium

General information: Cetylpyridium is an antiseptic used for oral hygiene to freshen and clean the mouth.

Available preparations: Mouthwash
Brand names: Merocet

Chlorhexidine

General information: Chlorhexidine is an antiseptic used for oral hygiene; it also has a specific effect in helping to prevent the formation of plaque on the teeth.

Available preparations: Mouthwash, spray, gel
Brand names: Chlorohex, Corsodyl, Eludril

Corticosteroids

General information: Corticosteroids are anti-inflammatories which can be used locally to treat mouth ulcers.

Available preparations: Oral paste, lozenges
Brand names: Adcortyl in Orabase, Corlan

Hexetidine

General information: Hexetidine is an antiseptic used for oral hygiene.

Available preparations: Mouthwash or gargle
Brand names: Oraldene

Hydrogen peroxide

General information: Hydrogen peroxide is used for oral hygiene. It froths in the mouth and helps to clean the mouth and treat gingivitis.

Available preparations: Mouthwash
Brand names: Peroxyl

Miconazole

General information: Miconazole is an antifungal which is used to treat oral thrush.

Precautions: Tell your doctor if you are pregnant or breastfeeding, or if you have liver disease or porphyria.
Side effects: Side effects are rare, but gastrointestinal disturbances and allergic reactions may occur.
Available preparations: Oral gel, denture lacquer
Brand names: Daktarin, Dumicoat

Nystatin

General information: Nystatin is an antifungal which is used locally to treat oral thrush.

Side effects: Nausea and mouth irritation may occur.
Available preparations: Oral suspension, pastilles
Brand names: Nystan

Pilocarpine

General information: Pilocarpine is used to treat dry mouth due to poor function of the salivary glands following radiotherapy for head and neck cancer.

Precautions: Tell your doctor if you are pregnant or breastfeeding, or if you have or have had asthma or any other lung disease or eye disease, liver or kidney disease, heart problems or peptic ulcer.
Side effects: Sweating, blurred vision, chills, nausea, diarrhoea, vomiting, dizziness, headache, runny nose, flushing, increased urinary frequency and indigestion may occur.
Warnings: Take care with driving as this medicine may cause blurred vision.
Interactions: Pilocarpine interacts with several other drugs. Check with your doctor or pharmacist before taking other medicines.
Available preparations: Tablets
Brand names: Salagen

Povidone-iodine

General information: Povidone iodine is an antiseptic used for oral hygiene.

Precautions: Tell your doctor if you are pregnant or breastfeeding, or if you have a thyroid condition or are taking lithium. It should not be used for longer than 14 days because of the risk of absorbing too much iodine.
Available preparations: Mouthwash
Brand names: Betadine

Salicylates

General information: Salicylates are related to aspirin and are mild painkillers. They are used locally to reduce the pain associated with mouth ulcers. Some products are available in the form of teething gels and can be used to alleviate infant teething.

Available preparations: Teething gels, liquid
Brand names: Various teething gels (eg Bonjela, Dinnefords) are available. Pyralvex is a liquid (containing salicylic acid) which is not suitable for teething or for children under 12 years.

Sodium perborate

General information: Sodium perborate is similar to hydrogen peroxide and is used for oral hygiene.

Available preparations: Mouthwash
Brand names: Bocasan

Thymol

General information: Thymol is used for oral hygiene.

Available preparations: Mouthwash
Brand names: None

Infection

MOST INFECTION DEVELOPS as a result of disease-causing (pathogenic) micro-organisms invading the body and multiplying. Found everywhere – in the air, water and soil – and often called germs, micro-organisms are tiny, living creatures which can be seen only with the aid of a microscope. Every day we eat, drink and breathe them. Not all of them cause disease – particularly if the individual is healthy. Many micro-organisms live on the skin, in the mouth, intestine, respiratory tract and genitals, and cause no ill effects. Indeed, some of these micro-organisms act as part of your defence against infection by helping to kill other organisms which could cause disease.

Whether a micro-organism causes infection depends on the actual type of micro-organism and the strength of the human body's defences. There are four types of micro-organisms – bacteria, fungi, viruses and protozoa – as well as the larger parasitic worms.

Infection is most often 'caught' from people round you. Body fluids are the most common sources of infection, which is why attention to hygiene is so important. Influenza, measles and mumps are transmitted by inhaling infected droplets from other sufferers, while hepatitis and AIDS are transmitted via seminal or vaginal fluid or the blood. Faeces and urine are common sources of infection such as cholera and typhoid. Infection can also be transmitted from the mother to her unborn child, and other infections (eg malaria) are transmitted by blood-sucking insects.

The body has several defences against infection, including the skin and the linings of the intestine, respiratory tract and genito-urinary tract, all of which act as natural barriers to invading organisms. Other defences, known collectively as the immune response, include certain types of white blood cells, and also antibodies which are produced by dedicated white cells in response to specific infections. Both of these are produced in large numbers during infection and help to immobilise hostile micro-organisms and kill them.

What can go wrong

Sometimes, however, the immune response may be overwhelmed by large numbers of micro-organisms or by other factors that reduce the person's defences (eg smoking, poor diet, the presence of other disease). Anti-infective drugs can aid the body's natural defences. They either kill micro-organisms or prevent them from multiplying.

There are five main types of anti-infective drugs. These are antibiotics, antifungal drugs, antiviral drugs, drugs for malaria and similar infections (antiprotozoals) and drugs for worm infestations (anthelmintics).

Infections and the drugs used to treat them

Site of infection	Example of drugs used
Gastrointestinal system	Ciprofloxacin, erythromycin, trimethoprim
Cardiovascular system	Various penicillins, gentamicin
Respiratory system	Amoxycillin, erythromycin, trimethoprim, tetracycline
Brain and nervous system	Benzylpenicillin, cefotaxime, chloramphenicol, amoxycillin, gentamicin
Urinary tract	Trimethoprim, amoxycillin, nitrofurantoin, cephalosporins
Genital system	Various penicillins, tetracyclines, metronidazole or erythromycin
Musculoskeletal system	Clindamycin, flucloxacillin, fusidic acid
Eye	Chloramphenicol or gentamicin eye drops
Ear, nose and throat	Various penicillins, tetracyclines, cephalosporins, erythromycin, metronidazole
Skin	Various penicillins, erythromycin, fusidic acid

ANTIBIOTICS

Antibiotics are drugs used to treat infection caused by bacteria. There are more than 50 antibiotics, and which one is used depends on several factors, such as where the infection is in the body and the likely organism that is causing it. Ideally, when you have symptoms of infection, your doctor should identify the micro-organism present by sending a sample of blood, urine, faeces or sputum – whichever is appropriate – to the laboratory before prescribing any drug for you. However, analysis of samples may take 24 hours or more and your doctor usually makes a guess as to the likely organism and prescribes accordingly. In practice, this usually means that the doctor will prescribe what is known as a broad spectrum antibiotic – in other words an antibiotic that is active against a wide range of bacteria. If laboratory tests later reveal that this antibiotic was inappropriate, then the drug will be changed. Other factors governing the choice of an antibiotic include the severity of the infection, the person's age, his or her kidney and liver function, history of allergies such as penicillin allergy, whether she is pregnant or breastfeeding, and what other medicines are being used.

Antibiotics have no effect on any other type of infection, including viruses. This is important because many infections, including those of the throat and upper respiratory tract, are caused by viruses and therefore cannot be treated by antibiotics. In the past, antibiotics have often been prescribed somewhat indiscriminately, and they are still among the most frequently prescribed medicines. This has contributed to the problem of antibiotic resistance, in which bacteria develop ways to counter the effects of antibiotics. When penicillin was first developed, for example, it was a powerful killer of Staphylococcus aureus, a bacterium causing skin and other infections. But within 20 years of penicillin usage, the bacterium had developed resistance to the antibiotic. A new antibiotic, methicillin, was developed, which again worked well for a time, but the bacterium has now developed new super strains that are resistant to the new drug too. Even the development of new antibiotics, therefore, does not always solve the problem. The risk of antibiotic resistance also increases if you do not take the drug properly. If you miss a dose or do not complete the course of antibiotics, resistant bacteria get the chance to grow and the infection will not be eliminated properly,

Most antibiotics are taken by mouth in the form of tablets, capsules or liquids, but occasionally – and this is usually the case with severe infections – the drugs are given by injection. Antibiotics fall into several categories – penicillins, cephalosporins, tetracyclines, aminoglycosides, macrolides, sulphonamides, quinolones and other miscellaneous drugs.

PENICILLINS

In use since the 1940s, the penicillins were one of the first types of antibiotics to be discovered. Unfortunately, many bacteria are now resistant to penicillins, which has led to the development of a whole range of these drugs with different activities. Some (eg amoxycillin, ampicillin) have a broad spectrum of activity, while others (eg benzylpenicillin) have a narrow, specific spectrum of activity. Penicillins are used for a wide range of bacterial infections of the ear, chest and urinary tract; they kill the bacteria by blocking synthesis of the bacterial cell wall.

How to use: Take the medicine exactly as prescribed by the doctor. If you miss a dose, take it as soon as you remember. Take the full course of antibiotics. Even if you feel better, the original infection may still be present and if you stop taking your antibiotic, your symptoms may return.

Precautions: Tell your doctor if you are pregnant, planning to become pregnant or are breastfeeding, but note that if you develop an infection during pregnancy, your doctor may prescribe a penicillin because these drugs are not known to cause harm to the foetus. Also tell your doctor if you have or have ever had penicillin or other allergy, kidney disease or porphyria.

Side effects: These drugs are generally very safe, but the following side effects may occur: skin rash, nausea, vomiting diarrhoea. If you develop a severe skin rash, itching, difficulty in breathing, wheezing, joint swelling or swollen mouth or tongue, this may indicate an allergic reaction. Stop taking the antibiotic immediately and contact your doctor.

Warnings: Drinking alcohol is not a problem with these drugs.

Interactions: Talk to your doctor if you are taking oral contraceptives because penicillins may reduce their effectiveness.

Amoxycillin

Available preparations: Capsules, sachets, liquid, injection
Brand names: Amoxil
Combination preparations: Augmentin (co-amoxiclav: amoxycillin and clavulanic acid)

Ampicillin

Available preparations: Capsules, liquid, injection
Brand names: Penbritin
Combination preparations: Magnapen (co-fluampicil: ampicillin and flucloxacillin)

Benzylpenicillin

Available preparations: Injection
Brand names: Crystapen

Flucloxacillin

General information: This drug is particularly effective against *staphylococcus aureus* infections, which cause conditions such as boils.

Available preparations: Capsules, liquid, injection
Brand names: Floxapen

Phenoxymethylpenicillin

Available preparations: Tablets, liquid
Brand names: None

Pivampicillin

Available preparations: Tablets
Brand names: Pondocillin

Procaine penicillin

Available preparations: Injection
Brand names: Bicillin

CEPHALOSPORINS

Cephalosporins are broad spectrum antibiotics, used in a variety of infections, including urinary tract infections, meningitis and pneumonia.

How they work: Cephalosporins, like penicillins, kill bacteria by interfering with cell wall synthesis.

How to use: Take the medicine exactly as prescribed by the doctor. If you miss a dose, take it as soon as you remember. Take the full course of antibiotics. Even if you feel better, the original infection may still be present and if you stop taking your antibiotic, your symptoms may return.

Precautions: Tell your doctor if you are pregnant or breastfeeding but note that if you develop an infection during pregnancy, your doctor may prescribe a cephalosporin because these drugs are not known to cause harm to the foetus. Also tell your doctor if you have or have ever had antibiotic or other allergy, kidney disease or porphyria. (About 10 per cent of people who are allergic to penicillins are also allergic to cephalosporins.)

Side effects: Side effects are uncommon but the following may occur: skin rash, nausea, vomiting and diarrhoea. If you develop a severe skin rash, itching, difficulty in breathing, wheezing, joint swelling or swollen mouth or tongue, this may indicate an allergic reaction. Stop taking the antibiotic immediately and contact your doctor.

Warnings: Drinking alcohol is not a problem with these drugs.

Interactions: Talk to your doctor if you are taking oral contraceptives because cephalosporins may reduce their effectiveness. Cephalosporins also interact with oral anticoagulants.

Cefaclor

Available preparations: Capsules, liquid
Brand names: Cefaclor, Distaclor, Distaclor MR

Cefadroxil

Available preparations: Capsules, liquid
Brand names: Baxan

Cefixime

Available preparations: Tablets, liquid
Brand names: Suprax

Cefpodoxime

Available preparations: Tablets, liquid
Brand names: Orelox

Cefprozil

Available preparations: Tablets, liquid
Brand names: Cefzil

Ceftibuten

Available preparations: Capsules, liquid
Brand names: Cedax

Cefuroxime

Available preparations: Tablets, sachets, liquid, injection
Brand names: Zinacef, Zinnat

Cephalexin

Available preparations: Tablets, capsules, liquid
Brand names: Ceporex, Keflex

Cephradine

Available preparations: Capsules, liquid, injection
Brand names: Velosef

TETRACYCLINES

Tetracyclines are antibiotics with a broad spectrum of activity, although bacterial resistance has now reduced their value. However, they are particularly useful for treating some cases of bronchitis, as well as certain chest infections caused by organisms that are unaffected by penicillin because they lack a cell wall. They are also used for pelvic inflammatory disease and certain skin conditions, including acne. Tetracycline itself is used, together with bismuth and another antibiotic called metronidazole, to get rid of *Helicobacter pylori* infection in the treatment of peptic ulcer (see page 117). Tetracyclines work by inhibiting the production of protein in bacteria. They prevent bacteria from multiplying, but do not kill them.

How to use: Take the medicine exactly as prescribed by the doctor. If you miss a dose, take it as soon as you remember. Take the full course of antibiotics. Even if you feel better, the original infection may still be present and if you stop taking your antibiotic, your symptoms may return. Milk and dairy produce may reduce the absorption of some of these drugs. These drugs are best taken on an empty stomach, or at least an hour before any food. Check the label or ask your pharmacist for instructions.

Precautions: Tell your doctor if you are pregnant, planning to become pregnant or are breastfeeding, or you have or have ever had antibiotic or other allergy, kidney disease, systemic lupus erythmatosus or porphyria. Tetracyclines are deposited in growing bones and teeth and cause staining. They should therefore not be taken by women who are pregnant or breastfeeding, or by children under 12.

Side effects: Side effects are uncommon but the following may occur: nausea, vomiting and diarrhoea. Some tetracyclines – particularly demeclocycline and doxycycline – cause the skin to be sensitive to sunlight, and it is best to avoid exposure to sunlight and/or sunlamps while taking these drugs. If you develop a severe skin rash, this may indicate an allergic reaction. Stop taking the antibiotic immediately and contact your doctor.

Warnings: Drinking alcohol is not a problem with these drugs.

Interactions: Talk to your doctor if you are taking oral contraceptives because tetracyclines may reduce their effectiveness. Tetracyclines also interact with a number of other medicines, including indigestion remedies and dietary supplements containing minerals (eg iron, calcium and zinc). Ask your doctor or pharmacist before taking any other medicines.

Demeclocycline

Available preparations: Capsules
Brand names: Ledermycin

Doxycycline

Available preparations: Tablets, capsules
Brand names: Vibramycin, Vibramycin-D

Lymecycline

Available preparations: Capsules
Brand names: Tetralysal 300

Minocycline

Available preparations: Tablets, capsules
Brand names: Minocin MR

Oxytetracycline

Available preparations: Tablets, capsules
Brand names: Terramycin

Tetracycline

Available preparations: Tablets, capsules
Brand names: Achromycin, Tetrachel
Combination preparations: Deteclo (tetracycline, chlortetracycline and demeclocycline)

MACROLIDES

Macrolides are broad spectrum antibiotics with a similar activity to the penicillins. They are often prescribed as an alternative to penicillins in people who are penicillin-allergic, and are used for respiratory tract infections, pelvic infections, skin and wound infections, middle ear infections and Legionnaire's disease (a rare type of pneumonia). They are also used in certain chest infections caused by organisms that are unaffected by penicillin because they lack a cell wall. In addition, erythromycin, the most frequently prescribed drug in this group, is used in acne. Macrolides work by inhibiting the production of protein in bacteria. They prevent bacteria from multiplying, but do not kill them.

How to use: Take the medicine exactly as prescribed by the doctor. If you miss a dose, take it as soon as you remember. Take the full course of antibiotics. Even if you feel better, the original infection may still be present and if you stop taking your antibiotic, your symptoms may return.

Precautions: Tell your doctor if you are pregnant or breastfeeding, if you have or have ever had antibiotic or other allergy, kidney, liver or heart disease. Note that if you develop an infection during pregnancy, your doctor may prescribe a macrolide because these drugs are not known to cause harm to the foetus. Also tell your doctor

Side effects: Side effects are uncommon, but nausea, diarrhoea and vomiting may occur, particularly with erythromycin. Allergic reactions are not uncommon and if you develop a skin rash, fever or jaundice (which may indicate a liver disorder), stop taking the antibiotic immediately and contact your doctor.

Warnings: Drinking alcohol is not a problem with these drugs.

Interactions: Macrolides interact with a number of other medicines, including some antihistamines (eg astemizole, terfenadine), carbamazepine, warfarin, theophylline and digoxin. Ask your doctor or pharmacist before taking any other medicines.

Azithromycin

Available preparations: Capsules, liquid
Brand names: Zithromax

Clarithromycin

Available preparations: Tablets, sachets, liquid, injection
Brand names: Klaricid, Klaricid XL

Erythromycin

Available preparations: Tablets, capsules, liquid, injection
Brand names: Erymax, Erymin, Erythrocin, Erythroped, Erythroped A, Ilosone, Tiloryth

SULPHONAMIDES

Sulphonamides were the first group of chemicals used as antibiotics. Used extensively until the 1960s, they have now been largely superseded by newer antibiotics possessing a lower risk of side effects and bacterial resistance and a broader spectrum of activity. Sulphonamides inhibit the production of folic acid by bacteria. Folic acid is a substance which is essential for the growth of bacteria; by inhibiting its production, bacterial multiplication is prevented.

How to use: Take the medicine exactly as prescribed by the doctor. If you miss a dose, take it as soon as you remember. Take the full course of antibiotics. Even if you feel better, the original infection may still be present and if you stop taking your antibiotic, your symptoms may return.

Precautions: Tell your doctor if you are pregnant, planning to become pregnant or are breastfeeding, or if you have or ever have had antibiotic or other allergy, kidney or liver disease, asthma, porphyria, blood disorders or glucose 6-phosphate dehydrogenase deficiency (G6PD deficiency). These drugs should be avoided in pregnancy.

Side effects: Side effects may include allergic rashes and severe skin eruptions with blistering, as well as damage to bone marrow resulting in a low white blood cell count. If you develop a skin rash, sore throat, fever or jaundice, this may indicate a liver disorder or an allergic reaction. Stop taking the antibiotic immediately and contact your doctor.

Warnings: Drinking alcohol is not a problem with these drugs.

Interactions: Sulphonamides interact with a number of other medicines, including some heart drugs, oral anticoagulants, drugs for diabetes, anticonvulsants, antimalarials and cyclosporin. Ask your doctor or pharmacist before taking any other medicines.

Co-trimoxazole

General information: Co-trimoxazole is a mixture of the sulphonamide, sulphamethoxazole with trimethoprim. It was at one time quite a popular drug, but it is now associated with serious side effects. Its use is therefore now limited to pneumocystitis pneumonia. It is not recommended for uncomplicated urinary tract infections, chronic bronchitis or ear infections in children.

Available preparations: Tablets, dispersible tablets, liquid, injection
Brand names: Septrin

Sulphametopyrazine

Available preparations: Tablets
Brand names: Kelfizine W

Sulphadiazine

Available preparations: Tablets, injection
Brand names: None

Sulphadimidine

Available preparations: Tablets
Brand names: None

QUINOLONES

Quinolones are active against a wide range of bacteria and are particularly useful for infections of the urinary tract, gastrointestinal tract and respiratory tract. They are normally reserved for the treatment of infections where other antibiotics do not work or the person is allergic to other antibiotics. Quinolones work by interfering with the internal structure of the bacteria, causing rapid death of bacteria.

How to use: Take the medicine exactly as prescribed by the doctor. If you miss a dose, take it as soon as you remember. Take the full course of antibiotics. Even if you feel better, the original infection may still be present and if you stop taking your antibiotic, your symptoms may return.

Precautions: Tell your doctor if you are pregnant, planning to become pregnant or are breastfeeding, or if you have or ever have had antibiotic or other allergy, kidney or liver disease, epilepsy, porphyria or glucose 6-phosphate dehydrogenase deficiency. These antibiotics are not suitable during pregnancy or breastfeeding, and are not recommended for children or adolescents.

Side effects: Nausea, vomiting, diarrhoea, stomach pain, dyspepsia, headache, dizziness, sleeping problems, rash and itching may occur. Other possible side effects include loss of appetite, drowsiness, depression, confusion, hallucinations, convulsions, disturbances in taste, vision, hearing and smell. Inflammation of the tendons, particularly in the elderly and in those taking corticosteroids, may also occur. If you develop any inflammation or pain in a joint, a rash, or any psychiatric disturbance, contact your doctor immediately.

Warnings: Avoid alcohol because it may increase the adverse effects of these drugs. Take care with driving and other similar activities until you know how you react to these drugs because they can cause dizziness.

Interactions: Quinolones interact with a number of other medicines, including some heart drugs, indigestion remedies, oral anticoagulants, beta-blockers, oral antidiabetic drugs, NSAIDs, cyclosporin and theophylline. Dietary supplements containing minerals (eg calcium, iron and zinc) may reduce the absorption of quinolones. Ask your doctor or pharmacist before taking any other medicines.

Cinoxacin

Available preparations: Capsules
Brand names: Cinobac

Ciprofloxacin

Available preparations: Tablets, liquid, injection
Brand names: Ciproxin

Grepafloxacin

Available preparations: Tablets
Brand names: Raxar

Levofloxacin

Available preparations: Tablets, injection
Brand names: Tavanic

Nalidixic acid

Available preparations: Tablets, sachets, liquid
Brand names: Mictral, Negram, Uriben

Norfloxacin

Available preparations: Tablets
Brand names: Utinor

Ofloxacin

Available preparations: Tablets, injection
Brand names: Tarivid

MISCELLANEOUS ANTIBIOTICS

In this section is included a list of several different antibiotics which do not easily fit into a readily definable group.

How to use: Take the medicine exactly as prescribed by the doctor. If you miss a dose, take it as soon as you remember. Take the full course of antibiotics. Even if you feel better, the original infection may still be present and if you stop taking your antibiotic, your symptoms may return.

Chloramphenicol

General information: Chloramphenicol is a powerful, broad spectrum antibiotic. However, it has serious side effects and it is usually reserved for the treatment of certain specific, life-threatening infections. It is also used in the form of eye drops for eye infections (see page 225).

How to use: As miscellaneous antibiotics (see page 255).
Precautions: Tell your doctor if you are pregnant, planning to become pregnant or are breastfeeding, or if you have or have had kidney or liver problems or porphyria.
Side effects: These may include nausea, vomiting, mouth ulcers, tingling of the eyes, hands and feet and various blood disorders. Note that allergic reactions can occur to chloramphenicol eye drops (see page 225).
Warnings: Alcohol is not a problem with this drug.
Interactions: Chloramphenicol interacts with oral anticoagulants, drugs for diabetes and anticonvulsants.
Available preparations: Capsules, injection
Brand names: Kemicetine

Clindamycin

General information: Clindamycin is used to treat infections of bones and joints, peritonitis and to help in the prevention of endocarditis. This antibiotic has limited use because of serious side effects, but it is safe to use as a lotion (see page 211) to treat acne.

How to use: As miscellaneous antibiotics (see page 255).
Interactions: Clindamycin interacts with few drugs; check with your doctor or pharmacist before taking any other medication.
Side effects: These may include diarrhoea, nausea, vomiting, jaundice and blood disorders.
Warnings: Alcohol is not a problem with this drug.
Precautions: Tell your doctor if you are pregnant, planning to become pregnant or are breastfeeding, or if you have or have had kidney or liver problems or if you are prone to diarrhoea. If you develop jaundice, tell your doctor immediately.
Available preparations: Capsules, liquid, injection
Brand names: Dalacin C

Colistin

General information: Colistin is a fairly toxic antibiotic and is used only rarely, primarily to sterilise the bowel. It is also used by inhalation (often via a nebuliser) in certain chest conditions that predispose to infections.

How to use: As miscellaneous antibiotics (see page 255).
Precautions: Tell your doctor if you are pregnant, planning to become pregnant or are breastfeeding, or if you have or have had myasthenia gravis.
Side effects: These may include numbness round the mouth, tingling in the hands

and feet, muscle weakness and breathlessness. Slurred speech, visual disturbances and confusion may also occur, but these effects are rare.

Warnings: Alcohol is not a problem with this drug.
Interactions: Colistin interacts with several drugs, but check with your doctor or pharmacist before taking any other medication.
Available preparations: Tablets, liquid, injection
Brand names: Colomycin

Fusidic acid

General information: Fusidic acid is a narrow spectrum antibiotic and is used fairly rarely. However, it is particularly effective against *staphylococcus aureus* infections. It is used – usually in combination with another antibiotic – to treat infections of the bone and endocarditis, and also in the form of eye drops to treat eye infections (see page 226). Fusidic acid is also employed in the form of a cream or a dressing to treat skin infections (see page 216).

How to use: As miscellaneous antibiotics (see page 255).
Precautions: None
Side effects: May include nausea, vomiting, rashes and jaundice.
Warnings: Alcohol is not a problem with this drug.
Interactions: None reported, but check with your doctor or pharmacist before taking any other medication.
Available preparations: Tablets, liquid, injection
Brand names: Fucidin

Hexamine

General information: Hexamine is used in the prevention and long term treatment of urinary tract infections. It is rarely used nowadays.

How to use: As miscellaneous antibiotics (see page 255).
Precautions: Tell your doctor if you are pregnant, planning to become pregnant or are breastfeeding, or if you have or have had kidney disease.
Side effects: Gastrointestinal disturbances, bladder irritation and rash may occur.
Warnings: Alcohol is not a problem with this drug.
Interactions: Hexamine interacts with few drugs, but check with your doctor or pharmacist before taking any other medication.
Available preparations: Tablets
Brand names: Hiprex

Metronidazole

General information: Metronidazole has a narrow spectrum of activity, but it has several types of use; firstly for bacterial infections of the vagina, dental infections, leg ulcers, pressure sores and for infection during surgery; secondly for an infection on the face known as acne rosacea; and thirdly for protozoal infections, especially trichomonas vaginitis, a vaginal infection, and also two protozoal infections that affect the gut (*Giardia lamblia* and *Entamoeba histolytica*).

How to use: As miscellaneous antibiotics (see page 255).

Precautions: Tell your doctor if you are pregnant, planning to become pregnant or are breastfeeding.

Side effects: Nausea, vomiting, unpleasant taste, furred tongue, rashes and itching may occur. Some people may experience drowsiness, headache, dizziness and darkened urine.

Warnings: Avoid alcohol with this drug as it causes very unpleasant side effects.

Interactions: Metronidazole interacts with several drugs, including anticoagulants and anticonvulsants.

Available preparations: Tablets, liquid, suppositories, injection

Brand names: Flagyl, Flagyl S, Metrolyl

Combination preparation: Flagyl Compak (metronidazole tablets with nystatin – an antifungal – pessaries)

Nitrofurantoin

General information: Nitrofurantoin is used for infections of the urinary tract.

How to use: As miscellaneous antibiotics (see page 255).

Precautions: Tell your doctor if you are pregnant, planning to become pregnant or are breastfeeding, or if you have or have had liver or kidney problems, glucose 6-phosphate deficiency, porphyria, anaemia, diabetes or lung disease.

Side effects: Loss of appetite, nausea, vomiting, diarrhoea, shortness of breath, tingling of the hands and feet, rash, itching and other allergic reactions may occur. Some people may experience darkened urine.

Warnings: Alcohol is not a problem with this drug.

Interactions: Nitrofurantoin interacts with few other drugs, but check with your doctor or pharmacist before taking other medicines.

Available preparations: Tablets, capsules

Brand names: Furadantin, Macrobid, Macrodantin

Spectinomycin

General information: Spectinomycin is used to treat gonorrhoea in people who are allergic to penicillin and/or in infections resistant to penicillin.

How to use: As miscellaneous antibiotics (see page 255).

Precautions: Tell your doctor if you are pregnant, planning to become pregnant or are breastfeeding.

Side effects: Nausea, dizziness, itching and fever may occur.

Warnings: Alcohol is not a problem with this drug.

Interactions: Spectinomycin interacts with few other drugs, but check with your doctor or pharmacist before taking other medicines.

Available preparations: Injection

Brand names: Trobicin

Teicoplanin

General information: Teicoplanin is reserved for use in serious infections, including endocarditis, peritonitis associated with dialysis and serious infections caused by *Staphylococcus aureus*.

How to use: As miscellaneous antibiotics (see page 255).
Precautions: Tell your doctor if you are pregnant, planning to become pregnant or are breastfeeding, or you have or have had liver or kidney problems.
Side effects: Nausea, vomiting, diarrhoea, ringing in the ears and mild hearing loss may be experienced. There may be serious allergic reactions including rash, itching, fever, and difficulty in breathing.
Warnings: Alcohol is not a problem with this drug.
Interactions: Teicoplanin interacts with few other drugs, but check with your doctor or pharmacist before taking other medicines.
Available preparations: Injection
Brand names: Targocid

Tinidazole

General information: Tinidazole is a similar drug to metronidazole, with a similar spectrum of activity.

How to use: As miscellaneous antibiotics (see page 255).
Precautions, side effects, warnings, interactions: As metronidazole (see above).
Available preparations: Tablets
Brand names: Fasigyn

Trimethoprim

General information: Trimethoprim is similar to the sulphonamides (see page 253). It is used particularly in infections of the urinary tract and in acute and chronic bronchitis.

How to use: As miscellaneous antibiotics (see page 255).
Precautions: Tell your doctor if you are pregnant, planning to become pregnant or are breastfeeding, or you have or have had liver or kidney problems.
Side effects: Rash, itching, nausea and vomiting may occur. However, more serious effects, especially blood disorders, may also occur, particularly if you are on long term treatment with this drug. Seek medical advice immediately if you develop symptoms such as fever, sore throat, rash, mouth ulcers, bruising or bleeding.
Warnings: Alcohol is not a problem with this drug.
Interactions: Trimethoprim interacts with several other drugs, including antimalarials and cyclosporin. Check with your doctor or pharmacist before taking other medicines.
Available preparations: Tablets, liquid, injection. It is also combined with sulphamethoxazole in co-trimoxazole (see page 253).
Brand names: Monotrim, Trimopan

Vancomycin

General information: Vancomycin is reserved for use in certain specific infections such as endocarditis and pseudomembranous colitis (a severe infection of the gastrointestinal tract which can occur as a result of antibiotic use).

How to use: As miscellaneous antibiotics (see page 255).

Precautions: Tell your doctor if you are pregnant, planning to become pregnant or are breastfeeding, or you have or have had kidney problems or hearing problems.

Side effects: These may include kidney damage, hearing problems, nausea and allergic reactions such as rash, itching and wheezing.

Warnings: Alcohol is not a problem with this drug.

Interactions: Several drugs interact with vancomycin to increase the risk of hearing loss and/or kidney problems.

Available preparations: Capsules, injection

Brand names: Vancocin

DRUGS USED TO TREAT TUBERCULOSIS

Tuberculosis (TB) is a chronic infectious disease, transmitted from person to person by inhalation of infected droplets from the air. Disease develops in only 5 to 15 per cent of infected people. It most commonly affects the respiratory tract, but the infection may spread to other parts of the body, such as the heart, gastrointestinal tract, genito-urinary tract, brain, bones, joints and skin. Symptoms appear gradually and include generally poor health, loss of appetite, weight, night sweats, recurrent fever and cough.

TB is treated using several drugs simultaneously. This helps to reduce the risk of the bacteria becoming resistant to one of the drugs. Treatment involves following a strict timetable with specialist supervision. The total duration of treatment is usually several months, and it is vital that the medicines are taken exactly as prescribed during the entire treatment period.

Treatment normally consists of two phases. The initial phase of treatment usually consists of three drugs – commonly isoniazid, rifampicin and pyrazinamide. If after a period of about two months, this first phase has proved to be successful, one of the three drugs will be stopped and treatment will continue with two drugs, often isoniazid and rifampicin. If the first phase is not successful, other drugs will be used.

How to use: Take all your medicines exactly as prescribed by the doctor. If you miss a dose, take it as soon as you remember. Take the full course of all the medicines prescribed. Even if you feel better, the original infection may still be present and if you stop taking your medication, your symptoms may return.

Capreomycin

General information: Capreomycin is used in the treatment of TB, usually when drugs normally prescribed have not worked or when the person is intolerant to their side effects.

How to use: As drugs for tuberculosis (see page 260).
Precautions: Tell your doctor if you are pregnant, planning to become pregnant or are breastfeeding, or you have or have had kidney or liver problems or hearing problems.
Side effects: Kidney damage, hearing loss with ringing in the ears and dizziness, and allergic reactions such as rash and itching may occur.
Warnings: Avoid excessive amounts of alcohol with this drug.
Interactions: Several drugs interact with capreomycin to increase the risk of hearing loss and/or kidney problems.
Available preparations: Injection
Brand names: Capostat

Cycloserine

General information: Cycloserine is used in the treatment of TB, usually when drugs normally prescribed have not worked or when the person is intolerant to their side effects.

How to use: As drugs for tuberculosis (see page 260).
Precautions: Tell your doctor if you are pregnant, planning to become pregnant or are breastfeeding, or you have or have had kidney problems, epilepsy, depression, anxiety, psychiatric problems or porphyria.
Side effects: These may include headache, dizziness, drowsiness, trembling, convulsions, depression and rash.
Warnings: Avoid alcohol with this drug because there is an increased risk of seizures.
Interactions: Cycloserine interacts with phenytoin.
Available preparations: Capsules
Brand names: None

Ethambutol

General information: Ethambutol is used in the treatment of tuberculosis.

How to use: As drugs for tuberculosis (see page 260).
Precautions: Tell your doctor if you are pregnant, planning to become pregnant or are breastfeeding, or you have or have had kidney problems.
Side effects: These may include eye pain, blurred vision, red/green colour blindness, tingling hands and feet, rash and itching. Report any visual changes or eye pain to your doctor immediately.
Warnings: Avoid excessive alcohol with this drug.
Interactions: None
Available preparations: Tablets
Brand names: None

Isoniazid

General information: Isoniazid is used in the treatment of tuberculosis. It is also used to prevent tuberculosis in people who are close to infected patients.

How to use: As drugs for tuberculosis (see page 260).
Precautions: Tell your doctor if you are pregnant, planning to become pregnant or are breastfeeding, or you have or have had kidney or liver problems, epilepsy or porphyria.
Side effects: One of the main side effects of isoniazid is damage to the nervous system, leading to symptoms of tingling and numbness in the hands and feet. Although such effects usually only occur with high doses, supplements of pyridoxine are normally prescribed with this drug to prevent them. Other side effects may include nausea, vomiting, tiredness, weakness and jaundice, and various allergic reactions including rash may occur. Tell your doctor immediately if you develop symptoms such as persistent nausea, vomiting, malaise or jaundice; these symptoms may indicate liver disorder.
Warnings: Avoid excessive alcohol with this drug.
Interactions: Isoniazid interacts with several drugs, particularly anticonvulsants.
Available preparations: Tablets, liquid, injection
Brand names: None

Pyrazinamide

General information: Pyrazinamide is used in the treatment of tuberculosis.

How to use: As drugs for tuberculosis (see page 260).
Precautions: Tell your doctor if you are pregnant, planning to become pregnant or are breastfeeding, or you have or have had kidney or liver problems or porphyria.
Side effects: Nausea, vomiting, fever, jaundice, tiredness, weakness, attacks of gout and various allergic reactions including rash may occur. Tell your doctor immediately if any of these side effects occur. This drug may also cause anaemia.
Warnings: Avoid excessive alcohol with this drug.
Interactions: Pyrazinamide interacts with few other drugs, but check with your doctor or pharmacist before taking other medicines.
Available preparations: Tablets
Brand names: Zinamide

Rifabutin

General information: Related to rifampicin, rifabutin is used in the treatment of tuberculosis. It is also used for the prevention and treatment of related infections in patients who are immunosuppressed (eg those with HIV infection).

How to use: As drugs for tuberculosis (see page 260).
Precautions: Tell your doctor if you are pregnant, planning to become pregnant or are breastfeeding, or if you have or have had kidney or liver problems, jaundice or porphyria, or if you wear contact lenses.

Side effects: Nausea, vomiting, fever, jaundice, flu-like symptoms, bone and joint pain, visual disturbance and various allergic reactions, including rash and fever, may occur. Tell your doctor immediately if any of these side effects occur. Rifabutin discolours soft contact lenses, and saliva and urine may be coloured orange-red.

Warnings: Avoid excessive alcohol with this drug. Rifabutin reduces the effectiveness of oral contraceptives. Use other non-hormonal methods of contraception while taking this drug.

Interactions: Rifabutin interacts with several other drugs, including calcium-channel blockers, corticosteroids, cyclosporin, oral contraceptives and some cytotoxic drugs.

Available preparations: Capsules

Brand names: Mycobutin

Rifampicin

General information: Rifampicin is used in the treatment of tuberculosis, and also for the treatment of other serious infections, including artificial heart valve infections (endocarditis), bone infections, legionnaire's disease and leprosy.

How to use: As drugs for tuberculosis (see page 260).

Precautions: Tell your doctor if you are pregnant, planning to become pregnant or are breastfeeding, or you have or have had kidney or liver problems, jaundice or porphyria, or if you wear contact lenses.

Side effects: Nausea, loss of appetite, vomiting, diarrhoea, fever, jaundice, flu-like symptoms, bone and joint pain, visual disturbance and various allergic reactions, including rash and fever, may occur. Tell your doctor immediately if any of these side effects occur. Rifampicin discolours soft contact lenses, and may turn saliva and urine orange-red.

Warnings: Avoid excessive alcohol with this drug. Rifampicin reduces the effectiveness of oral contraceptives. Use other non-hormonal methods of contraception while taking this drug.

Interactions: Rifampicin interacts with several other drugs, including calcium-channel blockers, corticosteroids, cyclosporin, oral contraceptives and some cytotoxic drugs.

Available preparations: Tablets, capsules, liquid, injection

Brand names: Rifadin, Rimactane

Combination preparations: Rifater (rifampicin, isoniazid, pyrazinamide); Rifinah (rifampicin, isoniazid), Rimactazid (rifampicin, isoniazid)

Streptomycin

General information: Streptomycin is used (nowadays very rarely) for the treatment of tuberculosis.

How to use: As drugs for tuberculosis (see page 260).

Precautions: Tell your doctor if you are pregnant, planning to become pregnant or are breastfeeding, or if you have or have ever had kidney disease or myasthenia gravis.

Side effects: Side effects can be serious and include damage to hearing, dizziness and loss of balance and kidney damage (which may lead to blood in the urine or cloudy urine). Nausea, vomiting and skin rash may also occur.
Warnings: None
Interactions: A wide range of drugs interact with streptomycin to increase the risk of hearing loss and/or kidney problems.
Available preparations: Injection
Brand names: None

ANTIFUNGAL DRUGS

Antifungal drugs are used in the treatment of fungal infections. We are continually exposed to fungi – from food, air and water – in our daily lives, but most fungi are harmless. Some, however, can grow in the mouth and gastrointestinal tract, the genital tract, the skin, hair and nails, causing unsightly changes or itching or irritation. Some fungi can cause serious disease.

The most common fungal infections are caused by the fungus known as Candida albicans. This fungus is normally present in the body, but overgrowth causes the infection known as thrush, which can occur in the mouth, vagina and skin. Another type of fungal infection is caused by Tinea organisms. These include tinea pedis (athlete's foot), tinea unguim (infection of the nail), tinea cruris (infection of the groin) and tinea capitis (scalp ringworm).

Antibiotics have no effect on fungal infections. This is because the structure of fungi is very different from that of bacteria. Different drugs – known as antifungal drugs – are therefore needed. Superficial fungal infections, such as those on the skin, nails and in the mouth and vagina, are usually treated topically with creams, pessaries, lozenges, pastilles and paints. Internal fungal infections, however, are treated systemically with tablets, capsules and sometimes injections. Antifungals damage the cell wall of the fungus, causing the contents of the cell wall to leak out. The fungus then dies.

How to use: Take the medicine exactly as prescribed by the doctor. If you miss a dose, take it as soon as you remember. Take the full course of treatment. Even if you feel better, the original infection may still be present and if you stop taking your medicine, your symptoms may return.

Amphotericin

General information: Amphotericin is a broad spectrum antifungal drug which is active against most yeasts and fungi. It is given orally for the treatment of candida infection in the intestine. It is also used locally to treat thrush infection in the mouth (see page 241).

How to use: As antifungal drugs (see above).
Precautions: Tell your doctor if you are pregnant, planning to become pregnant or are breastfeeding, or if you have or have had liver or kidney problems.
Side effects: Side effects from oral administration are rare. However, when the drug

is given by injection the following may occur: nausea, vomiting, diarrhoea, loss of appetite, stomach pain, headache and muscle and joint pain. Pain may also occur at the site of the injection.

Warnings: Alcohol is not a problem with these drugs.

Interactions: Amphotericin interacts with a number of drugs including digoxin, corticosteroids, cyclosporin and tacrolimus.

Available preparations: Tablets, lozenges, liquid, injection

Brand names: Abelcet, Ambisome, Amphocil, Fungilin, Fungizone

Fluconazole

General information: Fluconazole can be used to treat a wide range of fungal infections, including those of the mouth, gastrointestinal tract, respiratory tract, skin, head and feet. It is also used to prevent fungal infection in people who have a disease (eg AIDS) which predisposes them to infection.

How to use: As antifungal drugs (see page 264).

Precautions: Tell your doctor if you are pregnant, planning to become pregnant or are breastfeeding, or if you have or have had liver or kidney problems.

Side effects: Side effects are rare, but the following may occur: nausea, abdominal discomfort, diarrhoea, flatulence, rash and other allergic reactions.

Warnings: Alcohol is not a problem with this drug.

Interactions: Fluconazole interacts with a very wide range of other drugs. Check with your doctor or pharmacist before taking any other medication.

Available preparations: Capsules, liquid, injection; also available as a single dose over-the-counter preparation for thrush

Brand names: Diflucan

Flucytosine

General information: Flucytosine is used to treat various internal fungal infections, sometimes in conjunction with amphotericin.

How to use: As antifungal drugs (see page 264).

Precautions: Tell your doctor if you are pregnant, planning to become pregnant or are breastfeeding, or if you have or have had liver or kidney problems.

Side effects: Nausea, vomiting, diarrhoea and rash are the most common side effects, but confusion, convulsion, hallucinations, headache, drowsiness and dizziness may also occur.

Warnings: Avoid excessive alcohol with this drug. Take care with driving and other similar activities until you have learned how this drug affects you.

Interactions: None reported, but check with your doctor or pharmacist before taking any other medication.

Available preparations: Injection

Brand names: Alcoban

Griseofulvin

General information: Griseofulvin is used for fungal infections of the skin, scalp, hair and nails, where local therapy has failed or is not appropriate.

How to use: As antifungal drugs (see page 264). Take with food.
Precautions: Tell your doctor if you are pregnant, planning to become pregnant or are breastfeeding, or if you have or have had liver problems, lupus erythmatosus or porphyria.
Side effects: Nausea, vomiting, headache, sensitivity of the skin to sunlight and rash are the most common side effects, but confusion, poor co-ordination, tiredness, dizziness and tingling of the hands and feet may also occur.
Warnings: Avoid alcohol with this drug. Take care with driving and other similar activities until you have learned how this drug affects you. Avoid pregnancy while taking this drug and for one month after treatment has finished. Men should not father a child within 6 months of treatment.
Interactions: Griseofulvin interacts with several drugs, including oral anticoagulants and oral contraceptives. Use a non-hormonal method of contraception while taking this drug.
Available preparations: Tablets, liquid
Brand names: Grisovin

Itraconazole

General information: Itraconazole is a broad spectrum antifungal drug which is used to treat a wide range of fungal infections (eg in the mouth, vagina, skin), particularly where other antifungals are inappropriate or have failed to work. It is also used to prevent fungal infections in patients with AIDS.

How to use: As antifungal drugs (see page 264).
Precautions: Tell your doctor if you are pregnant, planning to become pregnant or are breastfeeding, or if you have or have had liver or kidney problems.
Side effects: Nausea, abdominal pain, indigestion, constipation, headache, dizziness, and various allergic reactions including rash. Loss of appetite, nausea, vomiting, abdominal pain, fever, tiredness and dark urine could indicate liver problems. Tell your doctor immediately if you experience any of these effects.
Warnings: Avoid excessive alcohol with this drug because it may increase the risk of adverse effects. Take care with driving and other similar activities until you have learned how this drug affects you.
Interactions: Itraconazole interacts with a wide range of other drugs, so check with your doctor or pharmacist before taking any other medication.
Available preparations: Capsules, liquid
Brand names: Sporanox

Ketoconazole

General information: Ketoconazole is a broad spectrum antifungal drug which is used to treat a wide range of fungal infections (eg in the mouth, vagina, skin). It is also used to prevent fungal infections in patients particularly prone to infection (eg those with AIDS).

How to use: As antifungal drugs (see page 264).

Precautions: Tell your doctor if you are pregnant, planning to become pregnant or are breastfeeding, or if you have or have had liver problems.

Side effects: Nausea, vomiting, abdominal pain, headache and various allergic reactions including rash and itching may occur. Loss of appetite, nausea, vomiting, abdominal pain, fever, tiredness and dark urine could indicate liver problems. Tell your doctor immediately if you experience any of these effects.

Warnings: Avoid excessive alcohol with this drug because it may increase the risk of adverse effects. Take care with driving and other similar activities until you have learned how this drug affects you.

Interactions: Ketoconazole interacts with a wide range of other drugs, so check with your doctor or pharmacist before taking any other medication.

Available preparations: Tablets, liquid. It is also available in the form of a shampoo to treat seborrhoeic dermatitis (dandruff – see page 201).

Brand names: Nizoral

Nystatin

General information: Nystatin is used to treat thrush infections of the mouth, gastrointestinal tract and vagina.

How to use: As antifungal drugs (see page 264).

Precautions: None

Side effects: Side effects are rare, but nausea, vomiting, diarrhoea and allergic reactions (including rash) may occur.

Interactions: None

Warnings: Alcohol is not a problem with this drug.

Available preparations: Tablets, liquid

Brand names: Nystan

Terbinafine

General information: Terbinafine is used for fungal infections of the nails, feet and head where oral, as opposed to local, treatment is needed.

How to use: As antifungal drugs (see page 264).

Precautions: Tell your doctor if you are pregnant, planning to become pregnant or are breastfeeding, or if you have or have had liver or kidney problems.

Side effects: Nausea, diarrhoea, abdominal pain, headache and various allergic reactions (including rash, itching and joint and bone pain) may occur. Tell your doctor immediately if you get a rash that spreads.

Warnings: Alcohol is not a problem with this drug.
Interactions: Terbinafine interacts with few drugs, but check with your doctor or pharmacist before taking any other medication.
Available preparations: Tablets, cream.
Brand names: Lamisil

ANTIVIRAL DRUGS

There are many different kinds of viral infection, ranging from the common cold, influenza and cold sores to more serious conditions such as measles, polio and HIV, the virus that causes AIDS. Viruses, as opposed to bacteria, are very difficult to treat. Antibiotics are useless for the treatment of viral infections. This is because viruses have quite a different structure to bacteria. Viruses contain only nucleic acid, rather than a clearly definable structure, and they survive and multiply by entering ordinary body cells using the cells' synthetic machinery to make more viral particles. Drugs that kill viruses therefore also tend to kill body cells. Immunisation (see page 319) is used to prevent various viral infections (eg measles, polio, influenza).

Antiviral drugs are used to treat specific types of viral infections, including herpes viruses (eg cold sores, shingles and genital herpes), human immunodeficiency virus (HIV) and cytomegalovirus, which is often found in AIDS patients and other people with a low resistance to infection.

How to use: Take the medicine exactly as prescribed by the doctor. If you miss a dose, take it as soon as you remember. Take the full course of treatment. Even if you feel better, the original infection may still be present and if you stop taking your medicine, your symptoms may return.

Aciclovir

General information: Aciclovir is used to treat herpes virus infection (eg cold sores, shingles, genital herpes and chickenpox). It is also used for prevention of herpes infection in people who are particularly prone to infection (such as AIDS patients). It can be used locally in the eye (see page 225) and also in the mouth (see page 240).

How to use: As antiviral drugs (see above).
Precautions: Tell your doctor if you are pregnant, planning to become pregnant or are breastfeeding, or have or have had kidney problems.
Side effects: Side effects are generally uncommon. Taken by mouth, aciclovir may cause gastrointestinal disturbances, headache, dizziness and fatigue. Used by injection, it may cause confusion and other psychotic symptoms and convulsions.
Warnings: Alcohol is not a problem with this drug.
Interactions: Aciclovir interacts with a few drugs, particularly those affecting the kidney. Check with your doctor or pharmacist before taking other medicines.
Available preparations: Tablets, liquid, injection; topical preparations (eg eye ointment and cream) are also available
Brand names: Zovirax

Amantadine

General information: Amantadine is used for the treatment of herpes zoster and for prevention of influenza type A in people who are at special risk (eg those in whom immunisation is not appropriate). It is also used in Parkinson's disease (see page 54 for further information on side effects, interactions, etc).

Cidofovir

General information: Cidofovir is used for the treatment of cytomegalovirus (CMV) in AIDS patients.

How to use: As antiviral drugs (see page 268).
Precautions: Tell your doctor if you are pregnant, planning to become pregnant or are breastfeeding, and if you have or have had liver or kidney problems or diabetes.
Side effects: This drug can cause kidney damage. Other side effects include fever, nausea and hair loss.
Warnings: No known problems with alcohol exist. You will be asked to attend for regular blood tests during treatment. Do not miss your appointments. Avoid pregnancy while taking this drug and after treatment has finished. Men should not father a child within three months of treatment.
Interactions: Cidofovir may interact with a range of other drugs. Check with your doctor or pharmacist before taking other medicines.
Available preparations: Injection
Brand names: Vistide

Didanosine

General information: Didanosine belongs to the group of drugs known as the nucleoside reverse transcriptase inhibitors. It is used in the treatment of AIDS in combination with other drugs.

How to use: As antiviral drugs (see page 268).
Precautions: Tell your doctor if you are pregnant, planning to become pregnant or are breastfeeding, or if you have or have had pancreatitis, gout, liver or kidney problems or peripheral neuropathy (tingling/numbness in the hands and feet).
Side effects: Side effects can be serious and include pancreatitis, increased uric acid levels (which may lead to gout) and peripheral neuropathy (numbness/tingling in the hands and feet). Diarrhoea, nausea, vomiting, dry mouth, diabetes, damage to the eye (especially in children) and liver problems may also occur.
Warnings: No known problems with alcohol. You will be asked to attend for regular blood tests during treatment. Do not miss your appointments.
Interactions: Didanosine may interact with a range of other drugs. Check with your doctor or pharmacist before taking other medicines.
Available preparations: Tablets
Brand names: Videx

Famciclovir

General information: Famciclovir is similar to aciclovir (see page 268) and is used to treat herpes infection (eg cold sores, shingles, genital herpes).

How to use: As antiviral drugs (see page 268).
Precautions, side effects, warnings, interactions: As aciclovir (see page 268).
Available preparations: Tablets
Brand names: Famvir

Foscarnet sodium

General information: Foscarnet is used for the treatment of cytomegalovirus retinitis in AIDS patients, and for herpes infections in patients who do not respond to aciclovir.

How to use: As antiviral drugs (see page 268).
Precautions: Tell your doctor if you are pregnant, planning to become pregnant or are breastfeeding, and if you have or have had kidney problems.
Side effects: Common side effects include nausea, vomiting, diarrhoea, abdominal pain, loss of appetite, headache, fatigue, mood changes, dizziness, confusion, convulsions, rash and a range of other effects.
Warnings: No known problems exist with alcohol. You will be asked to attend for regular blood tests during treatment. Do not miss your appointments.
Interactions: Foscarnet may interact with a range of other drugs. Check with your doctor or pharmacist before taking other medicines.
Available preparations: Injection
Brand names: Foscavir

Ganciclovir

General information: Ganciclovir is used for the treatment of cytomegalovirus (CMV) in AIDS patients and others who are immunosuppressed.

How to use: As antiviral drugs (see page 268).
Precautions: Tell your doctor if you are pregnant, planning to become pregnant or are breastfeeding, or if you have or have had kidney problems or blood disorders.
Side effects: Common side effects may include blood disorders, fever, rash, chills, infections, fluid retention and swelling, nausea, vomiting, diarrhoea, mouth ulcers, loss of appetite, swallowing difficulties, chest pain, mood changes, dizziness, confusion and a range of other effects.
Warnings: No known problems with alcohol. You will be asked to attend for regular blood tests during treatment. Do not miss your appointments. Avoid pregnancy while taking this drug and after treatment has finished. Men should not father a child within three months of treatment.
Interactions: Ganciclovir may interact with a range of other drugs. Check with your doctor or pharmacist before taking other medicines.
Available preparations: Capsules, injection
Brand names: Cymevene

Indinavir

General information: Indinavir belongs to the group of drugs known as protease inhibitors. It is used in the treatment of AIDS in combination with other drugs.

How to use: As antiviral drugs (see page 268).
Precautions: Tell your doctor if you are pregnant, planning to become pregnant or are breastfeeding, or if you have or have had liver or kidney problems or haemophilia.
Side effects: These may include nausea, vomiting, diarrhoea, abdominal discomfort, dry mouth, taste changes, headache, dizziness, insomnia, rash and other skin problems, kidney problems.
Warnings: No known problems with alcohol. You will be asked to attend for regular blood tests during treatment. Do not miss your appointments.
Interactions: Indinavir may interact with a range of other drugs. Check with your doctor or pharmacist before taking other medicines.
Available preparations: Capsules
Brand names: Crixivan

Inosine pranobex

General information: Inosine pranobex is used to treat herpes infections of the mucous membranes and surrounding areas. It is rarely used now because there is little evidence that it works.

How to use: As antiviral drugs (see page 268).
Precautions: Tell your doctor if you have or have had kidney problems or gout.
Side effects: Increase in uric acid levels which may cause gout.
Warnings: Alcohol is not a problem with this drug.
Interactions: None reported.
Available preparations: Tablets
Brand names: Immunovir

Lamivudine

General information: Lamivudine belongs to the group of drugs known as the nucleoside reverse transcriptase inhibitors. It is used in the treatment of AIDS in combination with other drugs.

How to use: As antiviral drugs (see page 268).
Precautions: Tell your doctor if you are pregnant, planning to become pregnant or are breastfeeding, or if you have or have had kidney problems.
Side effects: These may include nausea, vomiting, diarrhoea, abdominal pain, cough, headache, sleeping problems, fatigue, muscle and joint pain. Peripheral neuropathy (numbness/tingling in the hands and feet) and pancreatitis may occur, but these are rare.
Warnings: No known problems with alcohol. You will be asked to attend for regular blood tests during treatment. Do not miss your appointments.

Interactions: Lamivudine may interact with a range of other drugs. Check with your doctor or pharmacist before taking other medicines.
Available preparations: Tablets, liquid
Brand names: Epivir

Nelfinavir

General information: Nelfinavir belongs to the group of drugs known as protease inhibitors. It is used in the treatment of AIDS in combination with other drugs.

How to use: As antiviral drugs (see page 268).
Precautions: Tell your doctor if you are pregnant, planning to become pregnant or are breastfeeding, or if you have or have had liver or kidney problems, diabetes or haemophilia.
Side effects: Nausea, diarrhoea, flatulence, rash and liver problems may occur.
Warnings: No known problems with alcohol. You will be asked to attend for regular blood tests during treatment. Do not miss your appointments. Use a non-hormonal method of contraception while taking this drug.
Interactions: Nelfinavir may interact with a range of other drugs, including oral contraceptives. Check with your doctor or pharmacist before taking other medicines.
Available preparations: Tablets, powder
Brand names: Viracept

Nevirapine

General information: Nevirapine belongs to the group of drugs known as nonnucleoside reverse transcriptase inhibitors. It is used in the treatment of AIDS in combination with other drugs.

How to use: As antiviral drugs (see page 268).
Side effects: Rash is the most common symptom. In rare cases, this may be accompanied by fatigue, muscle and joint pain, itching, blistering, swelling, conjunctivitis and mouth ulcers. If you experience any of these symptoms, tell your doctor immediately. Nausea, headache and fever may also occur.
Precautions: Tell your doctor if you are pregnant, planning to become pregnant or are breastfeeding, or if you have or have had liver or kidney problems.
Warnings: No known problems with alcohol. You will be asked to attend for regular blood tests during treatment. Do not miss your appointments. Use a non-hormonal method of contraception while taking this drug.
Interactions: Nevirapine may interact with a range of other drugs, including oral contraceptives. Check with your doctor or pharmacist before taking other medicines.
Available preparations: Tablets
Brand names: Viramune

Ritonavir

General information: Ritonavir belongs to the group of drugs known as protease inhibitors. It is used in the treatment of AIDS in combination with other drugs.

How to use: As antiviral drugs (see page 268).
Precautions: Tell your doctor if you are pregnant, planning to become pregnant or are breastfeeding, or if you have or have had liver problems.
Side effects: Nausea, vomiting, diarrhoea, abdominal pain, taste changes, indigestion, loss of appetite, headache, numbness/tingling of hands and feet, dizziness, rash and other skin problems.
Warnings: No known problems exist with alcohol. You will be asked to attend for regular blood tests during treatment. Do not miss your appointments. Use a non-hormonal method of contraception while taking this drug.
Interactions: Ritonavir may interact with a range of other drugs, including oral contraceptives. Check with your doctor or pharmacist before taking other medicines.
Available preparations: Capsules, liquid
Brand names: Norvir

Saquinavir

General information: Saquinavir belongs to the group of drugs known as protease inhibitors. It is used in the treatment of AIDS in combination with other drugs.

How to use: As antiviral drugs (see page 268).
Precautions: Tell your doctor if you are pregnant, planning to become pregnant or are breastfeeding, or if you have or have had liver or kidney problems or haemophilia.
Side effects: Nausea, diarrhoea, abdominal discomfort, mouth ulcers, headache, numbness/tingling of hands and feet, rash and other skin problems.
Warnings: No known problems exist with alcohol. You will be asked to attend for regular blood tests during treatment. Do not miss your appointments.
Interactions: Saquinavir may interact with a range of other drugs. Check with your doctor or pharmacist before taking other medicines.
Available preparations: Capsules
Brand names: Invirase

Stavudine

General information: Stavudine belongs to the group of drugs known as the nucleoside reverse transcriptase inhibitors. It is used in the treatment of AIDS in combination with other drugs.

How to use: As antiviral drugs (see page 268).
Precautions: Tell your doctor if you are pregnant, planning to become pregnant or are breastfeeding, or if you have or have had pancreatitis, liver or kidney problems or peripheral neuropathy (tingling/numbness in the hands and feet).

Side effects: Side effects can be serious and include pancreatitis and peripheral neuropathy (numbness/tingling in the hands and feet). Diarrhoea, constipation, nausea, vomiting, abdominal discomfort, chest pain, breathlessness, headache, sleeping problems, dizziness, joint and bone pain, mood changes, rash and other allergic symptoms may occur.

Warnings: No known problems exist with alcohol. You will be asked to attend for regular blood tests during treatment. Do not miss your appointments.

Interactions: Stavudine may interact with a range of other drugs. Check with your doctor or pharmacist before taking other medicines.

Available preparations: Capsules, liquid

Brand names: Zerit

Tribavirin

General information: Tribavirin is used in severe bronchiolitis caused by respiratory syncytial virus in infants and children.

How to use: As antiviral drugs (see page 268).

Side effects: Reduced breathing capacity and other lung disorders, anaemia.

Warnings: None

Interactions: None reported.

Available preparations: Inhalation

Brand names: Virazid

Valaciclovir

General information: Valaciclovir is similar to aciclovir and is used to treat herpes infection (eg cold sores, shingles, genital herpes).

How to use: As antiviral drugs (see page 268).

Precautions, side effects, warnings, interactions: As aciclovir (see page 268).

Available preparations: Tablets

Brand names: Valtrex

Zalcitabine

General information: Zalcitabine belongs to the group of drugs known as the nucleoside reverse transcriptase inhibitors. It is used in the treatment of AIDS in combination with other drugs.

How to use: As antiviral drugs (see page 268).

Precautions: Tell your doctor if you are pregnant, planning to become pregnant or are breastfeeding, or if you have or have had pancreatitis, liver or kidney problems, heart failure or peripheral neuropathy (tingling/numbness in the hands and feet).

Side effects: Side effects can be serious and include pancreatitis and peripheral neuropathy (numbness/tingling in the hands and feet). Diarrhoea, nausea, vomiting, abdominal pain, loss of appetite, mouth ulcers, chest pain, sweating, fever, headache, dizziness, joint and bone pain, rash and other allergic symptoms may also occur.

Warnings: No known problems with alcohol. You will be asked to attend for regular blood tests during treatment. Do not miss your appointments.

Interactions: Zalcitabine may interact with a range of other drugs. Check with your doctor or pharmacist before taking other medicines.

Available preparations: Tablets

Brand names: Hivid

Zidovudine

General information: Zidovudine belongs to the group of drugs known as the nucleoside reverse transcriptase inhibitors. It is used in the treatment of AIDS in combination with other drugs.

How to use: As antiviral drugs (see page 268).

Precautions: Tell your doctor if you are pregnant, planning to become pregnant or are breastfeeding, or if you have or have had liver or kidney problems, or blood disorders.

Side effects: The most common side effect is anaemia, causing pallor, tiredness and shortness of breath. Other side effects include: nausea, vomiting, abdominal pain, loss of appetite, fever, headache, joint and bone pain, rash and other allergic symptoms.

Warnings: No known problems with alcohol. You will be asked to attend for regular blood tests during treatment. Do not miss your appointments.

Interactions: Zidovudine may interact with a range of other drugs. Check with your doctor or pharmacist before taking other medicines.

Available preparations: Tablets, capsules, liquid, injection

Brand names: Retrovir

Combination preparations: Combivir (zidovudine and lamivudine)

ANTIMALARIAL DRUGS

Malaria is one of the main killer diseases in tropical countries. However, there are also now over 2,000 cases of malaria in the UK each year, including a number of deaths. Almost all cases of malaria are caught while travelling abroad. The disease is caused by infection with the malaria parasite, known as *Plasmodium*, which lives for part of its life cycle in the female mosquito. The infection is transmitted to humans by the bite of the female mosquito.

A number of drugs are available for both the treatment and prevention of malaria. For treatment, the drug or drugs used will depend on the part of the world you have visited and the likely strain of malaria you may have caught. For prevention, again the area of the world you plan to visit will govern the drugs that you are recommended to take. Ask your doctor or pharmacist for advice.

How to use: Take the medicine exactly as prescribed by the doctor. If you miss a dose, take it as soon as you remember. For malaria prevention, start to take the medicine one week (2–3 weeks in the case of mefloquine) before you travel and continue for at least 4 weeks after. For malaria treatment, take the full course of treatment. Even if you feel better, the original infection may still be present and if you stop taking your medicine, your symptoms may return.

Remember that taking malaria tablets is not a guarantee of total protection. You must also take steps to prevent being bitten. Wear clothes with long sleeves and trousers, particularly after dusk, and always use a mosquito net impregnated with permethrin. Lotions, sprays and roll-ons containing diethyltoluamide (DEET) are effective when applied to the skin, but their effect lasts only a few hours and you must re-apply them frequently. In addition, if you develop a feverish illness within one year of your return (and especially in the first three months), you should seek medical advice. Tell your doctor exactly where you have been travelling, in case you have developed malaria.

Chloroquine

General information: Chloroquine is used in the prevention and treatment of malaria. It is also used in autoimmune disease such as rheumatoid arthritis (see page 145) and systemic lupus erythmatosus.

How to use: As antimalarials (see page 275).

Precautions: Tell your doctor if you are pregnant, planning to become pregnant or are breastfeeding, or if you have or have had liver or kidney problems, psoriasis, eye or vision problems, epilepsy, myasthenia gravis or glucose 6-phosphate dehydrogenase (G6PD) deficiency.

Side effects: Gastrointestinal disturbances (eg nausea, diarrhoea, abdominal pain) are the most common. Headache, dizziness, convulsions and rash may occur. If you experience any visual changes, tell your doctor immediately.

Warnings: Avoid excessive alcohol intake. Take care with driving and other similar activities until you know how the drug affects you.

Interactions: Chloroquine interacts with various other drugs such as digoxin, amiodarone, and cyclosporin. It also interacts with halofantrine, another drug used in the treatment of malaria. Tell your doctor or pharmacist if you are taking other medicines.

Available preparations: Tablets, liquid, injection
Brand names: Avloclor, Nivaquine

Halofantrine

General information: Halofantrine is used for the treatment of malaria.

How to use: As antimalarials (see page 275).

Precautions: Tell your doctor if you are pregnant, planning to become pregnant or are breastfeeding, or if you have or have had any heart disease.

Side effects: Diarrhoea, abdominal pain, vomiting, nausea, arrhythmias (abnormal heart beats), rash and other allergic reactions may occur.

Warnings: None

Interactions: Halofantrine interacts with several other drugs, including drugs used

for heart conditions, beta-blockers, antipsychotics and other sedatives and anhista-mines (astemizole and terfenadine).
Available preparations: Tablets
Brand names: Halfan

Mefloquine

General information: Mefloquine is used for the prevention and treatment of malaria.

How to use: As antimalarials (see page 275).
Precautions: Tell your doctor if you are pregnant, planning to become pregnant or are breastfeeding, or if you have or have had any heart disease, epilepsy or history of psychiatric disorders, including depression.
Side effects: Diarrhoea, abdominal pain, vomiting, nausea, dizziness, loss of balance, sleep disturbances, anxiety, panic attacks, depression, hallucinations, visual distur-bances, ringing in the ears, palpitations, muscle weakness, joint pain, fever, loss of appetite, rash and other allergic reactions may occur. If you experience severe side effects, seek medical advice before taking the next dose.
Warnings: Avoid pregnancy during treatment and for three months after.
Interactions: Mefloquine interacts with several other drugs, including drugs used for heart conditions, beta-blockers, antipsychotics and anticonvulsants.
Available preparations: Tablets
Brand names: Lariam

Primaquine

General information: Primaquine is used in the treatment of malaria with chloro-quine.

How to use: As antimalarials (see page 275).
Precautions: Tell your doctor if you are pregnant, planning to become pregnant or are breastfeeding, or if you have or have had glucose 6-phosphate dehydrogenase (G6PD) deficiency, rheumatoid arthritis or systemic lupus erythmatosus.
Side effects: Nausea, vomiting and abdominal pain may occur.
Warnings: None
Interactions: Primaquine interacts with few other drugs. Ask your pharmacist or doctor before taking any other medicines.
Available preparations: Tablets
Brand names: None

Proguanil

General information: Proguanil is used for the prevention of malaria in conjunction with chloroquine.

How to use: As antimalarials (see page 275).

Precautions: Tell your doctor if you are pregnant, planning to become pregnant or are breastfeeding, or if you have or have had kidney problems.

Side effects: Mild gastrointestinal disturbances and diarrhoea. Occasionally mouth ulcers, hair loss and rash may occur.

Warnings: None

Interactions: Proguanil interacts with oral anticoagulants. Ask your pharmacist or doctor before taking any other medicines.

Available preparations: Tablets

Brand names: Paludrine

Combination preparations: Paludrine/Avloclor (travel pack containing tablets of chloroquine and proguanil); Macaroon (proguanil and atovaquone – for malaria treatment)

Pyrimethamine

General information: Pyrimethamine is mainly used in combination with sulfadoxine to treat malaria and in combination with dapsone for malaria prevention.

How to use: As antimalarials (see page 275).

Precautions: Tell your doctor if you are pregnant, planning to become pregnant or are breastfeeding, or if you have or have had liver or kidney problems.

Side effects: Various blood disorders, insomnia and rash may occur.

Warnings: None

Interactions: Ask your pharmacist or doctor before taking any other medicines.

Available preparations: Tablets

Brand names: Daraprim

Combination preparations: Fansidar (pyrimethamine and sulfadoxine); Maloprim (pyrimethamine and dapsone)

Quinine

General information: Quinine is used for the treatment of malaria.

How to use: As antimalarials (see page 275).

Precautions: Tell your doctor if you are pregnant, planning to become pregnant or are breastfeeding, or if you have or have had heart problems, optic neuritis or glucose 6-phosphate dehydrogenase deficiency.

Side effects: These may include ringing in the ears, loss of hearing, nausea, abdominal pain, rash and flushed skin, visual disturbances and confusion.

Warnings: None

Interactions: Quinine interacts with several other drugs including digoxin, amiodarone, flecainide and some antihistamines (eg astemizole and terfenadine). Ask your pharmacist or doctor before taking any other medicines.

Available preparations: Tablets

Brand names: None

ANTIPROTOZOAL DRUGS

Protozoa are microscopic organisms, mostly found in soil and water, whose life cycles are extremely complicated. They may live in an insect or an animal for part of their life cycle and in a human for another part. They are transmitted to or in between humans by means of contaminated water, food, sexual contact or insect bites or other animal carriers. Several diseases, some of which are more common in tropical countries than in the UK, are caused by protozoa. Malaria (see page 275) is the best-known example, but others include amoebiasis and giardiasis, both of which are protozoal infestations of the bowel. Leishmaniasis affects the mucous membranes of the mouth, nose and throat, and sometimes the liver. Pneumocystitis pneumonia, a potentially fatal lung infection, generally affects only those with reduced resistance to infection, such as patients with AIDS. Other examples include trichomoniasis (an infection which commonly affects the vagina), trypanasomiasis (sleeping sickness) and toxoplasmosis.

Metronidazole (see page 218) and tinidazole (see page 259) are used for amoebiasis, giardiasis and trichomonas vaginitis. Other drugs used for protozoal infections are listed below.

How to use: Take the medicine exactly as prescribed by the doctor. If you miss a dose, take it as soon as you remember. Take the full course of treatment. Even if you feel better, the original infection may still be present and if you stop taking your medicine, your symptoms may return.

Atovaquone

General information: Atovaquone is used in the treatment of pneumocystitis pneumonia in patients who cannot tolerate co-trimoxazole.

How to use: As antiprotozoal drugs (see above).
Precautions: Tell your doctor if you are pregnant, planning to become pregnant or are breastfeeding, or have or have had liver or kidney problems.
Side effects: These may include diarrhoea, nausea, vomiting, headache, insomnia, fever and rash.
Warnings: None
Interactions: Atovaquone interacts with few other drugs. Check with your doctor or pharmacist before taking any other medication.
Available preparations: Liquid
Brand names: Wellvone

Diloxanide

General information: Diloxanide is used in the treatment of amoebiasis.

How to use: As antiprotozoal drugs (see above).
Precautions: None
Side effects: These may include vomiting, flatulence, itching skin.
Warnings, interactions: None
Available preparations: Tablets
Brand names: Furamide

Mepacrine

General information: Mepacrine is used in the treatment of giardiasis.

How to use: As antiprotozoal drugs (see page 279).
Precautions: Tell your doctor if you have or have had liver problems, psoriasis or any psychotic condition.
Side effects: These may include gastrointestinal disturbances (occasionally nausea and vomiting), dizziness, headache and mental disturbances. Prolonged treatment may cause yellowing of the skin and urine, skin disorders, blue-black discoloration of the nails and palate, and visual disturbances.
Warnings: None
Interactions: Mepacrine interacts with few other drugs. Check with your pharmacist or doctor before taking any other medication.
Available preparations: Tablets
Brand names: None

Pentamidine

General information: Pentamidine is used in the treatment of pneumocystitis pneumonia, leishmaniasis and trypanosomiasis. This drug is given under specialist supervision only.

How to use: As antiprotozoal drugs (see page 279).
Precautions: Tell your doctor if you are pregnant, planning to become pregnant or are breastfeeding, or have or have had liver or kidney problems, diabetes, high or low blood pressure or any blood disorders.
Side effects: Side effects can be severe and include low blood pressure, low blood sugar, pancreatitis, dizziness, flushing, rash and a range of other disturbances.
Warnings: None
Interactions: Pentamidine interacts with few other drugs. Check with your pharmacist or doctor before taking any other medication.
Available preparations: Injection, solution for inhalation
Brand names: Pentacarinat

Sodium stibogluconate

General information: Sodium stibogluconate is used in the treatment of leishmaniasis.

How to use: As antiprotozoal drugs (see page 279).
Precautions: Tell your doctor if you are pregnant, planning to become pregnant or are breastfeeding, or have or have had liver or heart problems.
Side effects: Loss of appetite, nausea, vomiting, abdominal pain, headache, lethargy and occasionally allergic reactions may occur.
Warnings: None
Interactions: Sodium stibogluconate interacts with few other drugs. Check with your pharmacist or doctor before taking any other medication.
Available preparations: Injection
Brand names: Pentostam

Trimetrexate

General information: Trimetrexate is used for the treatment of pneumocystitis pneumonia

How to use: As antiprotozoal drugs (see page 279).

Precautions: Tell your doctor if you are pregnant, planning to become pregnant or are breastfeeding, or have or have had liver or kidney problems.

Side effects: These may include vomiting, diarrhoea, mouth ulcers, fever, confusion, rash and other allergic reactions.

Warnings: Men should avoid fathering a child and women should avoid pregnancy for at least six months after treatment.

Interactions: Trimetrexate interacts with few other drugs. Check with your pharmacist or doctor before taking any other medication.

Available preparations: Injection

Brand names: Neutrexin

ANTHELMINTICS

Anthelmintics are drugs used in the treatment of worm infestations. Worms are parasites that live for part of their life cycle in animals and part in humans. Many worm infestations are transmitted to humans in contaminated food that carries the eggs of young worms. Most worms live in the intestine where they feed from the intestinal contents or blood supply.

Some worms cause fairly mild symptoms whereas others can cause a great deal of harm. The most dangerous infestations tend to occur in developing countries, but those that occur in Britain tend to be relatively harmless. The most common worm infestation in Britain is caused by threadworm.

Threadworm is easily transmitted through unwashed hands, etc. The worm grows in the intestine and passes out to the skin round the anus where it lays eggs during the night. This causes itching and if the area is scratched, the eggs lodge under the finger nails. If the hands are not washed and the nails not scrubbed, the eggs can easily be swallowed and enter the gut. Good hygiene is therefore essential to break the chain of infection.

Another worm infestation is caused by roundworm and a much rarer one by tapeworm. Most worm infestation can be effectively eliminated with drugs known as anthelmintics.

How to use: Take the medicine exactly as prescribed by the doctor. If you miss a dose, take it as soon as you remember. Take the full course of treatment. Even if you feel better, the original infection may still be present and if you stop taking your medicine, your symptoms may return.

Albendazole

General information: Albendazole is used for the treatment of strongyloidiasis (tropical threadworm) and other infestations.

How to use: As anthelmintics (see page 281).
Precautions: Tell your doctor if you are pregnant, planning to become pregnant or are breastfeeding.
Side effects: Side effects are rare, but the following may occur: gastrointestinal disturbances, headache, dizziness and rash.
Warnings: Avoid pregnancy and use a non-hormonal method of contraception during treatment and for one month afterwards.
Interactions: Albendazole interacts with few other drugs. Check with your pharmacist or doctor before taking any other medicines.
Available preparations: Tablets
Brand names: Eskazole

Mebendazole

General information: Mebendazole is used for threadworm, roundworm and other similar infestations.

How to use: As anthelmintics (see page 281). It is given as a single dose, which may be repeated after 2–3 weeks. It is often necessary to treat the whole family to avoid repeated infections.
Precautions: Tell your doctor if you are pregnant, planning to become pregnant or are breastfeeding. This drug is not recommended for pregnant women or children under the age of 2 years.
Side effects: Side effects are rare, but the following may occur: diarrhoea and abdominal pain, rash and other allergic reactions.
Warnings: None
Interactions: Mebendazole interacts with few other drugs. Check with your pharmacist or doctor before taking any other medicines.
Available preparations: Tablets, liquid
Brand names: Vermox

Piperazine

General information: Piperazine is used for roundworm and threadworm.

How to use: As anthelmintics (see page 281). For roundworm, it is given as a single dose, which may be repeated after 2–4 weeks, depending on the preparation and your doctor's instructions. For threadworm it may be given daily for one week (liquid only) or as a single dose (powder only) and repeated after 7–14 days, depending on the preparation and your doctor's instructions. It is often necessary to treat the whole family to prevent recurring infection.
Precautions: Tell your doctor if you are pregnant, planning to become pregnant or are breastfeeding, or if you have or have had epilepsy or kidney problems.

Side effects: Side effects are rare, but the following may occur: nausea, vomiting, diarrhoea and abdominal pain, dizziness, drowsiness, confusion, incoordination, rash and other allergic reactions.
Warnings: Take care with driving and other similar activities until you know how the drug affects you.
Interactions: Piperazine interacts with few other drugs. Check with your pharmacist or doctor before taking any other medicines.
Available preparations: Powder, liquid
Brand names: Pripsen (also contains senna, a laxative)

Niclosamide

General information: Niclosamide is used for tapeworm.

How to use: As anthelmintics (see page 281). Take the prescribed dose followed by a purgative two hours later (to empty the bowel and expel the tapeworm).
Precautions: None
Side effects: Side effects are rare, but the following may occur: nausea and retching, light-headedness and itching skin.
Warnings: None
Interactions: None
Available preparations: Tablets
Brand names: Yomesan

Thiabendazole

General information: Thiabendazole is used for the treatment of strongyloidiasis (tropical threadworm) and other infestations.

How to use: As anthelmintics (see page 281).
Precautions: Tell your doctor if you are pregnant or breastfeeding, or have or have had liver or kidney problems.
Side effects: These may include loss of appetite, nausea, vomiting, dizziness, drowsiness, diarrhoea, headache, itching skin and other allergic reactions.
Warnings: Take care with driving and other similar tasks until you know how the drug affects you.
Interactions: Thiabendazole interacts with few other drugs. Check with your pharmacist or doctor before taking any other medicines.
Available preparations: Tablets
Brand names: Mintezol

Allergy

AN ALLERGIC REACTION is an inappropriate or excessive reaction of the body's immune system to a substance from outside, which in most people is harmless. In a person who is allergic to the substance, however, it causes an unpleasant – and in some instances a dangerous – reaction. An allergic reaction involves antibodies, known as immunoglobulins – usually immunoglobulin E (IgE). IgE antibodies attach themselves to special body cells and when they encounter allergens in the blood, the cells release chemicals, including histamine, that damage surrounding tissues. An allergen can be almost anything, including food, dust, a drug or pollen, and is said to be an antigen which stimulates an allergic response.

Allergic reactions range from mild to severe. Most reactions are just a nuisance and consist of an itchy skin rash, itchy eyes or sneezing. At the other end of the spectrum, allergy can be life-threatening and may result in severe breathing difficulty and malfunctioning of the heart, leading to shock. Known as anaphylaxis, this type of reaction occurs in some people after eating certain foods (peanuts are a well known culprit) and after taking certain medicines or being stung by a wasp or bee.

Allergy sometimes runs in families. Hayfever, eczema and asthma are examples of allergic conditions that may be inherited, and the tendency is known as atopy.

The best treatment for an allergy is to avoid the offending substance, but this is often easier said than done. It may involve avoiding a certain food, banning a pet from the home or keeping the car windows shut in the summer when driving through the countryside. If house dust is suspected, the removal of carpets and the covering of mattresses and pillows with plastic protectors may help. However, because some allergens cannot be avoided, drugs – usually antihistamines – are sometimes used to block the allergic response and relieve the symptoms. Adrenaline is used in emergencies (see page 288).

ANTIHISTAMINE

Antihistamines are the drugs most commonly used in allergies such as hayfever and allergic rash, including allergic eczema. They are also used in the treatment of insect bites and stings. Some antihistamines are used for the prevention and treatment of travel sickness (see page 70).

There are nearly 20 antihistamines available for the treatment of allergy and they differ mainly in their duration of action and frequency of side effects. Many antihistamines have been on the market for a long time and these older antihistamines (eg chlorpheniramine) tend to be relatively short acting compared with the longer duration of action in newer ones (eg cetirizine, loratadine). All antihistamines can cause drowsiness, but the older ones are more sedating than the newer ones.

Many allergic reactions involve the production of the chemical called histamine. Histamine causes several adverse reactions, including itching of the skin, sneezing, and itching and watering of the eyes and nose – symptoms that are characteristic of eczema and hayfever. Antihistamines block the production of histamine and by so doing they inhibit the adverse effects.

How to use: Take antihistamines exactly as prescribed. If you miss a dose, take it as soon as you remember.

Precautions: Tell your doctor if you are pregnant, planning to become pregnant or are breastfeeding, or have or have had prostate enlargement, problems passing urine, glaucoma, liver problems, epilepsy, heart disease or porphyria.

Side effects: All the antihistamines can cause drowsiness, but some (eg chlorpheniramine, promethazine) do this more than others (eg cetirizine, loratadine). In addition, all the antihistamines can cause dry mouth, blurred vision, gastrointestinal disturbances and dizziness, but the older, more sedative antihistamines are more likely to do this than the newer, less sedating drugs. Some antihistamines – notably astemizole and terfenadine – can have adverse effects on the heart (eg rapid, irregular heart beat and palpitations). It is for this reason, and also because of the risk of dangerous interactions with other drugs, that astemizole and terfenadine have recently reverted to prescription-only status after several years of being available over the counter.

Warnings: Alcohol is best avoided with the more sedative antihistamines (see individual drugs listed below). Take care with driving or other similar activities until you know how the drug affects you, because it may cause drowsiness and dizziness.

Interactions: Other sedative drugs (eg antidepressants, hypnotics, drugs for anxiety) may increase the sedative effects of antihistamines. Other drugs (eg those used for various heart conditions and some antibiotics) can cause a dangerous interaction with the antihistamines astemizole and terfenadine.

Acrivastine

General information: Acrivastine is a relatively non-sedating antihistamine used for relief of allergies such as hayfever and itching skin.

Available preparations: Capsules
Brand names: Semprex

Astemizole

General information: Astemizole is a relatively non-sedating antihistamine used for relief of allergies such as hayfever and itching skin. It is particularly important that you ask your doctor or pharmacist before taking any other medicines while taking this drug. Interactions can cause serious effects in the heart.

Available preparations: Tablets, liquid
Brand names: Hismanal

Azatadine

General information: Azatadine is a sedative antihistamine used for relief of allergies such as hayfever and itching skin.

Available preparations: Tablets, liquid
Brand names: Optimine

Brompheniramine

General information: Brompheniramine is a sedative antihistamine used for relief of allergies such as hayfever and itching skin.

Available preparations: Tablets
Brand names: Dimotane, Dimotane LA

Cetirizine

General information: Cetirizine is a relatively non-sedating antihistamine used for relief of allergies such as hayfever and itching skin.

Available preparations: Tablets
Brand names: Zirtek

Chlorpheniramine

General information: Chlorpheniramine is a sedative antihistamine used for relief of allergies such as hayfever and itching skin.

Available preparations: Tablets, liquid, injection
Brand names: Piriton

Clemastine

General information: Clemastine is a sedative antihistamine used for relief of allergies such as hayfever and itching skin.

Available preparations: Tablets, liquid
Brand names: Tavegil

Cyproheptadine

General information: Cyproheptadine is a sedative antihistamine used for relief of allergies such as hayfever and itching skin.

Available preparations: Tablets
Brand names: Periactin

Fexofenadine

General information: Fexofenadine is a relatively non-sedating antihistamine used for relief of allergies such as hayfever and itching skin.

Available preparations: Tablets
Brand names: Telfast

Hydroxyzine

General information: Hydroxyzine is a sedative antihistamine used for relief of itching skin.

Available preparations: Tablets, liquid
Brand names: Atarax, Ucerax

Ketotifen

General information: Ketotifen is an antihistamine which is used in asthma (it is the only antihistamine for use in asthma and it is used rarely).

Available preparations: Tablets, capsules, liquid
Brand names: Zaditen

Loratadine

General information: Loratadine is a relatively non-sedating antihistamine used for relief of allergies such as hayfever and itching skin.

Available preparations: Tablets, liquid
Brand names: Clarityn

Mequitazine

General information: Mequitazine is a sedative antihistamine used for relief of itching skin.

Available preparations: Tablets
Brand names: Primalan

Mizolastine

General information: Mizolastine is a relatively non-sedating antihistamine used for relief of allergies such as hayfever and itching skin.

Available preparations: Tablets
Brand names: Mizollen

Phenindamine

General information: Phenindamine is a sedative antihistamine used for relief of allergy such as hayfever and itching skin. This drug may cause mild over-stimulation in some individuals.

Available preparations: Tablets
Brand names: Thephorin

Promethazine

General information: Promethazine is a sedative antihistamine used for relief of allergy such as hayfever and itching skin.

Available preparations: Tablets, liquid, injection
Brand names: Phenergan

Terfenadine

General information: Terfenadine is a relatively non-sedating antihistamine used for relief of allergies such as hayfever and itching skin. It is particularly important that you ask your doctor or pharmacist before taking any other medicines while taking this drug. Interactions can cause serious effects in the heart.

Available preparations: Tablets, liquid
Brand names: Triludan

Trimeprazine

General information: Trimeprazine is a sedative antihistamine used for relief of itching skin.

Available preparations: Tablets, liquid
Brand names: Vallergan

ADRENALINE

Adrenaline is not technically an anti-allergy drug. However, it is used in the emergency treatment of severe allergic reactions (anaphylactic shock) to drugs, insect bites and stings and other substances – notably peanuts. It can be life-saving in anaphylactic shock, since it is able to act as a bronchial dilator, dilating the airways of the lung. These become constricted by the release of histamine due to the allergic reaction, causing severe, asthma-like attack. People at risk of anaphylaxis are often given adrenaline in the form of a pen-like device to inject themselves. This device is pre-assembled and ready to use and should be injected intramuscularly.

How to use: Learn carefully how to use the injection before it is needed, and make sure that your friends and family know too. If it is a child that could be affected, make sure that school staff know about his or her condition, so that the preparation can be injected rapidly should the child collapse suddenly. When given by injection, adrenaline takes about 5 minutes to work and is life-saving.

Precautions: Tell your doctor if you have thyroid disease, diabetes, heart problems or high blood pressure.

Side effects: Nervousness, rapid or irregular heart beat, nausea, vomiting sweating. (When given for anaphylaxis any of these could also be symptoms of the allergic reaction.)

Warnings: None

Interactions: Adrenaline interacts with various drugs, but for anaphylaxis it is a life-saving drug. Check in advance with your doctor about other medicines you may be taking.

Available preparations: Intramuscular injection for self-medication

Brand names: EpiPen, EpiPen Junior

Cancer

CANCER IS ESSENTIALLY the disordered and uncontrolled growth of cells. In other words, the affected cells have lost their normal control mechanisms and their growth is therefore unregulated. Cancer can develop from any tissue within any organ. As cancer cells grow and multiply, they form a mass of cancerous tissue that invades nearby tissue and can spread (metastasis) round the body.

Cancer is extremely common. In the UK, one in three people will develop the disease at some time in their lives, and one in four will die from it. The incidence of specific cancers varies, but a few common cancers such as cancers of the lung, bowel and skin in both men and women, breast in women and prostate in men are responsible for a large proportion of the total. Although skin cancers are common, they account for only a small proportion of the deaths from cancer.

A host of genetic and environmental factors increase the risk of developing cancer. Age is an important factor and many cancers, including those of the prostate, colon and stomach, are most likely to occur after the age of 60. The increased risk of cancer with age is probably a combination of prolonged exposure to cancer-causing agents (carcinogens) and weakening of the body's immune system, both of which are associated with a longer life span. However, some cancers, such as acute lymphocytic leukaemia and Burkitt's lymphoma, occur almost exclusively in young people. Why these cancers occur in the young is not fully understood, but genetic predisposition is one factor. Cancer is the commonest cause of death in children between the ages of 3 and 13.

Genetics and family history play a role in the development of some adult cancers too. For example, a woman's risk of developing breast cancer increases more than twice if her mother or sister had breast cancer.

A number of environmental factors also increase the risk of cancer of which one of the most important is cigarette smoking. Smoking substantially increases the risk of developing cancers of the lung, mouth, throat, oesophagus and bladder.

Diet is another important factor, and it is thought that as many as one third of all cancers could be linked to poor diet. Current evidence suggests that a diet containing plenty of fruit and vegetables – five or more servings a day – reduces the risk of almost all cancers. A diet high in dietary fibre (eg wholemeal bread, brown pasta, brown rice, wholegrain and high fibre breakfast cereals, peas, beans and lentils) is thought to reduce the risk of colon cancer and a diet low in fat may help to prevent cancers of the breast, colon and prostate. People who drink large amounts of alcohol are at increased risk of cancers of the throat and oesophagus.

Several chemicals are known to cause cancer. For example, asbestos exposure may cause a type of lung cancer. Cancer may also be caused by certain viruses. Hepatitis B, for example, can cause liver cancer and the papilloma virus that causes genital warts is probably one cause of cervical cancer in women. Some human retroviruses, such as HIV (the virus that causes AIDS), can cause lymphomas and other cancers of the blood.

In general, early diagnosis and treatment of cancer improves the outcome. The signs and symptoms of cancer are many and various, so anything unusual should be reported to your doctor immediately to increase the chance of successful treatment. In particular, if you notice any of the following changes – particularly if they persist for more than two weeks – see your doctor. These could be a change in bowel or bladder habits, a nagging cough, hoarseness, indigestion, difficulty in swallowing, a lump in the breast, testicle, or anywhere else in the body, any unusual bleeding or discharge from the vagina, bladder, back passage or nipple, a noticeable change in a wart or mole or a sore in the mouth or on the skin which does not heal.

Screening programmes for some cancers have been set up to enable early changes to be detected. One example of this is the cervical smear test which is used to detect pre-cancerous cells in the cervix. The Breast Screening Programme has been established to try to reduce the number of women who die each year from breast cancer. A special X-ray called a mammogram can detect very small lumps or areas of abnormal cells in the breast before the lump can be felt by the individual.

If your doctor suspects you have cancer, you will usually be referred to a hospital specialist for various tests. A biopsy, which means taking a sample of the suspect tissue, is the most common method for confirming a diagnosis of cancer, but many other tests, including blood tests, X-rays and various other scanning techniques may be used to determine the extent and type of the cancer.

When the results of the tests and investigations have been obtained, you will be advised on the type of treatment you can have. Basically there are three types of treatment – surgery, radiotherapy and chemotherapy. In addition some cancers are dependent on sex hormones, so appropriate hormone treatment may be used.

CHEMOTHERAPY

Chemotherapy is treatment with drugs. These drugs, of which there are more than 50, are often known as cytotoxics. They are given to destroy or control the growth of cancer cells, and may also be prescribed to prevent development of further cancer in people who have already had some form of treatment for cancer (eg surgery or radiotherapy).

Cytotoxic drugs destroy cancer cells by interfering with their ability to grow and divide, often by targeting the cells' nucleic acids. Because normal cells grow and develop using similar mechanisms to cancer cells, rapidly dividing normal cells may be damaged too, especially in the bone marrow, gut, ovaries, testes, hair follicles and skin. As cancer cells can become resistant to drugs used in chemotherapy, combinations of drugs are often given, usually as courses of treatment with rest periods to allow for the recovery of normal tissue.

How they are used: Some cytotoxics are given by mouth in the form of tablets or capsules. Others are given by injection or drip (infusion) into a vein, although a few are given by injection into a muscle or under the skin.

A course of chemotherapy usually continues over several months and the specific treatment will be prescribed for you by a doctor who specialises in cytotoxic drug treatment (a medical oncologist). The chosen regime may be such that you have an injection one week, or tablets for one week, then three or four weeks off. The total length of treatment will depend on how well your disease responds to the drugs. This will be investigated by the use of blood tests, X-rays and various other tests.

Some cytotoxic drugs can be given over a few minutes while others must be given over several hours. You may therefore have to go into hospital for a period of 24–48 hours to have chemotherapy, but often you will be treated as an out-patient.

Precautions: These relate mainly to the side effects of the drugs (see below). In addition always discuss your treatment if you are pregnant or breastfeeding.

Side effects: Side effects are often encountered with cytotoxic drugs. However, the situation is continuously improving with the development of newer drugs that often cause fewer side effects than their predecessors. Individuals also differ in their experience of side effects. Some people suffer very little and are able to carry on much as usual, while others find the drugs influence their day-to-day activities considerably. The side effects you experience will also depend on the precise drug or drugs prescribed for you and your doctor or nurse will advise you what to expect.

The most well-known side effects of cytotoxics are nausea and vomiting. Not every drug will cause this, but platinum-based compounds and doxorubicin are more likely to have this effect. Some patients are more susceptible than others. Those most commonly affected include people under 50, women, anxious patients and those who experience travel sickness. Symptoms may occur within the first 24 hours of treatment or more than 24 hours after treatment. They may sometimes also be anticipatory – that is, sickness starts before a dose of chemotherapy is given. This is particularly common if your chemotherapy has made you vomit before. If your doctor thinks that you are at risk of nausea and vomiting, you will be given an anti-emetic drug (see page 70) to help, and certain modern anti-emetics are particularly effective.

Another side effect of chemotherapy is bone marrow suppression. The bone marrow is the place where your blood cells are made and cytotoxic drugs can affect their production. This may in turn lead to anaemia and a reduction in blood cell counts. People on chemotherapy therefore have regular blood counts to make sure that their bone marrow is not being too badly affected. If the blood counts fall too low, the doctor will adjust the dose of the drug regimen.

Usually the count is at its lowest 10–14 days after chemotherapy, and many people feel quite tired and depressed at this time. However, your bone marrow normally starts to recover and your blood count will increase again, which will usually make you feel better. If your blood count is still very low by the time you are ready for the next dose of chemotherapy, the doctor may delay giving you more of the drug until your count has fully recovered.

It is important to watch out for symptoms of a low blood count. A drop in your red cell count will mean that you become anaemic, and you may feel tired or short of breath. A drop in the white cell count will make you more prone to infection. If you experience a sore throat or a mouth sore that does not heal, or any other signs of infection, tell your doctor immediately. If your platelet count falls too low, you will often find that you bruise more easily and that your gums bleed, particularly when you brush your teeth. Report any of these signs to your doctor.

Another possible side effect of chemotherapy is hair loss. This is not inevitable and it is always reversible. In other words your hair will grow again, although it may grow back a slightly different colour or texture. Treat your hair very gently. Use a soft brush and a gentle shampoo, and if you are out in the sun, cover your head. If your doctor thinks that you are likely to lose a lot of hair, he or she will recommend a wig and you can arrange to have one made before your treatment starts.

ANTI-CANCER DRUGS

Aclarubicin

General information: Aclarubicin is used in acute lymphocytic leukaemia (in patients who have relapsed or are resistant to first-line chemotherapy).

Side effects: As above; this drug may also affect the heart.
Available preparations: Injection
Brand names: Aclacin

Aldesleukin

General information: Aldesleukin is used in kidney cancer.

Side effects: As above; this drug may have effects upon the nervous system, liver, kidney and cause thyroid toxicity.
Available preparations: Injection
Brand names: Proleukin

Altretamine

General information: Altretamine is used in acute ovarian cancer where other treatments have failed.

Side effects: As above; this drug may also cause toxicity to the nervous system, kidney and liver, as well as rash and itching.
Available preparations: Capsules
Brand names: Hexalen

Amsacrine

General information: Amsacrine is used in acute myeloid leukaemia.

Side effects: As above; this drug may also affect the heart, particularly if it is used in high doses.
Available preparations: Infusion
Brand names: Amsidine

Bleomycin

General information: Bleomycin is used in squamous cell carcinoma, lymphomas and certain solid tumours. It is given by injection into a vein or a muscle.

Side effects: As above; may also include progressive lung damage, skin pigmentation, and allergic reactions.
Available preparations: Injection
Brand names: None

Busulphan

General information: Busulphan is used almost exclusively to treat chronic myeloid leukaemia.

Side effects: As above; may also include hyperpigmentation of the skin and damage to the lungs, although this latter effect is rare. Monitoring of the blood cells is essential, as this drug can cause irreversible damage to the bone marrow.
Available preparations: Tablets
Brand names: Myleran

Carboplatin

General information: Carboplatin is used in ovarian cancer and small cell lung cancer.

Side effects: As above; may also cause damage to the kidneys, nerves and ear.
Available preparations: Injection
Brand names: Paraplatin

Cisplatin

General information: Cisplatin is used in certain solid tumours (eg ovarian cancer and testicular teratoma).

Side effects: As above; may cause damage to the kidneys, nerves and ear.
Available preparations: Injection
Brand names: None

Carmustine

General information: Carmustine is used most commonly for myeloma, lymphoma and brain tumours.

Side effects: As above, may also include damage to the kidneys and lungs.
Available preparations: Injection
Brand names: BiCNU

Chlorambucil

General information: Chlorambucil is used commonly for chronic lymphocytic leukaemia, Hodgkin's disease, indolent non-Hodgkin's lymphomas and ovarian cancer.

Side effects: Rare, apart from bone marrow suppression. However, rashes develop occasionally and these can become quite severe. If that happens, the drug must be stopped and another substituted.
Available preparations: Tablets
Brand names: Leukeran

Cladribine

General information: Cladribine is used in hairy cell leukaemia, and also in chronic lymphocytic leukaemia (in patients who have failed to respond to standard therapy).

Side effects: As above; may also cause nerve damage and severe damage to the bone marrow.
Available preparations: Injection
Brand names: Leustat

Crisantaspase

General information: Crisantaspase is used almost exclusively in acute lymphoblastic leukaemia. It may be given by injection under the skin or into a muscle.

Side effects: As above; may also include allergic reactions, central nervous system toxicity, raised blood sugar, changes in liver function and blood fats.
Available preparations: Injection
Brand names: Erwinase

Cyclophosphamide

General information: Cyclophosphamide is widely used for chronic lymphocytic leukaemia, lymphomas and solid tumours.

Side effects: As above; may also include a serious type of cystitis, but this is rare. You may be advised to increase your fluid intake for 24–48 hours after having the drug.
Available preparations: Tablets, injection
Brand names: Endoxana

Cytarabine

General information: Cytarabine is used mainly in the induction of remission of acute myeloblastic leukaemia. It may be given intravenously, subcutaneously or intrathecally (an injection into the fluid that bathes the spinal cord).

Available preparations: Injection
Brand names: Cytostar

Dacarbazine

General information: Dacarbazine is used in melanoma, soft tissue sarcomas and Hodgkin's disease.

Side effects: As above; may also include intense nausea and vomiting and damage to the bone marrow.
Available preparations: Injection
Brand names: DTIC-Dome

Dactinomycin

General information: Dactinomycin tends to be used mainly in children.

Available preparations: Injection
Brand names: Cosmegen Lyovac

Daunorubicin

General information: Daunorubicin is used in acute leukaemias. A new formulation (DaunoXome) is available for AIDS-related Kaposi's sarcoma.

Available preparations: Injection, infusion
Brand names: Cerubidin, DaunoXome

Docetaxel

General information: Docetaxel is a relatively new drug and is used in breast cancer resistant to standard therapy.

Side effects: As above; may also include allergic reactions, and a corticosteroid or an antihistamine may be given to prevent this. This drug may also affect the heart and fluid retention can be a particular problem.
Available preparations: Intravenous infusion
Brand names: Taxotere

Doxorubicin

General information: Doxorubicin is used in acute leukaemias, lymphoma and certain solid tumours. It is given intravenously and by bladder instillation. A new formulation (Caelyx) is available for AIDS-related Kaposi's sarcoma.

Side effects: As above; may also affect the heart, particularly if it is used in high doses.
Available preparations: Injection, infusion
Brand names: Caelyx, Doxorubicin

Epirubicin

General information: Epirubicin is used in acute leukaemias, lymphoma and certain solid tumours. It may be given intravenously and by bladder instillation. Side effects include those listed above, but this drug may also affect the heart, particularly if it is used in high doses.

Available preparations: Injection
Brand names: Pharmorubicin

Estramustine

General information: Estramustine has both a cytotoxic and a hormonal action. It is used mainly in prostate cancer.

Available preparations: Capsules
Brand names: Estracyt

Etoposide

General information: Etoposide is used in small cell carcinoma of the bronchus, lymphomas and testicular cancer.

Available preparations: Capsules, injection
Brand names: Etopophos, Vepesid

Fludarabine

General information: Fludarabine is used in B-cell chronic lymphocytic leukaemia (when initial treatment with standard therapy has failed).

Available preparations: Injection
Brand names: Fludara

Fluorouracil

General information: Fluorouracil is used in solid tumours such as gastrointestinal, breast and colo-rectal cancer. It is usually given intravenously, but may also be given topically in malignant and pre-malignant skin conditions.

Available preparations: Capsules, injection, cream
Brand names: Efudix (cream only)

Gemcitabine

General information: Gemcitabine is used in non-small lung cancer or pancreatic cancer.

Side effects: May include gastrointestinal disturbances, rashes, kidney impairment and influenza-like symptoms.
Available preparations: Injection
Brand names: Gemzar

Hydroxyurea

General information: Hydroxyurea is used mainly in the treatment of chronic myeloid leukaemia, but occasionally for polycythaemia.

Available preparations: Capsules
Brand names: Hydrea

Idarubicin

General information: Idarubicin is used in acute leukaemia, and also in advanced breast cancer (where standard chemotherapy has failed). It may be given by mouth or intravenously.

Side effects: As above; may also affect the heart, particularly if it is used in high doses.
Available preparations: Capsules, injection
Brand names: Zavedos

Ifosfamide

General information: Ifosfamide is related to cyclophosphamide (see page 295) and has similar uses.

Available preparations: Injection
Brand names: Mitoxana

Interferon alpha

General information: Interferon alpha is used in certain leukaemias, lymphomas and solid tumours.

Side effects: May include nausea, depression, lethargy, flu-like symptoms, cardiovascular problems and damage to the eye, liver and kidney.
Available preparations: Injection
Brand names: Intron A, Roferon A, Viraferon, Wellferon

Irinotecan

General information: Irinotecan is used in colon cancer.

Available preparations: Intravenous infusion
Brand names: Campto

Lomustine

General information: Lomustine is used mainly in Hodgkin's disease and certain solid tumours. It is generally given at intervals of 4–6 weeks (because bone marrow toxicity is delayed).

Side effects: Permanent bone marrow damage is a risk with prolonged use and severe nausea and vomiting are common.
Available preparations: Capsules
Brand names: CCNU

Melphalan

General information: Melphalan is used mainly to treat myeloma and occasionally lymphomas and solid tumours. It is generally given at intervals of 4–6 weeks (because bone marrow toxicity is delayed) and is usually given by mouth, but sometimes intravenously.

Available preparations: Tablets, injection
Brand names: Alkeran

Mercaptopurine

General information: Mercaptopurine is used almost exclusively to control the progress of acute leukaemias.

Available preparations: Tablets
Brand names: Puri-Nethol

Methotrexate

General information: Methotrexate is used to control the progress of childhood acute lymphoblastic leukaemia, and also of choriocarcinoma, non-Hodgkin's lymphoma and a number of solid tumours. In these situations it may be given by mouth, or by injection into a vein or muscle. It is also used in therapy of established meningeal cancer or lymphoma. In these situations it is given by injection. Methotrexate is also used in severe cases of rheumatoid arthritis (see page 145) and in severe cases of the skin condition known as psoriasis (see page 208).

Available preparations: Tablets, injection
Brand names: None

Mitomycin

General information: Mitomycin is used in upper gastrointestinal and breast cancer (when it is given intravenously) and in superficial bladder tumours (when it is given by bladder instillation). It is generally given at six-weekly intervals (because bone marrow toxicity is delayed).

Side effects: Bone marrow damage can be permanent with prolonged use, and there may also be damage to the lungs and the kidneys.
Available preparations: Injection
Brand names: Mitomycin C Kyowa

Mitozantrone

General information: Mitozantrone is used in breast cancer.

Available preparations: Infusion
Brand names: Novantrone

Mustine

General information: Mustine is used for Hodgkin's disease (but is now used very rarely).

Side effects: Mustine tends to cause severe vomiting.
Available preparations: Injection
Brand names: None

Octreotide

General information: Octreotide is used in various specific cancers of the gastrointestinal tract.

Precautions: Tell your doctor if you are pregnant or breastfeeding.
Side effects: Gastrointestinal disturbances, including loss of appetite, nausea, vomiting, abdominal pain, wind and diarrhoea are the most common side effects.
Available preparations: Injection
Brand names: Sandostatin, Sandostatin LAR

Paclitaxel

General information: Paclitaxel is a relatively new drug and is used in ovarian cancer and breast cancer.

Side effects: As above; may include allergic reactions, and a corticosteroid or an antihistamine may be given to prevent this. This drug may also affect the heart.

Available preparations: Intravenous infusion
Brand names: Taxol

Pentostatin

General information: Pentostatin is used in hairy cell leukaemia.

Available preparations: Injection
Brand names: Nipent

Procarbazine

General information: Procarbazine is used most often in Hodgkin's disease.

Warnings: Do not drink alcohol with this drug.
Available preparations: Capsules
Brand names: None

Raltitrexed

General information: Raltitrexed is used in colon cancer.

Side effects: Gastrointestinal side effects are particularly common.
Available preparations: Injection
Brand names: Tomudex

Razoxane

General information: Razoxane is used for leukaemias.

Available preparations: Tablets
Brand names: None

Rituximab

General information: Rituximab is used for non-Hodgkin's lymphoma.

Available preparations: Injection
Brand names: Rabthera

Thioguanine

General information: Thioguanine is used to induce remission in acute myeloid leukaemia.

Available preparations: Tablets
Brand names: Lanvis

Thiotepa

General information: Thiotepa is used mainly in bladder cancer and occasionally in breast cancer.

Available preparations: Injection
Brand names: None

Topotecan

General information: Topotecan is used in ovarian cancer (when first line or subsequent therapy has failed).

Available preparations: Intravenous infusion
Brand names: Hycamtin

Treosulfan

General information: Treosulfan is used to treat ovarian cancer. It can be given by mouth or intravenously.

Side effects: As above; may also include skin pigmentation. Rarely, damage to the lung and a serious type of cystitis may occur.
Available preparations: Capsules, injection
Brand names: None

Tretinoin

General information: Tretinoin is used for induction of remission in acute promyelocytic leukaemia. It is also used in acne (see page 213).

Available preparations: Capsules
Brand names: Vesanoid

Vinblastine

General information: Vinblastine is used in acute leukaemias, lymphomas and certain solid tumours (eg breast and lung cancer).

Side effects: As above; may also include neurological toxicity (commonly manifested as pins and needles, numbness in the arms and legs, loss of tendon reflexes, muscle weakness); abdominal pain and constipation; and severe irritation at injection site. If symptoms occur, the dose should be reduced and the development of severe muscle weakness means that treatment should be stopped.
Available preparations: Injection
Brand names: Velbe

Vincristine

General information: Vincristine is used in acute leukaemias, lymphomas and certain solid tumours (eg breast and lung cancer).

Side effects: As above; may also include neurological toxicity (commonly manifested as pins and needles, numbness in the arms and legs, loss of tendon reflexes, muscle weakness); abdominal pain and constipation; and severe irritation at injection site.
Available preparations: Injection
Brand names: Oncovin

Vindesine

General information: Vindesine is used in acute leukaemias, lymphomas and certain solid tumours (eg breast and lung cancer).

Side effects: As above; may also include neurological toxicity (commonly manifested as peripheral paraesthesia, loss of deep tendon reflex, abdominal pain and constipation); muscle weakness and severe irritation at injection site.
Available preparations: Injection
Brand names: Eldisine

Vinorelbine

General information: Vinorelbine is used in advanced breast cancer where other treatment has failed, and also for advanced non-small cell lung cancer.

Side effects: As above; may also include neurological toxicity (commonly manifested as peripheral paraesthesia, loss of deep tendon reflex, abdominal pain and constipation); muscle weakness and severe irritation at injection site.
Available preparations: Injection
Brand names: Navelbine

SEX HORMONES

Various sex hormones are used in the treatment of cancer. They are used to treat cancers that are dependent on sex hormones, for example breast, uterus, ovaries and prostate. Sometimes male hormones are used to treat cancers in women and vice versa.

Ethinyloestradiol

General information: Ethinyloestradiol is an oestrogen and is used (rarely) in breast cancer.

Precautions: Tell your doctor if you have a heart problem or liver disease.
Side effects: Fluid retention and jaundice are possible.
Warnings: Tell your doctor immediately if you experience any pain in the chest or in the calf of your leg because of the risk of deep-vein thrombosis.
Available preparations: Tablets
Brand names: None

Fosfesterol

General information: Fosfesterol is an oestrogen used in prostate cancer.

Precautions: Tell your doctor if you have a heart problem or liver disease.
Side effects: Fluid retention, nausea, vomiting and jaundice are possible.

Warnings: Tell your doctor immediately if you experience any pain in the chest or in the calf of your leg because of the risk of deep-vein thrombosis.
Available preparations: Tablets, injection
Brand names: Honvan

Gestronol

General information: Gestronol is a progestogen used in breast cancer and endometrial cancer. It is similar to medroxyprogesterone.

Precautions, side effects, warnings: As medroxyprogesterone (see below).
Available preparations: Injection
Brand names: Depostat

Medroxyprogesterone

General information: Medroxyprogesterone is a progestogen used in breast cancer and endometrial cancer. It is also used in menstrual disorders, including endometrioisis (see page 187).

Precautions, side effects, warnings: As progestogens (see pages 186–7).
Available preparations: Tablets, injection
Brand names: Depo-Provera, Farlutal, Provera

Megesterol

General information: Megesterol is a progestogen used in breast cancer and endometrial cancer. It is similar to medroxyprogesterone.

Precautions, side effects, warnings: As progestogens (see pages 186–7).
Available preparations: Tablets
Brand names: Megace

Norethisterone

General information: Norethisterone is a progestogen used in breast cancer and endometrial cancer. It is also used in various menstrual disorders (see page 187).

Precautions, side effects, warnings: As progestogens (see pages 186–7).
Available preparations: Tablets
Brand names: Primulot N

Stilboestrol

General information: Stilboestrol is an oestrogen used in prostate cancer (rarely used) and occasionally in breast cancer.

Precautions: Tell your doctor if you have a heart problem or liver disease.
Side effects: Fluid retention and jaundice are possible.

Warnings: Tell your doctor immediately if you experience any pain in the chest or in the calf of your leg because of the risk of deep-vein thrombosis.
Available preparations: Tablets
Brand names: None

Polyestradiol

General information: Polyestradiol is an oestrogen used in prostate cancer.

Precautions: Tell your doctor if you have a heart problem or liver disease.
Side effects: Fluid retention and jaundice are possible.
Warnings: Tell your doctor immediately if you experience any pain in the chest or in the calf of your leg because of the risk of deep-vein thrombosis.
Available preparations: Injection
Brand names: Estradurin

HORMONE ANTAGONISTS

Hormone antagonists are used in the treatment of breast cancer and prostate cancer. In breast cancer, various anti-oestrogens are used, the most widely used of which is tamoxifen. It is increasingly used in women with breast cancer (both pre and post the menopause) whose cell walls have receptors that bind oestrogen (known as 'positive oestrogen receptor status').

In prostate cancer, various antiandrogens are used, including bicalutamide, cyproterone acetate and flutamide. These drugs antagonise the male sex hormone testosterone, and are useful in tumours that are dependent on this hormone. Alternatively, a gonadorelin analogue (see page 190), such as buserelin, goserelin, leuprorelin or triptorelin, may be given. Gonadorelin analogues switch off any stimulus by the pituitary gland to the testes, and lowers the concentration of testosterone in the blood.

Aminoglutethimide

General information: Aminoglutethimide is used in advanced breast or prostate cancer, and also in Cushing's disease (overactivity of the adrenal glands) when this is caused by cancer.

Precautions: Tell your doctor if you are pregnant, planning to become pregnant or are breastfeeding, or if you have porphyria.
Side effects: Side effects are common with this drug and include drowsiness, lethargy and rash.
Warnings: Take care with driving and similar activities until you know how this drug affects you.
Available preparations: Tablets
Brand names: Orimeten

Anastrozole

General information: Anastrozole is an anti-oestrogen used in advanced breast cancer in postmenopausal women.

Precautions: Tell your doctor if you are pregnant, planning to become pregnant or are breastfeeding, or if you have liver or kidney disease.
Side effects: These include hot flushes, vaginal dryness, vaginal bleeding, hair thinning, anorexia, nausea. vomiting, diarrhoea, headache and rash.
Warnings: Take care with driving and similar activities until you know how this drug affects you.
Available preparations: Tablets
Brand names: Arimidex

Bicalutamide

General information: Bicalutamide is an anti-androgen used in advanced prostate cancer.

Precautions: Tell your doctor if you have liver disease.
Side effects: These include hot flushes, skin itching, breast tenderness and swelling (in men), drowsiness and jaundice.
Warnings: Take care with driving and similar activities until you know how the drug affects you.
Available preparations: Tablets
Brand names: Casodex

Flutamide

General information: Flutamide is an anti-androgen used in advanced prostate cancer.

Precautions: Tell your doctor if you have a heart problem or liver disease.
Side effects: These include breast swelling (in men), nausea, vomiting, diarrhoea, decreased appetite, sleep disturbances and tiredness.
Available preparations: Tablets
Brand names: Drigenil

Formestane

General information: Formestane is an anti-oestrogen used in advanced breast cancer in postmenopausal women.

Side effects: These include nausea, vomiting, rash, itching and hot flushes.
Available preparations: Injection
Brand names: Lentaron

Letrozole

General information: Letrozole is an anti-oestrogen used in advanced breast cancer when other hormone antagonists have not worked.

Precautions: Tell your doctor if you are pregnant, planning to become pregnant or are breastfeeding, or if you have severe liver disease.
Side effects: These include hot flushes, nausea, vomiting, indigestion, constipation, diarrhoea, loss of appetite, weight gain and rash.
Available preparations: Tablets
Brand names: Femara

Tamoxifen

General information: Tamoxifen is an anti-oestrogen used in hormone-dependent breast cancer in both postmenopausal and premenopausal women.

Precautions: Tell your doctor if you are pregnant, planning to become pregnant or are breastfeeding, or if you have porphyria. Use a non-hormonal method of contraception, if appropriate, while taking this drug.
Side effects: There is a risk of endometrial changes, including polyps and even cancer. Tell your doctor if you have bleeding, discharge or pain. Other side effects include hot flushes, suppression of menstruation (in premenopausal women), dizziness, rash, fluid retention, hair loss and visual disturbances.
Available preparations: Tablets
Brand names: Nolvadex

Toremifine

General information: Toremifine is an anti-oestrogen used in hormone-dependent metastatic breast cancer in postmenopausal women.

Precautions: Tell your doctor if you have severe liver disease or a history of circulatory or heart disease.
Side effects: There is a risk of endometrial changes, including polyps and even cancer. Tell your doctor if you have bleeding, discharge or pain. Other side effects include hot flushes, dizziness, fluid retention, sweating, nausea, vomiting, chest or back pain, headache, weight gain, constipation and insomnia.
Available preparations: Tablets
Brand names: Fareston

DRUGS THAT SUPPRESS THE IMMUNE SYSTEM (IMMUNOSUPPRESSANTS)

The immune system is made up of special cells and tissues that help to protect the body against attack from bacteria and viruses. These defence mechanisms also help to get rid of cells which could develop abnormally and so cause cancer.

Sometimes, however, the immune system becomes very active and starts to attack the body's own normal cells. This happens in diseases known as autoimmune disorders, such as rheumatoid arthritis and systemic lupus erythmatosus (SLE). In these situations, the activity of the immune system needs to be dampened down. Immune system activity also needs to be reduced after organ transplantation. This is because the immune system recognises the new organ as foreign and starts to attack it. All immunosuppressant drugs therefore work by altering the activity of the immune system. They work by killing certain blood cells, including the white blood cells. They also kill cancer cells.

How to use: These drugs are often used under the supervision of specialists. Take the drug exactly as prescribed.

Azathioprine

General information: Azathioprine is used mainly to prevent rejection of transplanted organs and for a wide range of autoimmune diseases (eg SLE, chronic inflammatory bowel disease). Corticosteroids (eg prednisolone) are often prescribed in these conditions too, and azathioprine is useful when corticosteroids on their own have failed to work properly. This enables the dose of corticosteroids to be reduced with a consequent reduction in side effects.

Precautions: Tell your doctor if you are pregnant, planning to become pregnant or are breastfeeding, if you have long term liver or kidney problems, if you have an infection, or you have recently had shingles or chickenpox.
Side effects: Nausea, vomiting and various allergic reactions (eg rashes) are quite common. This drug may also cause blood disturbances and jaundice.
Tell your doctor immediately if you experience a sore throat, fever or any sign of an infection or unusual bleeding or bruising. Muscular pains and weakness are quite common.
Warnings: You will be asked to attend for full blood counts at regular intervals. Do not miss your appointments.
Interactions: Allopurinol, co-trimoxazole and trimethoprim interact with this drug.
Available preparations: Tablets, injection
Brand names: Imuran

Cyclosporin

General information: Cyclosporin is used to prevent rejection of transplanted organs. It is also used in rheumatoid arthritis and various skin conditions, such as dermatitis and psoriasis. It does not damage the bone marrow, but can damage the kidney.

Precautions: Tell your doctor if you are pregnant, planning to become pregnant or are breastfeeding.
Side effects: The most common side effects are increased body hair, tremor, swelling of the gums, fatigue, gastrointestinal disturbances and burning in the hands and feet.

Warnings: You will be asked to attend for various investigations while taking this drug. Keep your appointments.
Interactions: Cyclosporin interacts with a large number of drugs. Always check with your doctor or pharmacist before taking any other medication.
Available preparations: Capsules, liquid, injection
Brand names: Neoral, Sandimmnun

Mycophenolate

General information: Mycophenolate is used to prevent rejection of transplanted organs. It is given under specialist supervision.

Precautions: Tell your doctor if you are pregnant, planning to become pregnant or are breastfeeding, or if you have any gastrointestinal disease.
Side effects: Diarrhoea, vomiting, constipation, nausea and abdominal pain are quite common. Shortness of breath, dizziness, cough, insomnia, headache and allergic reactions may also occur. Tell your doctor if you experience a sore throat or any sign of infection.
Warnings: You will be asked to attend for full blood counts at regular intervals. Do not miss your appointments.
Interactions: Antacids may reduce the absorption of this drug.
Available preparations: Capsules, tablets
Brand names: CellCept

Tacrolimus

General information: Tacrolimus is a relatively new drug used mainly to prevent rejection of transplanted organs.

Precautions: Tell your doctor if you are pregnant, planning to become pregnant or are breastfeeding.
Side effects: Nausea, indigestion, peptic ulcers and a wide range of other side effects, including heart problems, have been reported with this drug.
Warnings: You will be asked to attend for various investigations while taking this drug. Do not miss your appointments.
Interactions: Tacrolimus interacts with various other drugs such as ibuprofen, some antibiotics and cyclosporin.
Available preparations: Capsules, injection
Brand names: Progral

Anaemias and other Nutritional Deficiencies

GOOD NUTRITION IS ESSENTIAL for health, and minerals (eg iron, calcium and magnesium) and vitamins (eg vitamins A, B, C, D and E) are an important part of this. Deficiencies of minerals and vitamins are relatively rare in the UK, although they can occur in some people with disease or inadequate diet. On NHS prescription, vitamins and minerals can only be given to treat a deficiency diagnosed by a doctor, or to prevent such a deficiency if the doctor thinks that a patient is at particular risk. Vitamins and minerals are not available on the NHS as general dietary supplements, and these, if wanted, must be bought over the counter. This section will therefore deal only with vitamins and minerals available on prescription, and discuss the conditions that they are used to treat.

What can go wrong

Nutritional deficiencies can cause a range of problems in the body, and they may also be symptoms of a particular ailment. Anaemia is the condition where there is less haemoglobin, which may be due to fewer red blood cells in the blood than is normal for a person's age and sex. If production of red blood cells is impaired in any way, or red blood cells are destroyed or lost from the body (as occurs, for example, in haemorrhage), then anaemia will develop. Red blood cell production requires the presence in the body of several vitamins and minerals, of which the main ones are iron, folic acid (a B vitamin) and vitamin B12. An insufficient amount of any of these can consequently cause anaemia. Such deficiencies can arise as a result of a dietary lack, poor absorption from an adequate diet, or increased loss of the nutrient from the body. Any disease (eg peptic ulcer) or drug (eg aspirin) which could cause blood loss may lead to anaemia. Kidney impairment can also cause this condition.

There are, in fact, several types of anaemia, of which iron-deficiency anaemia is the most common. Another type, megaloblastic anaemia, is a condition where there are large deformed blood cells. It is caused by lack of folic acid or vitamin B12 or both. There is also a special type of megaloblastic anaemia (known as pernicious anaemia) in which the vitamin B12 deficiency is caused by a disease process. In this condition, the body's immune system attacks the stomach's lining and prevents it from producing a substance – intrinsic factor – essential for absorption of vitamin B12.

Treatment of anaemia therefore involves a diagnosis of the specific deficiency – iron, vitamin B12 or folic acid – and then giving the appropriate preparation.

Common conditions and drugs used to treat them

Anaemias – iron, vitamin B12, folic acid (dependent on the type of anaemia)

Nutritional deficiencies – various vitamins and minerals

PREPARATIONS FOR IRON-DEFICIENCY ANAEMIA

There are several different types of iron preparations used for the treatment of iron-deficiency anaemia. They work by replacing natural iron that is either deficient in the diet or lost from the body. Ferrous sulphate is the most commonly prescribed.

How to use: Use exactly as prescribed. If you miss a dose, take it as soon as you remember.

Precautions: Tell your doctor if you are pregnant or breastfeeding, or if you have peptic ulcer or any other gastrointestinal disorder.

Side effects: Gastrointestinal irritation, black stools, nausea and indigestion are common side effects with iron preparations. They may also cause constipation, particularly in older people, and, in patients with inflammatory bowel disorders (eg Crohn's disease), they may cause diarrhoea.

Interactions: Iron reduces the absorption of levodopa (see page 56) and penicillamine (see page 153). Antacids and some antibiotics (eg tetracyclines and ciprofloxacin) may reduce the absorption of iron. Zinc can also reduce the absorption of iron, and vice versa.

Ferrous sulphate

Available preparations: Tablets, capsules, paediatric liquid
Brand names: Feospan, Ferrograd, Slow-Fe
Combination preparations: Ferrous sulphate with folic acid: Fefol, Ferrograd Folic, Fortespan, Slow Fe Folic; Ferrous sulphate with folic acid and zinc: Dencyl; Ferrous sulphate with vitamins: Ditemic, Ferrograd C, Fesovit Z

Ferrous fumarate

Available preparations: Tablets, capsules, syrup
Brand names: Fersaday, Fersamal, Galfer
Combination preparations: Ferrous fumarate with folic acid: Folex-350, Galfer FA, Meterfolic, Pregaday; Ferrous fumarate with vitamins: Galfer

Ferrous gluconate

Available preparations: Tablets
Brand names: None

Ferrous glycine sulphate

Available preparations: Syrup
Brand names: Plesmet

Ferric ammonium citrate

Available preparations: Syrup
Combination preparations: Ferric ammonium citrate with folic acid: Lexpec with Iron-M, Lexpec with Iron

Iron sorbitol

Available preparations: Injection
Brand names: Jectofer

Polysaccharide-iron complex

Available preparations: Capsules, liquid
Brand names: Niferex, Niferex-150

Sodium ironedetate

Available preparations: Liquid
Brand names: Sytron

PREPARATIONS FOR MEGALOBLASTIC ANAEMIA

Most megaloblastic anaemias are caused by a lack of folic acid or vitamin B12 or both, and it is essential to establish the correct deficiency before taking either vitamin. This is because, in cases of vitamin B12 deficiency, taking folic acid on its own can improve the symptoms of the anaemia without curing the underlying deficiency.

Folic acid is also given to help prevent neural tube defects (eg spina bifida), which can occur during the baby's development before birth. It should be taken by women from the time they start to plan a pregnancy until the 12th week of pregnancy. Women who have not taken a supplement from the time of conception should start to take one as soon as they realise that they are pregnant.

Cyanocobalamin (vitamin B12)

General information: Cyanocobalamin is given for dietary deficiency of vitamin B12.

Available preparations: Tablets, liquid, injection
Brand names: None

Folic acid

General information: Folic acid is given for prevention and treatment of megaloblastic anaemia and to pregnant women for the prevention of neural tube defects in babies.

Available preparations: Tablets, syrup
Brand names: None

Hydroxocobalamin (vitamin B12)

General information: Hydroxocobalamin is given for pernicious anaemia (a particular type of megaloblastic anaemia in which there is a difficulty in absorbing vitamin B12), and also in vitamin B12 deficiency.

Side effects: Itching, fevers, chills, hot flushes, nausea and dizziness may occur.
Available preparations: Injection
Brand names: None

PREPARATIONS USED IN ANAEMIA DUE TO RENAL FAILURE

Erythropoeitin

General information: Erythropoeitin is a hormone produced by the kidney to stimulate red cell production by the bone marrow. The synthetic version is used to treat anaemia, which often occurs in severe kidney disease.

Precautions: Tell your doctor if you are pregnant or breastfeeding, or if you have high blood pressure, circulatory or heart disease, liver disease, history of convulsions or cancer. Your doctor will check through tests that you have enough iron and folate in your blood and will monitor the effect of treatment.
Side effects: Allergic reactions including skin rashes may occur. Erythropoeitin may also cause an increase in blood pressure. If you experience a migraine-like headache, call your doctor immediately.
Available preparations: Injection
Brand names: Eprex, NeoRecormon

CALCIUM PREPARATIONS

Calcium preparations are usually only prescribed where dietary calcium intake is deficient. The requirement for calcium is relatively greater at certain times in our lives, for example in childhood, adolescence, pregnancy, lactation (breastfeeding) and old age. Calcium supplements (sometime prescribed with vitamin D) can also be beneficial in the prevention and treatment of osteoporosis, particularly in the elderly.

Side effects: Side effects are rare with calcium preparations, but gastrointestinal disturbances may occur.

Interactions: Calcium reduces the absorption of some antibiotics (eg tetracyclines and ciprofloxacin) and bisphosphonates (eg etidronate).

Available preparations: Calcium gluconate tablets, effervescent tablets and injection; Calcium lactate tablets

Brand names:
Cacit (calcium carbonate) – effervescent tablets
Calcichew (calcium carbonate) – chewable tablets
Calcidrink (calcium carbonate) – effervescent granule
Calcium-500 (calcium carbonate) – tablets
Calcium-Sandoz (calcium glubionate, calcium lactobionate) – syrup
Ossopan (hydroxyapatite: contains calcium) – tablets
Ostram (calcium phosphate) – tablets
Sandocal (calcium lactate gluconate, calcium carbonate) – effervescent tablets

PHOSPHATE SUPPLEMENTS

Oral phosphate supplements are sometimes given in a type of rickets (see page 145) where blood phosphate levels are low. They may also be given to reduce blood calcium levels.

Available preparations: Effervescent tablets

Brand names: Phosphate-Sandoz

PREPARATIONS TO REDUCE PHOSPHATE LEVELS

People with kidney disease sometimes have increased levels of phosphate in their blood, and medicines are available to reduce these levels. These medicines basically consist of aluminium and calcium salts, which are also used as antacids. Both aluminium and calcium attach themselves to phosphate in the blood and reduce the phosphate levels.

Aluminium hydroxide

Available preparations: Capsules, liquid
Brand names: Alu-Cap

Calcium salts

Available preparations: Tablets
Brand names: Calcichew, Calcium-500, Phosex, Titralac

FLUORIDE PREPARATIONS

Fluoride helps to protect the teeth against dental decay, particularly in children. In the UK, tap water has small quantities of fluoride added by many health authorities and you should be able to find information about the tap water in your area from your dentist, doctor, pharmacist or local health authority. If your tap water contains less than 1mg fluoride per litre (1 part per million), you may want to consider using a fluoride supplement. These can be bought over the counter and are also available on prescription, but should not be taken during pregnancy.

In addition, dentists now think that application of fluoride directly to the teeth has a greater protective action than the more general taking of fluoride by mouth. If you or your child are particularly prone to dental caries, you can ask your dentist to apply a coating of fluoride gel to your or your child's teeth. Alternatively, there are various gels for home use that contain a lower dose of fluoride than the stronger preparations used by the dentist. In addition, there are also various fluoride mouthwashes available which also help to protect the teeth.

The main thing to remember about fluoride is that, like any other medicine, it is safe if used in the correct dose, but it is a potentially toxic substance if used excessively. The teeth may turn yellowish-brown in colour if too high a dose is used. Read the labels very carefully and note that different doses are appropriate for children of different ages.

Available preparations:
En-De-Kay, Fluor-a-day, Fluorigard – tablets
En-de-Kay, Fluorigard – oral drops
En-de-Kay, Fluorigard – mouthwashes
Fluorigard – gel

ZINC

Zinc supplements are only prescribed on the NHS when the doctor thinks there is good evidence of zinc deficiency. Such a deficiency can occur when the diet is of poor quality, or if there is malabsorption of the mineral from an adequate diet. In particular, patients with severe burns and wounds may be prescribed zinc, as it helps with the body's healing process.

Side effects: These are rare, but indigestion and abdominal pain may occur.

Available preparations: Effervescent tablets, capsules

Brand names: Solvazinc, Z span

VITAMINS

Various vitamins are available on prescription, but there is a much larger range available over the counter. Vitamins are only prescribed on the NHS when the doctor thinks there is good evidence of deficiency or a definite risk of deficiency. Doctors do not prescribe vitamins as general 'pick-me-ups' or as dietary supplements. For these purposes, a huge range of products is available over the counter.

Vitamin A

Vitamin A deficiency is rare in Britain and the most common causes for prescribing it are probably liver disease and cystic fibrosis. In addition, the Department of Health recommends that babies from the age of 6 months up to 5 years should take supplements of vitamin A, but also vitamins C and D, if their diet is not sufficiently varied. Vitamin drops containing these vitamins are available free of charge from welfare clinics and also on prescription, but they can also be bought over the counter.

Vitamin A can be toxic in overdose and it is particularly important not to exceed the stated dose. This applies especially in pregnancy. Indeed, the Department of Health recommends that vitamin supplements containing vitamin A are avoided in pregnancy as well as foods high in vitamin A (eg liver, liver pâté).

Available preparations: Vitamin A injection; Vitamin A and D capsules; Halibut Liver oil (vitamin A and D) capsules; Halycitrol (vitamin A and D) oral liquid

Vitamin B group

Vitamins of the B group (eg thiamine, riboflavine, pyridoxine, nicotinamide) are rarely prescribed on the NHS. Deficiency of thiamine is a risk in chronic alcoholics; it can lead to damage to the peripheral nerves and the brain, resulting in weakness of the legs and numbness and unsteadiness, as well as confusional states. These conditions are treated with thiamine, other B vitamins and often vitamin C. An injection containing the B vitamins and vitamin C is available for this purpose.

Pyridoxine (vitamin B6) is prescribed for people taking isoniazid (see page 262). Isoniazid is a drug used in tuberculosis, which can cause vitamin B6 deficiency. In addition, there are various vitamin B tablets available on prescription which are prescribed occasionally for elderly people who may be eating poor diets.

Available preparations: Thiamine tablets; Nicotinamide tablets; Pyridoxine tablets; Vitamin B tablets compound (nicotinamide, ribloflavine, thiamine); Vitamin B tablets compound strong (nicotinamide, riboflavine, pyridoxine, thiamine)

Brand names:
Orovite Complement B6 tablets; Pabrinex (vitamins B and C) injection; Vigranon B (thiamine, riboflavine, nicotinamide, pyridoxine, pantothenol) syrup

Vitamin C

Vitamin C is prescribed in cases of scurvy, the disease arising from deficiency of vitamin C. Scurvy occurs occasionally in Britain and mild forms are fairly common, particularly in the elderly. Vitamin C is not available on prescription for the prevention of colds.

Available preparations: Ascorbic acid tablets

Vitamin D

Vitamin D is obtained from the diet, and it is also made in the skin when the skin is exposed to sunlight. Vitamin D deficiency is therefore a risk in anyone who does not go out of doors much, particularly older people. It occurs more commonly in northern than southern Britain, because of the relative lack of sunlight in the north.

In addition, people with dark skins (eg Asian people) seem to be at particular risk of deficiency in Britain and other northern latitudes. This is partly because of the relatively low strength of the sun in Britain compared with that in their countries of origin. Many people from the Indian subcontinent are also vegans, and their diet may consequently be low in vitamin D and calcium.

People with cystic fibrosis, and other conditions where there is severe gastrointestinal malabsorption, kidney and liver disease may also become vitamin D deficient. Additional vitamin D is thus often prescribed for these patients. However, vitamin D can be toxic in excessive dosage, like vitamin A. It is therefore particularly important not to exceed the stated dose, and to attend regularly for blood tests.

There are several forms of vitamin D available on prescription. These are known as ergocalciferol (vitamin D2), cholecalciferol (vitamin D3), alfacalcidol, calcitriol and dihydrotachysterol. Which one is prescribed for you depends on your individual requirement, but in general preparations containing ergocalciferol and cholecalciferol tend to be prescribed for vitamin D deficiency caused by poor diet or lack of sunlight. It may also be used in the prevention of osteoporosis. Other preparations tend to be prescribed more in patients with severe kidney disease, including those on dialysis.

Available preparations: Ergocalciferol or cholecalciferol; Calcium and ergocalciferol (vitamin D2) tablets

Brand names:
Cacit D3 (calcium carbonate, cholecalciferol) – tablets
Calceos (calcium carbonate, cholecalciferol) – tablets
Calcichew D3 (calcium carbonate, cholecalciferol) – tablets
Calcichew D3 Forte (calcium carbonate, cholecalciferol) – tablets

Alfacalcidol

Brand names: Alfa-D – capsules; One-Alpha – capsules, solution, injection

Calcitriol

Brand names: Calcijex – injection; Rocaltrol – capsules

Dihydrotachysterol

Brand names: AT10 solution

Vitamin E

Vitamin E is prescribed mainly in conditions such as cystic fibrosis where there is gastrointestinal malabsorption.

Available preparations: Tablets, liquid

Vitamin K

Vitamin K is necessary to help the blood to clot and also for the health of the bones. Like vitamins A, D and E, it is prescribed in people who have gastrointestinal malabsorption conditions (eg cystic fibrosis).

Vitamin K is also prescribed to prevent haemorrhage in newborn babies. In recent years there has been some controversy as to the use of vitamin K in newborn babies because some research showed that the injection was linked with an increased risk of cancer, whereas giving the vitamin by mouth was not. However, more recent research has shown that the fears about vitamin K were somewhat unfounded. No definite recommendations have yet been made as to the use of the injection versus oral vitamin K in babies, so you should discuss this matter with your general practitioner or paediatrician before your baby is born.

Menadiol

General information: Menadiol is a form of vitamin K available on prescription.

Available preparations: Menadiol tablets

Phytomenadione

General information: Phytomenadione is a form of vitamin K available on prescription.

Brand names: Konakion – tablets and injection; Konakion MM – injection; Konakion MM Paediatric – injection

Multivitamins

Various multivitamins are available on prescription to treat or prevent multiple vitamin deficiencies.

Available preparations: Vitamin capsules (vitamin C, B group vitamins, vitamin A)

Brand names:
Abidec (vitamin A, B group, C and D) – drops
Dalivit (vitamin A, B group, C and D) – drops
Forceval (vitamin A, B group, C, D, E with minerals and trace elements) – capsules
Forceval junior (vitamin A, B group, C, D, E with minerals and trace elements) – capsules
Ketovite (vitamin C, B group, E, K) – tablets
Ketovite (vitamin A, D, B12, choline) – liquid

MISCELLANEOUS

Penicillamine

General information: Penicillamine is used as a disease-modifying drug in rheumatoid arthritis, in cystinuria and also in Wilson's disease. Wilson's disease is an inherited condition in which quantities of copper build up in the body because the person cannot excrete it satisfactorily. Penicillamine works by attaching itself to copper and then eliminating it from the body through urination.

Precautions, side effects, warnings, interactions, preparations: See page 153.

CHAPTER 3

VACCINATIONS

VACCINATION IS ONE of the great triumphs of modern medicine. Diseases which in living memory caused untold misery have been eradicated (smallpox) or significantly tamed (polio, tetanus, tuberculosis, measles or rubella). In addition, the development of new vaccines offers the only realistic hope of eradicating HIV, the virus that can lead to AIDS and that has infected millions of people worldwide since the first cases were identified in 1983.

HOW VACCINES WORK

The body has an intricate system, known as the immune system, which enables it to recognise foreign proteins or organisms – bacteria, viruses, fungi and protozoa – and destroy them. Vaccination or immunisation works by priming the immune system in advance. This means that when the system encounters an infectious agent within the body, it has already learnt to recognise it and can stop it spreading. Specialised cells in the immune system, known as lymphocytes, target foreign cells or proteins and deal with them, either by making antibodies (immunoglobulins) or by killing the cells directly.

An antibody is a large complex molecule. It is produced specifically by lymphocytes in response to a particular protein or antigen (a substance that stimulates the production of antibodies). The antibody locks on to a foreign protein or antigen by means of a specialised binding site into which the antigen fits like a key into a lock. As it does so, it triggers other white cells and proteins in the blood which will engulf or destroy the foreign protein or prevent it entering other cells. There are several types of immunoglobulin, but the one present in the plasma in large amounts is IgG. This plays an important role in fighting bacterial infections. IgG is also able to cross the placenta into an unborn baby's bloodstream, and so give it temporary protection against infection.

The key features of the immune system are that it has a *memory* (which can last for many years after the original exposure), that it has to be *primed* – protection is not instant as cells have to be recruited – and that there is a *heightened response* on subsequent exposure.

Active and passive immunisation

In **active** immunisation the immune system is stimulated by injecting a part or the whole of an organism into the body. It may be a weakened (attenuated) strain of the organism, sufficient to multiply in the body without producing a clinical illness. In such a case, immunity is long-lasting at the price of a small risk of causing disease (eg paralytic polio after polio immunisation). Examples of such weakened organisms include many viruses, such as polio, mumps, measles and rubella, but only two bacteria – tuberculosis and oral typhoid. Inactivated vaccines, by contrast, contain killed whole organisms, or extracts of their cell walls or toxins, that have been shown to produce protective antibodies. Inactivated vaccines tend to require a course of injections followed by boosters to stimulate and maintain immunity, but they have no risk of producing infection.

In **passive** immunisation, pre-formed antibodies from a donor are present in the bloodstream and give temporary immunity. We have experienced this as babies in the womb; immunoglobulin from our mothers crossed the placenta into our circulation, so that when we were born we already had a temporary degree of protection from common infections in our community. In passive immunisation, immunoglobulin prepared from donor plasma is given by injection. Passive immunisation results in immediate immunity that lasts just for those few months that the immunoglobulins persist in the body. There is no long-term immunity because the priming process has been bypassed.

WARNINGS PRIOR TO VACCINATION

Vaccines are safe and effective products, but there are situations in which vaccination should be withheld or postponed.

1. You or your child should not have a vaccination during an acute feverish illness. It is safe to go ahead during a minor illness in which the child is generally well.

2. You should not go ahead if there has been a definite severe reaction to a previous dose. Such reactions include anaphylaxis with collapse, hives, wheeze and swelling of the lips and mouth. In addition, the vaccine should not be given if there has been a severe local or general reaction to a preceding dose. A severe local reaction is manifested by extensive redness or swelling that becomes thickened and involves most of the front and side of the thigh or upper arm. A general reaction is a fever of 39.5°C (103°F) within 48 hours of the vaccine being given. It may include collapse, severe wheezing and, in babies, prolonged unresponsiveness, inconsolable screaming or fits within 72 hours. If a child has a febrile convulsion following immunisation, the case should be discussed with a specialist before another dose is given.

3. You or your child should not have the vaccine if you are allergic to the antibiotics or preservatives in some vaccinations, such as the neomycin or kanamycin in MMR (mumps, measles and rubella) or hepatitis A vaccine. Similarly, an allergy to eggs means you cannot have vaccines grown in eggs – this mainly applies to the influenza vaccines.

4. Pregnancy is a time to avoid routine immunisations. Live vaccines should only be given if there is a real risk of exposure, such as yellow fever in someone who has to travel. The rubella vaccines (either alone or as the combined MMR vaccine) must not be given during pregnancy, and you should avoid becoming

pregnant for a minimum of one month after the vaccination. Oral typhoid should not be given, and many of the inactivated vaccines should also be avoided. If there is a significant risk of exposure to infection, you should seek advice from your doctor. Tetanus vaccine is safe in pregnancy.

5. You should not have live (attenuated) vaccines if your immune system is weakened, either by disease or by treatments that affect it. Such treatments include radiotherapy, chemotherapy or treatment with high doses of corticosteroids (not the lower doses in steroid creams or puffers used to treat eczema or asthma). You need to wait at least three months after stopping steroids and six months after completing chemotherapy before having live vaccines. You should also avoid live vaccines if you have cancers affecting the immune system, such as leukaemias or lymphomas. If you have HIV, you may have MMR and oral polio, but you must not have BCG, yellow fever or oral typhoid vaccinations. If your immune system is weakened by disease or treatments you should take advice from your specialist before having any immunisation.

TIMETABLE OF ROUTINE IMMUNISATIONS

There is a national recommended schedule for routine immunisations. If a dose is missed or is late, then have it as soon as possible and carry on with the course. There is no need to start the course from the beginning. Because the risk of side effects with pertussis (whooping cough) is less in babies under six months, you should aim to complete the first set of routine immunisations by then. Schedules vary from country to country; if you or your child are going to live abroad for less than a year, you should try to adhere to the schedule of your home country. If you or your child are going to live abroad for more than a year, however, you should switch to the vaccination schedule of your host country.

Vaccination is generally safe. Because immunisation is a matter of public policy, however, the government does run a scheme to compensate those few people who are believed to have sustained severe mental or physical disability as a result of routine immunisations. Details may be obtained via the Department of Social Security.

Table of routine immunisations in the UK

Age	Vaccine
up to 6 weeks	Tuberculosis (BCG) – only for infants at risk
2 months	Diphtheria, tetanus, whooping cough, polio, *Haemophilus influenzae*
3 months	Diphtheria, tetanus, whooping cough, polio, *Haemophilus influenzae*
4 months	Diphtheria, tetanus, whooping cough, polio, *Haemophilus influenzae*
12–18 months	Measles, mumps, rubella (MMR)
1–2 years	*Haemophilus influenzae*, if not previously given
4–5 years	Diphtheria, tetanus, polio, MMR booster

continued

Age	Vaccine
10–14 years	Tuberculosis (unless given in infancy)
15–19 years	Diphtheria, tetanus, polio
Adults	Tetanus and polio if previously unimmunised; women of child-bearing age should also be vaccinated against rubella if a blood test shows that they are not immune to the disease

For further details see under the specific conditions.

POST-VACCINE CARE

Serious reactions after vaccinations are rare. However, you may be advised to stay in the surgery or clinic for 20 minutes after the injection in case of an acute reaction.

Some children may get a slight fever after the injection, in which case your GP may suggest that you give them a low dose of paracetamol. Dress children in light clothes, encourage them to drink, and possibly bathe their foreheads and arms with a tepid sponge. If your child has a tendency to febrile convulsions, discuss this with your doctor prior to the immunisation and make sure that you have paracetamol on hand.

If you notice the following symptoms contact your doctor immediately:
• high fever – above 39.5°C (103°F)
• convulsions
• inconsolable crying for more than three hours, or an unusually high-pitched cry
• hoarseness and difficulty in breathing; swelling of the lips

As the oral polio virus may be excreted in the stools for a month or more after immunisation, you should be scrupulous about washing your hands after changing your baby and disposing of the nappy.

ADVICE TO TRAVELLERS

If you are travelling to northern Europe, North America, or Australia and New Zealand, you do not require additional vaccinations above those recommended in the UK national schedule. You may well require additional vaccinations, for example typhoid, yellow fever, rabies or hepatitis, if you are going to underdeveloped countries. It is important that you plan well in advance as some vaccines require more than one dose, and certain vaccines cannot be given together (eg oral polio and oral typhoid). Also, most vaccines take a week or two before they will elicit protective antibodies. The situation on what is needed abroad changes quite frequently, so obtain up-to-date advice from your doctor or a travel clinic prior to travelling. Remember that you must also take other routine precautions, such as food and water hygiene, protection against the sun and against malaria if indicated.

PHARMACEUTICAL PRECAUTIONS

Vaccines and immunoglobulins are biological products. They are much less robust than the tablets or medicines that you obtain over the counter or on prescription.

With the exception of oral polio and typhoid vaccines, they are given by injection. All vaccines need to be stored in a fridge at a temperature of between 2°C and 8°C. The diluent used, dose, depth (into muscle or skin) and site of injection (buttock, thigh or upper arm) are all specified by the manufacturer.

DIRECTORY OF ILLNESSES AND THEIR VACCINES

Diphtheria

Diphtheria is an infectious disease caused by a bacterium, *Corynebacteria diphtheriae*. It mainly affects the throat, where it causes inflammation and a greyish membrane that can obstruct breathing; a toxin produced by the organism can also cause damage to the heart and nerves. Virtually eradicated from the UK, diphtheria still occurs in Asia and Africa. There has recently been an epidemic in the former Soviet Union and parts of Eastern Europe.

Protection against diphtheria is provided by injections of purified toxin that has been rendered harmless by treatment with formaldehyde (toxoid). To boost antibody levels, it is either absorbed on to an aluminium compound, or combined with the pertussis (whooping cough) vaccine.

In infancy, the toxoid is given combined with tetanus and pertussis, or with the vaccine to *Haemophilus influenzae*. The course consists of three doses one month apart, starting at two months. A booster of diphtheria combined with tetanus is given at school entry and again at age 15. Low-dose preparations for adults and adolescents are available either alone or combined with tetanus for primary immunisation or boosters. Boosters are recommended for adults who completed primary immunisation more than 10 years previously and who are either travelling to areas where diphtheria is endemic or have been in contact with a case of diphtheria.

Side effects: Swelling and redness at the injection site are common, and there is occasionally a transient fever. A painless nodule may form at the injection site, but this always settles without treatment.

Warnings: As warnings prior to vaccination (see page 320). Diphtheria vaccine should not be given to people allergic to aluminium or the preservative thiomersal.

Haemophilus influenzae

Haemophilus influenzae is an organism that commonly colonises the respiratory tract. It is a cause of bronchitis or otitis media (ear infections). However, certain strains are much more aggressive. They can cause severe infections, including meningitis and epiglottitis (a form of overwhelming throat infection), in young children, especially those in the first year of life.

Haemophilus influenzae vaccine (HiB) consists of capsular polysaccharides of *Haemophilus influenzae* type B conjugated to a protein carrier. A primary course of three doses (either alone or more usually combined with diphtheria, tetanus and pertussis), spaced a month apart and starting at two months, is given in infancy.

Children over 13 months are considered to be at lower risk and require only a single dose of vaccine.

For those over four years of age, only people lacking a spleen or with conditions increasing their chances of invasive disease, such as sickle cell disease or cancer, are offered immunisation. Children under four years who have been in contact with a case of invasive *H. influenzae* disease should be offered immunisation.

Side effects: Transient swelling and redness at the injection site after the first dose, starting at 3–4 hours and resolving by 24 hours, have been reported. Reactions are usually less with subsequent doses and are not considered a reason to stop vaccination. Reactions to the combined vaccine (HiB and triple) do not appear to be worse than to either component on its own.

Warnings: As warnings prior to vaccination (see page 320).

Hepatitis A virus

Hepatitis A virus is one cause of viral hepatitis. It used to be known as 'infectious hepatitis', as the virus multiplies in the liver and is passed out of the body via the stools. Spread is mainly from person to person or via contaminated food and water. The illness is characterised by a period of tiredness, nausea and poor appetite followed by jaundice. Sufferers usually recover completely after a few weeks. Deaths are rare and cases without jaundice common, especially in young children. Although the disease is declining in the UK, travellers to less developed countries, especially the Indian subcontinent and the Far East, Africa, Latin America and Eastern Europe, are at risk.

The most durable protection against hepatitis A is provided by active immunisation with the inactivated virus. However, immediate temporary protection can be given by an injection of normal immunoglobulin (see page 325).

Active immunisation is recommended for travellers to high-risk areas, sewage workers, staff and residents of homes for people with severe learning difficulties, some groups of haemophiliacs, patients with chronic liver disease and individuals whose sexual behaviour puts them at high risk.

Hepatitis A vaccine is prepared from formaldehyde-inactivated hepatitis A virus. The virus is grown in human cells and absorbed on to aluminium hydroxide. It is given into the deltoid muscle of the upper arm, as antibody levels are better at this site. After a delay of about two weeks, protective antibodies appear and persist for at least one year. A booster dose given 6–12 months after the first dose will offer immunity for up to 10 years. The vaccine is also available combined with that for hepatitis B (see page 325).

Side effects: These are generally mild, but occasionally there may be redness and swelling at the injection site. Some people have a short-lived fever or feel generally unwell.

Warnings: As warnings prior to vaccination (see page 320). Take advice for children under one or two (age varies with different preparations).

Normal immunoglobulin

General information: Normal immunoglobulin is prepared from the plasma of routine blood donors, screened for hepatitis B and C and HIV. It is given by intramuscular injection into the buttock. Until the development of the vaccine, normal immunoglobulin was the only means of prevention against hepatitis A.

Normal immunoglobulin may be used for travellers to high risk areas who are going for a short time (that is, less than 4 months) and who are leaving before active immunisation may take effect. In those circumstances immunisation with hepatitis A vaccine and immunoglobulin may be performed simultaneously (protective antibody levels will be lower and a booster will still be required). Offered early to contacts in outbreaks, it gives some protection and is effective in reducing the numbers of new cases.

Side effects: The main side effect is discomfort at the injection site. Allergic reactions are rare, and most frequently occur in people who have previously reacted to blood products.

Warnings: As warnings prior to vaccination (see page 320). Not to be given to anyone who suffered a severe reaction to a previous dose.

Hepatitis B virus

Hepatitis B virus is one of the major causes of viral hepatitis. Its former name of 'serum hepatitis' indicates one of its main routes of transmission by the injection of blood or blood products or the sharing of contaminated needles by drug addicts, tattooists or acupuncturists. The virus is present in semen and may be spread by sexual contact, both heterosexual and homosexual. Transmission also occurs by blood splashes on the eye, mouth or fresh cuts and abrasions on the skin. A mother who is a carrier of hepatitis B may pass her infection on to her child at birth.

Although the incidence in the UK is relatively low, there are about 300 million carriers in the world and 4 million new infections a year. Areas where the disease is common include Africa, Asia, parts of Latin America, Southern and Eastern Europe and the former Soviet Union.

After an incubation period of 40–160 days, the illness starts with flu-like symptoms, fever, nausea, vomiting and abdominal pains. In a few days jaundice develops and the patient starts to feel better. Some infections do not display symptoms. Less than 1 per cent of cases develop severe hepatitis and die, and between 2 and 10 per cent of adults get better but continue to carry the virus. Children are more likely to become carriers and 90 per cent of infected newborns will become carriers. This is also important because 20–25 per cent of carriers go on to develop chronic liver disease, and some of them will develop liver cancer.

The most durable protection against hepatitis B is provided by active immunisation with the inactivated virus. However, temporary protection after exposure to the virus can be given by an injection of specific hepatitis B immunoglobulin combined with active immunisation to give active/passive immunity.

Members of high-risk groups should consider active immunisation with hepatitis B vaccine. Such groups include injecting drug users and their partners, individuals who change their partners frequently (especially homosexual and bisexual men and prostitutes), sexual partners and household contacts of a case or carrier, haemophiliacs, families adopting children from a high-risk country, patients with chronic renal failure, staff and residents of residential accommodation for people with severe learning disabilities and inmates of custodial institutions. It is the responsibility of occupational health departments to ensure all healthcare workers who have direct contact with patients' body fluids are immunised against hepatitis B. People planning to remain for long periods in areas where the disease is common should consider immunisation; short term tourists are not at great risk in these circumstances unless through their sexual behaviour. If a pregnant woman falls into a high-risk category she should consider immunisation.

Hepatitis B vaccine is inactivated hepatitis B virus surface antigen absorbed on to aluminium hydroxide. It is prepared biosynthetically and does not carry any risk at all of transmitting infection. A course of primary immunisation requires three doses (one month and six months after the first dose) given into the deltoid muscle of the upper arm. It takes up to six months to confer adequate protection. Not everyone develops protective antibody levels after a primary course, and a blood test is taken to identify those who need a further injection. A booster dose after five years is recommended for people at continuing risk. Preparations include hepatitis B in different strengths for adults, children and renal patients, as well as combined with hepatitis A.

Side effects: Redness and soreness at the injection site are common. Other occasional reactions include fever, rash and flu-like illnesses. Sometimes a painless nodule may form at the injection site, but this settles without treatment.

Warnings: As warnings prior to vaccination (see page 320). Hepatitis B vaccine should not be given if there is severe allergy to a component of the vaccine such as aluminium, thiomersal or yeast.

Specific hepatitis B immunoglobulin

General information: Specific hepatitis B immunoglobulin is prepared from the plasma of routine blood donors with a high level of protective antibody. It should be given as soon as possible (ideally within 48 hours, but in some circumstances up to a week) after exposure in order to reduce the chances of infection. The immunoglobulin will help prevent severe illnesses and the carrier state. It can be combined with active immunisation into the other arm using hepatitis B vaccine so that protection is ongoing. The course should be completed in the usual way. People known to have completed a primary course simply need a booster dose of vaccine unless they are already known to have protective levels of antibody.

Side effects: The main side effect is discomfort at the injection site. Allergic reactions are rare, and most frequently occur in people who have previously reacted to blood products.

Warnings: As warnings prior to vaccination (see page 320). Not to be given to anyone who suffered a severe reaction to a previous dose.

Influenza

Influenza is a common viral infection of the respiratory tract with a short incubation period of 1–3 days enabling it to spread rapidly within families and institutions. Starting abruptly, often in winter, with high fever, aching in the limbs and back, sore throat and dry cough, the illness usually clears up after 2–7 days. It may, however, be complicated by ear and chest infections in vulnerable people.

People at risk who should be offered immunisation include patients with chronic chest diseases (including asthma), heart disease, diabetes mellitus, chronic renal failure, immunosuppression, residents of nursing and residential homes and long-stay institutions, and people aged over 75. Elderly people with any of the other illnesses listed are particularly at risk. Immunisation against influenza results in a worthwhile reduction in deaths, hospital admissions and cases of pneumonia.

Unlike many other viruses which remain stable in structure, the common strains that cause epidemics have a propensity to change the surface structures that the body recognises and to which it makes antibodies. As a result, influenza vaccines must be prepared afresh each year, using monitoring of current strains to predict the likely dominant strains. Patients at risk are advised to have an annual 'flu jab'.

Influenza vaccine is prepared by chemically inactivating and purifying influenza viruses grown in hens' eggs. There are two types of preparation ('split virus' and 'surface antigen'), but both contain the same three current strains and produce good levels of protective antibody with a low incidence of side effects.

The vaccine is effective if given a month (but at least 10 days) before exposure to the virus. Antibody levels decline over 3–6 months. Most general practices offer a flu immunisation programme during October and November.

In adults there is usually sufficient residual immunity from previous exposure that a single annual injection suffices. At-risk children may require two doses.

Side effects: The main side effect is soreness at the injection site. Occasionally a flu-like illness starts 12–16 hours after the injection has been given. Very rarely there is an allergic reaction, with hives, swelling of the lips and mouth and wheezing, which is probably due to allergy to residual egg protein.

Warnings: As warnings prior to vaccination (see page 320). The virus is grown in hens' eggs and should not be given to people who are allergic to eggs.

Measles

Measles is a highly transmissible viral infection with an incubation period of about 8–14 days. It causes an unpleasant illness with high fever, cough, conjunctivitis and then a rash. Chest and ear infections commonly follow, and there is a risk of febrile convulsions and more rarely encephalitis and even death. Since the implementation of a national policy of active immunisation the number of new cases in the UK has fallen to very low levels. Nevertheless, population immunity must be maintained because importation of the disease from areas where it is common still occurs.

Measles vaccine, which is a live attenuated vaccine, is given combined with mumps and rubella vaccine as MMR (see page 333) to children over 12 months. When given early in the incubation period to those who have been in contact with a case, it will abort an attack of measles.

Side effects: Reactions to measles vaccine include transient rashes, fever and a mild measles-like illness with fever and a rash a week after injection. Feverish convulsions usually 6–11 days after injection do occur, but at a lower rate than after natural measles. Other complications are rare.

Normal immunoglobulin

General information: Normal immunoglobulin prepared from the plasma of routine blood donors, screened for hepatitis B and C and HIV, will give immediate temporary protection to children with compromised immunity after exposure to measles.

Side effects: The main side effect is discomfort at the injection site. Allergic reactions are rare, and most frequently occur in people who have previously reacted to blood products.

Warnings: As warnings prior to vaccination (see page 320). Not to be given to anyone who suffered a severe reaction to a previous dose.

Mumps

Mumps is a viral infection that largely attacks school-age children and young adults. It is transmitted through the air and has an incubation period of 14–21 days. Generally it causes a fever and swelling of the parotid glands (large salivary glands situated in front of, and below, each ear). Complications of the illness can include testicular problems, viral meningitis and deafness.

Mumps vaccine consists of the Jeryl Lynn strain of live attenuated virus grown in chick-embryo tissue culture. It is now given combined with measles and rubella as MMR (see page 333) at 13 months of age and four plus, as part of the routine childhood immunisation programme.

Side effects: Reactions to mumps vaccine include parotid swelling the weeks after the injection (ie minor mumps-like illness). Other reactions are rare.

Warnings: As warnings prior to vaccination (see page 320).

Neisseria meningitidis

The bacterium *Neisseria meningitidis*, which many of us carry in our noses, can cause severe overwhelming meningitis (infection of the membranes lining the brain) and septicaemia (infection of the blood) with fever, headache, vomiting, collapse, bleeding into the skin and even death occurring within hours.

Epidemics occur in the UK on an irregular basis, and the disease is common in parts of the Indian subcontinent and much of Africa, especially the 'meningitis belt' of sub-Saharan Africa. Children under five are particularly at risk, followed by adolescents and young adults, especially in communities such as schools or colleges. The vaccine contains polysaccharide antigens from two of the three strains of *Neisseria meningitidis* (meningococci): Group A (which is common abroad) and Group C (which accounts for only about a third of circulating strains in the UK). Antibodies are detectable in 90 per cent of people 5–7 days after vaccination, and immunity lasts 3–5 years. Infants have a poorer response and shorter duration of immunity. Currently there is no successful vaccine directed against Group B meningococci, which account for many of the infections in the UK.

People who should consider meningococcal vaccines include travellers for more than a month to high-risk areas including Delhi, Nepal, Bhutan, Pakistan and sub-Saharan Africa. It is also required for travellers to Saudi Arabia during the annual pilgrimage to Mecca. Travellers who have had a spleen removed should have a single dose of vaccine prior to travelling to high risk areas. Family or close contacts of a case of Group C disease should be offered immunisation, in addition to antibiotics. Outbreaks of Group C disease in schools or colleges may be cut short by a programme of mass vaccination of fellow students.

Side effects: These may include a fever, and a swelling at the injection site.

Warnings: As warnings prior to vaccination (see page 320).

Pertussis (whooping cough)

Pertussis (whooping cough) is a respiratory infection caused by the bacterium *Bordetella pertussis*. After an incubation period of 7–10 days, the illness starts with what appears to be a bad cold with a fever and runny nose. During this time the patient is infectious. After a week, spasms of coughing begin (often ending with vomiting or the classical 'whoop' on breathing in) and continue for 2–3 months. Complications include pneumonia, weight loss and occasionally fits in young babies due to a lack of oxygen reaching the brain. It sometimes results in death.

Pertussis vaccine is a suspension of killed *Bordetella pertussis* organism absorbed on to aluminium hydroxide. It is usually given combined with diphtheria and tetanus ('triple' vaccine) and *Haemophilus influenzae* type B for primary immunisation against whooping cough. The course for primary immunisation consists of three doses one month apart starting at two months. Boosters are not given.

Acellular pertussis vaccine consists of highly purified antigens and pertussis toxin from *Bordetella pertussis* which are absorbed on to aluminium hydroxide. It is available on a 'named patient' basis to immunise children whose course of pertussis vaccine was not given or completed as part of their triple vaccine course. Adverse reactions occur less frequently with acellular pertussis vaccine than to the whole cell vaccine.

Warnings: As warnings prior to vaccination (see page 320). Asthma or eczema, febrile convulsions or a stable neurological disorder such as spina bifida is not a reason to deny a child protection against whooping cough. However, if epilepsy or a progressive neurological disorder is involved, this must be discussed with the consultant.

Side effects: Reactions to the combined vaccine (HiB and triple) do not appear to be worse than to either on its own. Local and general reactions (see page 320) are rare. Large population studies have generally failed to show evidence of brain damage or epilepsy following pertussis immunisation, although giving the third dose after six months of age does appear to be associated with a higher rate of febrile convulsions. The current consensus is that the risks associated with the vaccine are much lower than the risks associated with the disease.

Polio

Poliomyelitis is an acute illness caused by an infection by one of three strains of polio virus. After an incubation period of 3–21 days, the virus, which colonises the gut, may spread to attack those grey cells in the brain and spinal cord which control muscles and this results in muscle paralysis and wasting. Often the infection is symptomless, but there may be fever, headache, neck and back stiffness and muscle pain followed by paralysis. Of the people infected, 1 in 75 adults and 1 in 1,000 children will develop paralysis. The infection, which is transmitted either via the stools or throat secretions, spreads rapidly through a household.

The introduction of universal childhood immunisation against polio has virtually eradicated the disease from Europe and the USA. There are two types of vaccine: oral polio vaccine, which contains live attenuated (weakened) virus that colonises the gut but does not spread to the central nervous system, and killed polio virus, which is given by injection. The advantages of the oral polio vaccine include the fact that it may be given by mouth and that, by colonising the gut, it helps drive the wild type virus out of the community. Unfortunately, however, there is a small risk that the virus will revert to causing paralysis and there is an average of one case of paralysis in a recipient of the vaccine and one case in a contact for every 2 million doses of oral polio vaccine given. The killed virus is safe in this regard, but it must be given by injection and will not eradicate wild strains from the community. For primary immunisation three doses are recommended to obtain immunity to all three strains.

Immunisation should be offered to all infants and children. For routine immunisations three doses of the oral vaccine a month apart, starting at two months, are given, usually at the same time as diphtheria/tetanus/pertussis and HiB vaccine. A booster dose is given at school entry combined with diphtheria/tetanus and second MMR injection. A further booster should be given on leaving school at 15–19.

As with children, primary immunisation in adults consists of three doses of polio vaccine one month apart; routine boosters for adults are not recommended. Adults born before 1958 may never have been offered immunisation and they should receive a course. Travellers to areas outside northern and western Europe, North America, Australia and New Zealand should be offered either primary immunisation if previously unimmunised or a booster dose if they have not received a booster dose in the previous 10 years. Health workers should also maintain their levels of immunity. Unimmunised parents of children receiving oral polio vaccine should be offered a dose when their child is immunised.

Either live (oral) or inactivated vaccine can complete a course begun with the other unless there are contra-indications.

Oral polio virus containing live attenuated polio virus types 1, 2 and 3 is the mainstay of the immunisation programme in the UK. The virus may be offered to breastfeeding babies and the dose should be repeated if the baby vomits.

Precautions: The vaccine stain of virus may be shed in the stools for up to six weeks after a dose of vaccine (longer in a baby with HIV) and carers must be scrupulous about washing their hands immediately after changing the baby's nappy. There is a very small risk of paralytic polio in a contact or carer after immunisation. If a carer has never been vaccinated against polio s/he should receive a dose (unless there are contra-indications) at the same time as the baby is immunised.

Side effects: There is a small risk (of the order of one case in a recipient and one case in a contact for every two million doses of vaccine given) that the virus will revert to causing paralysis.

Warnings: As warnings prior to vaccination (see page 320). Not only should the vaccine not be given to people who are immunosuppressed but it must not be given to their household contacts either. The vaccine should not be given at the same time as oral typhoid vaccine.

Rabies

Rabies (hydrophobia) is an acute viral infection which, after an incubation period of two to eight weeks, attacks the brain and is almost universally fatal. The virus is transmitted via a bite from a rabid animal. The rabies virus is endemic in dogs in Asia, Africa and Latin America whereas the main reservoir in Europe is in foxes. Rabies does not occur in the UK. The vaccine contains inactivated virus grown in human tissue culture and is used to protect people who might come into contact with rabies virus (pre-exposure prophylaxis) and those who may have had a recent exposure to the virus (post-exposure prophylaxis).

For pre-exposure prophylaxis, the vaccine is recommended for people who may come into contact with rabies as part of their work (eg staff at quarantine kennels). People living or travelling in remote areas where the virus is present in animals should also consider vaccination.

For post-exposure prophylaxis, the vaccine may help to prevent the illness if given early in the incubation period, and travellers who experience a bite or contamination of a mucosal surface should clean the wound immediately by scrubbing with soap and water under a running tap for five minutes and then seek medical assistance locally or immediately on their return to the UK. Under certain circumstances the vaccine may be combined with human rabies specific immunoglobulin.

Rabies vaccine consists of freeze-dried inactivated Wistar rabies virus cultivated in human diploid cells. For primary pre-exposure prophylaxis three doses are given, the second one week and the third one month after the first injection. Travellers who are not animal handlers and where post-exposure prophylaxis is available will get a degree of immunity from two injections one month apart followed by a third dose 6–12 months later. For detailed advice consult your doctor or occupational health adviser.

Side effects: These may include fever, malaise and soreness at the injection site. Occasionally there are more severe reactions.

Warnings: None

Specific rabies immunoglobulin

General information: Specific rabies immunoglobulin is prepared from the plasma of blood donors known to have a high level of protective antibody in their plasma. It is screened for hepatitis B and C and HIV. Under certain circumstances it is given in conjunction with rabies vaccine.

Side effects: The main side effect is discomfort at the injection site. Allergic reactions are rare, and most frequently occur in people who have previously reacted to blood products.

Warnings: As warnings prior to vaccination (see page 320). Not to be given to anyone who suffered a severe reaction to a previous dose.

Rubella

Rubella is a mild self-limiting viral infection that causes fever, a red raised rash and, occasionally, arthritis and joint pains. A pregnant woman who contracts the infection may pass it on to her unborn child, who may then suffer abnormalities that include deafness, blindness, heart disease and brain damage. Rubella is not a distinctive illness and infections may not be obvious, so the aim is to ensure that all women are immune prior to starting a pregnancy and also to immunise all young children to reduce circulating the virus in the community. Because of the previous programme targeting teenage girls, the main reservoir in the community now is young men.

Rubella vaccine is a live attenuated virus grown in human tissue culture cells. On its own it is used to immunise women of child-bearing age who have been shown by a blood test to lack protective antibodies to rubella. Rubella combined with measles and mumps as MMR (see page 333) is given at 13 months and four plus as part of the routine childhood immunisation programme.

Side effects: Reactions to rubella vaccine include rash, a fever 5–12 days after vaccination and joint pains (more common in adults). Serious reactions are rare.

Warnings: As warnings prior to vaccination (see page 320). The vaccine should not be given in pregnancy and the woman must not get pregnant for at least a month after being vaccinated.

Normal immunoglobulin

General information: Normal immunoglobulin prepared from the plasma of routine blood donors, screened for hepatitis B and C and HIV, contains antibody to rubella. Given as soon as possible after contact to a non-immune pregnant woman who would refuse a termination, it will not prevent the infection but may reduce the severity of the illness and offer some protection to her unborn baby. Protection is by far inferior to active immunisation.

Side effects: The main side effect is discomfort at the injection site. Allergic reactions are rare, and most frequently occur in people who have previously reacted to blood products.

Warnings: As warnings prior to vaccination (see page 320). Not to be given to anyone who suffered a severe reaction to a previous dose.

Measles/mumps/rubella combined vaccine

General information: Measles/mumps/rubella combined vaccine (MMR) was introduced in an attempt to eradicate those three illnesses from the population and to obtain better coverage than from the separate measles and rubella programme. The vaccine is a freeze-dried preparation of live attenuated measles, mumps and rubella virus which has to be reconstituted with a special diluent.

In the UK the first dose is delayed until after the age of one, usually between 13 and 15 months, to ensure any maternal antibody which could interfere with the immune response has been cleared from the child's circulation. Over 90 per cent of children given the vaccine will develop protective antibodies lasting many years. Unfortunately, the fact that vaccination coverage is not complete and that a proportion of children who are vaccinated fail to develop immunity to all components brings the overall level of immunity in the population down and means there will be sufficient non-immune people in the population to maintain epidemics. Therefore a second dose is given at four plus. Doses may also be offered to older children who missed the routine doses or at entry to institutions of further education and to people with chronic diseases. People with HIV should discuss MMR with their consultant.

The vaccine should be offered to all eligible people regardless of a history of measles, mumps or rubella. It is not harmful to people who are already immune and will not transmit the viruses to others.

Side effects: Local reactions include redness, pain or burning at the injection site; occasional hives at the injection site. General reactions are similar to those listed under the individual components and are not worse with the combined vaccine.

Warnings: As warnings prior to vaccination (see page 320). Remember, the vaccine must not be given in pregnancy and pregnancy must be avoided for at least one month after injection. Because of reduced effectiveness, do not give within three months of an injection of immunoglobulin. A history of severe allergic reactions to eggs, with facial swelling, hives, and wheezing, does not appear to be a contra-indication to MMR, even though it might be better to have the injection under supervision in hospital. In any case dislike or refusal to eat eggs is not a reason not to have the vaccination.

Streptococcus pneumoniae

Streptococcus pneumoniae (the pneumococcus) is an encapsulated bacterium that causes a range of severe infections including pneumonia, meningitis, bacteraemia (infections in the blood). It may follow a flu-like illness and commonly causes infection in the young, the elderly or people with impaired immunity, including those without a spleen. At least 84 strains have been identified on the basis of polysaccharide capsular antigens and immunity depends in part on the presence of antibodies to these antigens. Current vaccines contain purified polysaccharide from the 23 strains of pneumococci that together account for over 90 per cent of infections in the UK. The vaccine should be offered to patients with sickle cell disease, absent spleens, immunosuppression including HIV, chronic heart, lung, renal or liver disease, diabetes and coeliac disease.

Most healthy adults develop a good antibody response by three weeks, but the response in children under two, the elderly and those who are immunosuppressed is not so good.

Side effects: Soreness and thickening at the injection site, occasional fever. Revaccination is not recommended within 5–10 years.

Warnings: As warnings prior to vaccination (see page 320). Not to be given in pregnancy or to women who are breastfeeding.

Tetanus

Tetanus is an acute disease characterised by painful muscle spasm and rigidity. The cause is a powerful neurotoxin, *tetanospasmin*. This is produced by the organism *Clostridia tetani*, whose spores are everywhere in the environment and soil. After a wound has been contaminated by spores they germinate. The multiplying bacteria produce *tetanospasmin* which travels via the blood and peripheral nerves to the brain and spinal cord. Here *tetanospasmin* blocks inhibitory neurones and leads to over-excitability of the motor neurones and muscle spasm.

Clostridia cannot survive in the presence of normal amounts of oxygen, so tetanus-prone wounds are those where there is tissue damage (eg burns, wounds with damaged or dying tissue) or foreign bodies (puncture wounds while gardening, the classical rusty nail). Such wounds create a space without oxygen in the body where the organism can survive.

For primary immunisation in infancy three doses starting at two months with a month between each dose are recommended (usually given with diphtheria, pertussis and HiB). A booster at school entry (combined with diphtheria) and at school leaving age (combined with diphtheria) complete the course. Unimmunised adults require three injections each a month apart with two further boosters 10 and 20 years after primary immunisation. If five injections of toxoid have been given then no further routine booster injections are required, although a booster may be required at the time of a tetanus-prone wound. A single dose of booster in a previously immunised person will give a rapid rise in antibody levels.

Patients with tetanus-prone wounds will require active immunisation with tetanus toxoid and in some cases immediate protection with human tetanus immunoglobulin. If you have such a wound or you have impaired immunity, you should seek immediate advice from your doctor or local casualty department.

Tetanus toxoid

General information: Tetanus toxoid is available on its own for primary immunisation or boosters in adults. It is also available combined with diphtheria and pertussis ('triple vaccine') or with *Haemophilus influenzae* type B in addition for primary immunisation in infants. It is also available with two strengths of diphtheria for booster doses in childhood and adolescence.

Side effects: Local reactions include pain, redness and swelling around the injection site and sometimes a nodule at the injection site. Occasionally, people experience a flu-like illness with fever. More severe reactions are rare.

Warnings: As warnings prior to vaccination (see page 320).

Specific tetanus immunoglobulin

General information: Specific tetanus immunoglobulin is prepared from the plasma of blood donors known to have a high concentration of antibody to tetanus toxoid in their plasma. It is screened for hepatitis B and C and HIV. Given in conjunction with tetanus toxoid it will provide immediate temporary protection to patients with a tetanus-prone wound.

Side effects: The main side effect is discomfort at the injection site. Allergic reactions are rare, and most frequently occur in people who have previously reacted to blood products.

Warnings: As warnings prior to vaccination (see page 320). Not to be given to anyone who suffered a severe reaction to a previous dose.

Tuberculosis

Tuberculosis is a chronic infection caused by *Mycobacterium tuberculosis*. In the UK it is spread by droplets coughed up by an infected person. The spectrum of infection is very wide and after the initial infection the organism may lie dormant in the body and become active years later. However, cell mediated immunity to *M. tuberculosis* develops after 6–8 weeks and can be detected by a skin test (Mantoux or Heaf Test). TB mainly affects the lung with cough and fever, but may spread to other parts of the body. The disease is associated with poverty and is 20–50 times more common in underdeveloped countries than in the UK. *M. tuberculosis* is held in check by the immune system and immunosuppressant drugs or diseases such as HIV which impair the immune system lead to reactivation of the disease.

Immunisation against TB is with Bacillus Calmette-Guérin vaccine (BCG) which is a freeze-dried live attenuated bacterial vaccine prepared from a related strain to TB, *Mycobacterium bovis*, and named after the microbiologists who developed the original strain. The vaccination must not be given to someone who is already immune to TB as there will be a severe reaction, so everyone over three months of age must have a skin test (Mantoux or Heaf) prior to vaccination. Immunity after immunisation develops 2–3 months after immunisation and lasts about 15 years. It does not give complete immunity to TB, but does protect against the more severe forms of the disease.

People who should have the vaccine are children between 10 and 14 years of age, health workers (including students), contacts of patients with active pulmonary TB, immigrants from countries with a high incidence of TB and their UK-born children, staff in prisons, residential homes and hostels and those intending to stay for more than a month in countries with a high incidence of TB.

Precautions: BCG may be given at the same time as another live vaccine, but if they are not given simultaneously then three weeks should elapse between them, except in the case of babies where primary immunisation can proceed as normal. Except in babies under three months, the vaccination should not be given without a prior skin test. No other vaccine should be given in that arm for three months after BCG injection.

Side effects: A papule develops at the injection site within 2–4 weeks. It may scale or crust before healing to form a depressed scar by about six weeks. In dark-skinned people a keloid (thickened raised purple scar) may result. Sometimes there is a discharging ulcer which mostly requires no further treatment. Occasionally there is enlargement of the local lymph nodes. More severe reactions are very rare.

Warnings: As warnings prior to vaccination (see page 320). Septic skin conditions or eczema at the injection site may also occur. Do not take the vaccine if you have a positive skin test or have recently been given the live virus vaccine.

Typhoid

Typhoid fever is an unpleasant feverish illness caused by a bacterium, *Salmonella typhi*, which is one species of a large group of organisms well known for causing gastroenteritis and food poisoning. After an incubation period of one to three weeks, patients develop a fever, rash and constipation followed by bloody diarrhoea. The organism is shed in the stool for up to three months after the acute illness and sometimes for much longer. New cases result when food or water contaminated by infected stools is eaten or drunk; typhoid occurs mainly in countries with low standards of sanitation and hygiene. About 80 per cent of infections in the UK are contracted abroad, mainly from Asia.

Typhoid vaccine comes in two forms – a live attenuated strain taken by mouth and a killed vaccine containing the Vi (from *virulence*) polysaccharide antigen from the capsule. Neither vaccine gives complete protection, and travellers to high-risk areas should still take stringent precautions to prevent infection.

People who should consider vaccination are travellers to countries in Africa, Asia, South and Central America, the Caribbean and some parts of Eastern Europe where sanitation is poor. Immunisation is recommended for laboratory workers handling specimens that may contain typhoid organisms.

Live oral vaccine

General information: Live attenuated *Salmonella typhi* (Ty 21a) in an enteric coated capsule. The dose for adults and children over six is one capsule on days one, three, and five. The capsule should be swallowed as soon as possible after being placed in the mouth with a cold or lukewarm drink and the capsules should be stored in the refrigerator. Protection develops 7–10 days after the last dose and lasts up to three years in those repeatedly exposed to infection but occasional travellers will require annual doses.

Side effects: Less than 1 per cent of vaccinees experience mild gastroenteritis, with nausea, vomiting, cramps and diarrhoea.

Warnings: As warnings prior to vaccination (see page 320). The vaccine is not suitable for children under six years of age, during a febrile illness or if there is diarrhoea or vomiting. Oral polio and typhoid should be given three weeks apart. Antibiotics may interfere with oral typhoid and should not be taken at the same time. Ideally the vaccine course should be completed three days before malaria prophylaxis with mefloquine is begun.

Polysaccharide vaccine for injection

General information: Vi capsular polysaccharide typhoid vaccine contains the virulence polysaccharide antigen of *Salmonella typhi*. After a delay of about two weeks, a single dose gives protection in over 77 per cent of recipients lasting up to three years. Three yearly boosters are recommended for people who are still exposed to the risk of infection.

Side effects: Up to 20 per cent of recipients get redness and swelling in the arm and up to 3 per cent of recipients may develop a flu-like illness.

Warnings: As warnings prior to vaccination (see page 320). There is no data about its safety in pregnancy. Children under 18 months do not develop a good antibody response to this vaccine and protection is questionable.

Yellow fever

Yellow fever is an acute viral infection found in tropical Africa and South America where it is transmitted by bites from local mosquitoes, with monkeys in the jungle acting as reservoirs of infection. After an incubation period of 3–6 days, symptoms develop with, at its worst, a severe flu-like illness with fever and muscle pains, haemorrhage and, as its name suggests, jaundice. The death rate in locals is about 5 per cent, but during epidemics or in unimmunised adults visiting an area it can approach 50 per cent. There is no treatment for the disease. Apart from measures to protect against insect bites, the main protection is provided by immunisation with a live attenuated viral vaccine.

People who should consider vaccination are travellers over the age of nine months going to areas that are infected or living outside urban areas in those areas where yellow fever is potentially endemic. Protection against yellow fever, attested by a valid International Certificate of Vaccination, is a requirement for entry into some countries, either for all travellers or those coming from infected areas. Travellers should seek up-to-date advice. It is important not to be vaccinated at the border by potentially unsterile needles and travellers who on medical grounds must not be vaccinated should get a letter from their doctor and discuss the situation with the embassy of the country concerned.

Immunity develops 10 days after the injection and is probably life-long, but booster injections after 10 years are recommended for travel.

Yellow fever vaccine consists of a suspension of chick embryo proteins containing attenuated 17D strain of the yellow fever virus. The vaccine contains traces of the antibiotics polymyxin and neomycin.

Side effects: These include local pain and swelling lasting 2–5 days in 5 per cent of recipients. A mild flu-like illness develops in 2–5 per cent of vaccinees. More severe reactions are rare but babies under 9 months are more likely to develop an encephalitis (involvement of the brain).

Warnings: As warnings prior to vaccination (see page 320). The vaccine is not recommended routinely in pregnancy or for babies under 9 months unless the risk of yellow fever is unavoidable. Other live virus vaccines can be given simultaneously with yellow fever or after a delay of three weeks. Human normal immunoglobulin can be given at the same time as yellow fever as the UK preparation is unlikely to contain antibodies to yellow fever.

INDEX

A
Ababact 218
Abelcet 264-5
Abidec 318
acarbose 167-8
Accolate 142
accuhaler 134
Accupro 89
Accuretic 89
ACE (angiotensin-
  converting enzyme)
  inhibitors 7, 86-9
acebutolol 84
aceclofenac 147
acemetacin 147
acetazolamide 229
acetylcholine 41, 52, 138
acetylcholinesterase 58
acetylcysteine 232
Achromycin 251
aciclovir 215, 224, 225, 240,
  268
Aci-Jel 188
acipimox 100-1
acitretin 208
Aclacin 293
aclarubicin 293
alcometasone 205
acne 201, 211-13
acne rosacea 218
Acnecide 212
Acnidazil 212
Acnisal 213
acrivastine 285
Actinac 212
Acupan 61
Adalat/ Adalat LA/ Adalat
  Retard 96
adapalene 211-12
Adcortyl 151, 208
  Adcortyl in Orabase 242
  Adcortyl with Graneodin
  208
Addison's disease 163-5,
  172
ADH see anti-diuretic
  hormones
Adipine MR 96
Adizem-60/ Adizem-SR/
  Adizem-XL 95
adrenal glands 162-5, 172,
  174
adrenaline 162, 229, 288-9
adrenoceptor stimulants
  135-8
AeroBec 140
Aerocrom 141
Aerolin 137
agitation, severe 40-5
agonists 6-7
AIDS 245, 268-75, 296
Airomir 137
Akineton 53
albendazole 282

Alcoban 265
Alcoderm 202
alcohol 12, 14, 15, 16, 19,
  23, 78, 290
Aldactone 82
aldesleukin 293
Aldomet 91
aldosterone 162, 164
alendronic acid 159
alfacalcidol 317
Alfa-D 317
alfuzosin 197
Algesal 150
Algicon 114
alginates 113, 114
Algitec 119
Alkeran 299
allergens 132, 134, 284
allergic reactions, severe
  284, 288-9
allergies 284, see also asthma,
  eczema; hayfever
  nasal 234, 237-9
  see also antihistamines
allopurinol 153, 154
Alomide 228
alpha-blockers 90-2, 196-7
Alphaderm 207
Alphagan 229
Alpha Keri Bath 202
Alphosyl 209
  Alphosyl HC 207
alprazolam 27
alprostadil 194-5
Altacite Plus 114
altretamine 293
Alu-Cap 114, 314
aluminium chloride 222
aluminium hydroxide 114,
  314
Alupent 137
Alvercol 115
alverine 115
Alzheimer's disease 25, 26,
  58-9
amantadine 54, 269
Ambisome 264-5
Amias 87
amiloride 82, 84
aminoglutethimide 305
aminophylline 139
aminosalicylates 124-6
amiodarone 106
amisulpride 42
amitriptyline 3, 32, 33
amlodipine 95
Ammonia and Ipecacuanha
  Mixture 143
amoebiasis 279
amorolfine 215
amoxapine 32, 33
Amoxil 248
amoxycillin 120, 248
Amphocil 264-5

amphotericin 241, 264-5
ampicillin 248
amsacrine 293
Amsidine 293
amylobarbitone 29
Amytal 29
anabolic steroids 174-5
anaemias:
  iron-deficiency 310, 311-12
  megaloblastic (pernicious)
  310, 312-13
  from renal failure 313
anaesthetics, local 241
Anafranil/Ananfranil SR 33
analgesics 26, 59
  non-opioid 59-61
  opioid 62-5
anaphylactic shock/
  anaphylaxis 284, 288-9
  from vaccines 320
anastrozole 306
Androcur 189
Andropatch 189
Angettes 75 104
angina 4, 7, 77, 78
  beta-blockers 82-6
  calcium channel blockers
  94-6
  nitrates 93-4
angioedema, hereditary 175
Angiopine 40 LA 96
angiotensin-converting
  enzyme inhibitors see
  ACE inhibitors
angiotensin-II-receptor
  antagonists 86, 87, 88, 89
Angitil SR 95
Anhydrol Forte 222
anion-exchange resins 100
ankylosing spondylitis 145,
  147, 149
Anquil 42
antacids 113-15, 118
antagonists 7, 70, 86, 87, 88,
  89
antazoline 228
Antepsin 122
anthelmintics 281-3
anti-adrenal drugs 174
anti-arrhythmics 105-9
antibacterials 5
antibiotics 6, 8, 245, 246-60
  topical 211-13, 215, 216-19
anticoagulants 102-3
anticonvulsants 47-51
antidepressants 20, 32-40
  MAOIs 38-9
  NARIs 39-40
  SSRIs 36-8
  tricyclics 32-5
antidiabetic drugs, oral 167-9
anti-diuretic hormones
  (ADH) 162, 164, 175-6
anti-emetics 70-5

antifungal drugs 8, 215-20,
  245, 264-8
antihistamines 6, 29, 284-8
antihypertensives 4
anti-infective skin prep-
  arations 215-20
antimalarial drugs 245, 275-8
antimanic drugs 46
antimuscarinic broncho-
  dilators 138
antiperspirant 222
antiplatelet drugs 102, 104-5
antiprotozoal drugs 279-81
antipsychotic drugs 40-5
antirheumatic drugs,
  disease-modifying 151-3
antiseptics 215
antispasmodics 115-17
antiviral drugs 8, 215, 217,
  218, 245, 268-75
Anturan 155
Anugesic HC cream/
  suppositories 130
Anusol ointment/
  suppositories 130
anxiety 25, 29-31, 37, 82
apomorphine 54
Apresoline 91
Aprovel 88
Aquadrate 202
Aquasept 220
aqueous cream 202
Aredia 160-1
Aricept 58
Arimidex 306
Arpicolin 53
arrhythmia 78, 82-6, 96,
  103, 105-10
arteries 77
arthritis 144, 146
  osteoarthritis 144-5
  rheumatoid arthritis see
  rheumatoid arthritis
  Still's disease 145
Arthrotec 121, 148
Arythmol 108-9
Asacool 125
ascorbic acid 316
Asendis 33
Aserbine cream/solution
  215
Asilone 114
Asmabec 140
Asmasal 137
aspirin 20, 59, 60, 104, 112,
  133
Assantin Retard 104-5
astemizole 285
asthma 14, 15, 132-3,
  135-42, 284
  inhalers 134-5
AT10 solution 317
Atarax 287
atenolol 3, 84

atherosclerosis 77
athlete's foot 201, 216, 264
Ativan 28
atorvastatin 98
atovaquone 279
Atromid S 99
Atrovent 138
Audicort 236
Augmentin 248
auranofin 152
Aureocort 208
Aureomycin 216, 225
Autohalers 134
autonomic nervous system 25
Aveeno 202
Avloclor 276
Avomine 74
Axid 119
azapropazone 147
azatadine 286
azathioprine 308
azelaic acid 212
azelastine 228, 237
azithromycin 252

B
baclofen 157
Bactroban 218, 240
baldness, male 222
Balmosa 150
Balneum/Balneum Plus 203
  Balneum with Tar 209
balsalazide 125
Baltar 209
Bambec 136
bambuterol 136
Baratol 91
barbiturates 29
barrier preparations 204
bath additives 202–4
Baxan 249
Baycaron 81
BCG vaccination 321, 336
Becloforte 140
beclomethasone 140, 205, 237
Becodisks 140
Beconase 237
Becotide 140
bed sores 204, 217
bedwetting 32, 33, 34, 35, 176
Behcet's disease 175
bendrofluazide 80, 84, 85, 86
Benemid 155
Benoral 60
benperidol 42
benserazide 55
Benzamycin 212
benzhexol 52–3
benzodiazepines 26–9, 46
benzoic acid 215
benzoyl peroxide 212, 216
benzthiazide 82
benztropine 53
benzydamine 150, 241
benzyl benzoate 220
benzylpenicillin 248
Berotec 136
beta stimulants 135–8
Beta-Adalat 84
beta-blockers 7, 29, 82–6
Betacap 206
Betacardone 86
Betadine 188, 218, 243
Betagan 231
betahistine 70–1
Betaloc/Betaloc SA 85

betamethasone 173, 205, 227, 235, 237
betaxolol 84, 229
bethanecol 197, 198
Betim 86
Betnelan 173
Betnesol 173, 235, 237
  Betnesol N 227, 235, 240
Betnovate 130, 206
Betoptic 229
Bettamousse 206
bezafibrate 99
Bezalip/Bezalip Mono 99
bicalutamide 306
Bicillin 248
BiCNU 294
BiNovum 180
Bioplex 241
Biorphen 53
biperiden 53
bisacodyl 127, 128
bismuth chelate 117, 118, 120–1
bisoprolol 84
blackheads 201
bladder, the 196
  cancer 300, 301
  see also urinary problems
bleomycin 294
Blocadren 86
blood 77
blood clots 77, 78, 102
blood clotting *see* anti-coagulants; antiplatelet drugs
blood vessels 77
  vasodilators 90–2
Bocasan 244
Bonefos 161
bones 144
  disorders 144–6, 158–61
brain, the 24–5
brain tumours 294
bran 126, 127
Brasivol 213
breast cancer 193, 290, 291, 296, 297, 300, 302–7
breastfeeding 14, 22
breathing problems 132–3
Brevibloc 85
Brevinor 180
Bricanyl/Bricanyl SA 137
brimonidine 229
Britaject 54
Broflex 52–3
Brolene 226
bromazepam 27
bromocriptine 54–5, 190
brompheniramine 286
bronchiolitis 274
bronchitis 133, 139, 250, 323
Bronchodil 137
bronchodilators 133, 134, 135–9, 140
Brufen 3, 148
  Brufen Retard 148
bruising 222
Buccastem 44
Budenofalk 124
budesonide 124, 141, 237
bulimia nervosa 36, 37
bumetanide 80
buprenorphine 62
Burinex 80
  Burinex A 82
  Burinex K 80
Buscopan 116
buserelin 190
Buspar 30

buspirone 30
busulphan 294
Butacote 149
butobarbitone 29

C
Cabaser 55
cabergoline 55, 191
Cacit 314
  Cacit D3 317
Caelyx 296
Cafergot 66
calamine 204
Calceos 317
Calcicard CR 95
Calcichew 314
  Calcichew D3/Calcichew D3 Forte 317
Calcidrink 314
Calcijex 317
calcipotriol 208
Calcitare 159–60
calcitonin 159–60, 162
calcitriol 317
Calcium-500 314
calcium channel blockers 8, 94–6
calcium preparations 313–14
calcium salts 314
Calcium-Sandoz 314
Calcort 173
calluses 201, 214
Calmurid 203
  Calmurid HC 207
Calsynar 159–60
Camcolit 46
Campto 299
cancer 290–309
  see also specific cancers
candesartan 87
Candida albicans 264
Canesten 188, 216, 235
  Canesten HC 207
Capasal 209
capillaries 77
Capostat 261
Capoten 87
capreomycin 260–1
Caprin 104
captopril 87
Carace/Carace Plus 88
carbachol 197, 198, 230
Carbalax 129
carbamazepine 46
carbaryl 220
carbazepine 47–8
carbenoxolone 121, 241
carbimazole 7, 171
Carbo-Dome 209
carbomers 232
carboplatin 294
Cardene/Cardene SR 96
Cardilate MR 96
Cardura 91, 197
Carisoma 157
carisoprodol 157
carmellose 241
carmustine 294
carteolol 230
carvedilol 84
Carylderm 221
Casodex 306
Catapres 90
Caverject 195
CCNU 299
Cedax 250
Cedocard Retard 94

cefaclor 249
cefadroxil 249
cefixime 249
cefpodoxime 249
cefprozil 249
ceftibuten 250
cefuroxime 250
Cefzil 249
Celance 57
Celectol 84
Celevac 127
celiprolol 84
CellCept 309
cephalexin 250
cephalosporins 248–50
Ceporex 250
cerivastatin 98
Cerubidin 296
Cerumol 236
cetirizine 284, 286
cetylpyridium 242
CFC-free inhalers 135
chemotherapy 291–3, 321
  nausea from 70, 72–5
chenodeoxycholic acid 131
Chenofalk 131
chest infections 134, 250, 252
chickenpox 217
chilblains 222
chloral 30
chlorambucil 295
chloramphenicol 225, 235, 256
chlordiazepoxide 27
chlorhexidine 216, 242
chlormethiazole 30
Chlormycetin 225
chlorofluorcarbon–free inhalers 135
Chlorohex 242
chloroquine 151, 276, 278
chlorothiazide 80
chlorpeniramine 284, 286
chlorpromazine 42, 70
chlorpropamide 168
chlortetracycline 216, 225
chlorthalidone 81, 84
cholecalciferol 317
cholesterol 78, 97
  see also lipid-lowering drugs
cholestyramine 100
chorionic gonadotrophin 191
Chroagon 191
Cicatrin 218
cidofovir 269
Cidomycin 226, 235
  Cidomycin Topical 217
cilazapril 88
Cilest 180
Ciloxan 225
cimetidine 119
cinnarizine 71
Cinobac 255
cinoxacin 255
Cipramil 37
ciprofibrate 99
ciprofloxacin 225, 255
Ciproxin 255
cisapride 117
cisplatin 294
citalopram 37
cladribine 295
clarithromycin 120, 252
Clarityn 287
clemastine 286
clickhaler 134
Climagest 184

Climaval 184
Climesse 184
clindamycin 188, 212, 256
Clinitar 209
Clinoril 150
clobazam 48
clobetasol 206
clobetasone 206, 227
Cloburate 227
clofibrate 99
Clomid 192
clomiphene 192
clomipramine 32, 33
clonazepam 48
clonidine 69, 90
clopamide 85
clopidogrel 104
Clopixol 45
    Clopixol Accuphase 45
clorazepate 27
Clotam 68
clotrimazole 188, 216, 235
clozapine 42
Clozaril 42
coal tar 209
co-amilofruse 82
co-amilozide 82, 86
co-amoxiclav 248
Cobadex 207
Co-beneldopa 55
Co-Betaloc/Co-Betaloc SA 85
Co-careldopa 55
co-codamol 61
Cocois 209
Codafen Continus 148
Co-danthromer 128
Co-danthrusate 128
codeine 7, 15, 20, 61, 63, 123
    Codein Linctus 143
co-fluampicil 248
Cogentin 53
Colazide 125
colchicine 153, 154
cold sores 201, 215, 217,
    219, 240, 268, 270
Colestid 100
colestipol 100
Colifoam 124
colistin 256-7
colitis see ulcerative colitis
Colofac 116
Colomycin 219, 256-7
colon cancer 297, 299, 301
Colpermin 117
Combivent 138
Combivir 275
Comtess 56
Concordin 35
Condrotec 149
Condyline 214
conjunctivitis 224, 227-8
Conotrane 204
constipation 112, 113
    see also laxatives
contraceptives
    combined oral 178-81
    emergency ('morning
        after' pill) 182-3
    progestogen-only 181-2
Convulex 51
co-phenotrope 123
co-prenozide 85
co-proxamol 61
Coracten 96
Cordarone X 106
Cordilox 96
Corgard 85
Corgaretic 85
Corlan 242

Coroday MR 96
coronary heart disease 77,
    178
coronary thrombosis 102
Coro-Nitro Pump Spray 93
Corsodyl 242
corticosteroids 124, 134,
    139-41, 151, 171-3, 308
    eye preparations 226-7
    mouth preparations 242
    topical 205-8, 212
cortisol 162
cortisone 173
Cortisyl 173
Corwin 110
Cosmegen Lyovac 296
Cosopt 230
co-triamterzide 82
co-trimoxazole 253
coughs 133
cough suppressants 133, 143
Coversyl 89
Cozaar/Cozaar-Comp 88
Creon 131
Crinone gel 187
crisantaspase 295
Crixivan 271
Crohn's disease 112, 113,
    123-6
Cromogen 141
cromoglycate 141, 238
cromones 141
crotamiton cream 204
Crystapen 248
Cuplex 214
Curatoderm 211
Cushing's syndrome 164, 174
Cutivate 207
CX Antiseptic Dusting
    Powder 216
cyanocobalamin 312
Cyclimorph 64
cyclizine 71
Cyclogest pessaries 187
cyclopenthiazide 81, 85
cyclophosphamide 295
Cyclo-Progynova 184
cycloserine 261
cyclosporin 208, 308-9
Cymevene 270
cyproheptadine 286
Cyprostat 189
cyproterone acetate 189
cystic fibrosis 113, 131, 142,
    315, 317
cystitis 196
Cystrin 199
cytarabine 295
Cytostar 295
Cytotec 121
cytotoxics 291-3

D
dacarbazine 296
dactinomycin 296
Daktacort 207
Daktarin 218, 242
Dalacin 188
    Dalacin C 256
    Dalacin T 212
Dalivit 318
Dalmane 28
danazol 192
dandruff 201, 210, 218
Danol 192
danthron 128
Dantrium 157-8
dantrolene 156, 157-8

Daonil 168
dapsone 278
Daraprim 278
daunorubicin 296
DaunoXome 296
DC Skin Cleanser 217
DDAVP 176
Decadron 151, 173
    Decadron Shock-Pak 173
Deca-Durabolin 175
De-capeptyl 194
declofenac 150
decongestants 133, 135, 143
deflazacort 173
Deltastab 151
demeclocycline 251
dementia 25, 40
    see also Alzheimer's disease
demulcents 143
Dencyl 311
De-Nol 120-1
De-Noltab 120-1
Dentinox 114
Depixol 42
Depomedrone 151
    Depomedrone with Lidocaine
        151
Deponit 93
Depo-Provera 182, 304
Depostat 304
depot injections 9
depression 25, 46
    see also antidepressants
Derbac C 221
Derbac M 221
Dermamist 203
dermatitis 200-1, 308
Dermestril 184
Dermol 500 203
Dermovate/Dermovate NN
    206
Deseril 69
desmopressin 175, 176
Desmospray 176
Desmotabs 176
desoxymethasone 206
Destolit 151
Deteclo 251
Detrunorm 199
Detrusitol 199
dexamethasone 151, 173,
    227, 236, 238
Dexarhinaspray Duo 238
dextromoramide 63
dextropropoxyphene 61, 63
DF118 63
DHC Continus 63
diabetes (mellitus) 7, 78, 86,
    164, 167-9, 175, 224
    diabetes insipidus 164, 175,
        176
    and hypoglycaemia 169
Diamicron 168
diamorphine 63
Diamox/Diamox SR 229
Dianette 189
Diarrest 123
diarrhoea 112, 113, 122-3
diazepam 28, 156
diclofenac 121, 148, 153
Diclomax Retard 148
Diclomax SR 148
Diconal 63
dicyclomine 116
didanosine 269
Didronel/Didronel PMO 160
Differin 211-12
Difflam 150, 241
Diflucan 188, 265

diflucortolone 206
diflunisal 148
digestive system 111
digoxin 11, 109-10
dihydrocodeine 61, 63
dihydroergotamine 66
dihydrotachysterol 317
Dilcardia SR 95
diloxanide 279
diltiazem 95
Dilzem SR 95
Dilzem XL 95
dimenhydrinate 72
dimethicone 114
Dimetriose 193
Dimotane/Dimotane LA 286
Dindevan 103
Diocalm Junior 123
Dioctyl 128
Dioderm 207
Dioralyte/Dioralyte Relief 123
Diovan 89
Diovol 114
Dipentum 125
diphenhydramine 29
diphtheria vaccine 321,
    322, 323
dipipanone 63
dipivefrine 230
Diprobase 203
Diprobath 203
Diprosalic 206
Diprosone 206
dipyridamole 104-5
Dirythmin SA 106
Disipal 53
Diskhalers 134
disopyramide 106-7
disposing of old medicines
    19
Disprin CV 104
Distaclor/Distaclor MR 249
Distamine 153
distigmine 156, 197, 198
Ditemic 311
dithranol 209-10
Dithrocream 209-10
Ditropan 199
Diumide-K Continus 80
diuretics 79-82
Diurexan 81
diverticular disease/diver-
    ticulitis 112
    see also antispasmodics
Dixarit 69
dizziness 70-5
docetaxel 296
docusate 128
Docusol 128
Dolmatil 45
Dolobid 148
Doloxene 63
Domperamol 66
domperidone 70, 72
donepezil 58
dopamine 40, 52
Doralese 197
dornase alpha 142
dorzolamide 230
dosages 15, 16, 22
Dostinex 191, 194
dothiepin 32, 33
Dovonex 209
doxazosin 90, 91, 196, 197
doxepin 32, 34
doxorubicin 296
doxycycline 251
Dozic 43
Dramamine 72

Drapolone 204
Driclor 222
Drigenil 306
Droleptan 42
droperidol 42
DTIC-Dome 296
Dulco-Lax 128
Dumicoat 242
Duofilm 214
Duovent 136
Duphaston/Duphston HRT 187
Durogesic 64
Duromine 76
Dutonin 37
Dyazide 82
dydrogesterone 183, 187
Dyspamet 119
dyspepsia 111–12
    see also antacids
Dytide 82

E
E45 203
ears 234
    infections 234, 235–6, 246
ear wax 234, 236
Econacort 207
econazole 188, 216
Ecostatin 188, 216
eczema 200, 201, 202, 208–11, 284–8
Edecrin 80
Edronax 39–40
Efalith 210
Efcortelan 207
Efcortesol 173
Efexor/Efexor XL 44
eformoterol 136
Efudix 297
Elantan/Elantan LA 94
Eldepryl 58
Eldisine 303
Electrolade 123
elixirs 9
Elleste-Duet 184
Elleste-Solo/Elleste Solo MX 184
Elocon 208
Eludril 242
embolisms 102
Emcor 84
Emeside 48–9
Emflex 147
Emmolate 203
emollients 202
emphysema 133, 135–8
    inhalers 133–5
Emulsiderm 203
emulsifying ointment 202
emulsions 9
En-de-Kay 315
enalapril 88
endocrine glands 162–4
endometrial cancer 183
endometriosis 178, 186, 191–4
Endoxana 295
enemas 128, 129, 130
entacapone 56
Entocort 124
enzymes 7, 86, 111
Epaderm 203
Epanutin 50
ephedrine 240
epiglottitis 323
epilepsy 14, 25, 47–51
Epilim 51
EpiPen/EpiPen Junior 288–9

epirubicin 297
Epivir 271–2
Epogam 210
Eppy 229
Eprex 313
Equagesic 31
Erecnos 195
ergocalciferol 317
ergotamine 66
erthropoeitin 313
Erwinase 295
Eryacne 212
Erymax 252
Erymin 252
Erythrocin 252
erythromycin 212, 252
Erythroped/Erythroped A 252
Eskamel 213
Eskazole 282
esmolol 85
Estracombi 184
Estracyt 297
Estraderm MX 184
Estraderm TTS 184
Estradurin 305
estramustine 297
Estrapak 50 184
Estring 186
ethacrynic acid 80
ethambutol 261
ethinyloestradiol 178, 180–1, 303
Ethmozine 108
ethosuximide 48–9
etidronate 160
etodolac 148
Etopophos 297
etoposide 297
Eucardic 84
Eucerin 203
Euglucon 168
Eugynon 30 180
Eumovate 206
euphoria 40
Eurax 204
    Eurax Hydrocortisone 207
evening primrose oil 210
Evista 185–6
Evorel 184
    Evorel Conti/Evorel Pak/
        Evorel Sequi 185
Exelderm 220
Exelon 59
Exocin 226
Exorex 209
expectorants 133, 143
Exterol 236
eye, the 223
    problems and infections 223–33, 246
eye drops 17
eye ointments 18
    tear deficiency 232–3
    tear production 233

F
famciclovir 270
famotidine 119
Famvir 270
Fansidar 278
Fareston 307
Farlutal 304
Fasigyn 259
Faverin 37
Fefol 311
felbinacs 150
Feldene 150
felodipine 95

Femapak 185
Femara 307
Fematrix 184
Femeron 188
Femodene/Femodene ED 180
Femoston 185
FemSeven 184
Femulen 182
Fenbid 148
fenbufen 148
fenofibrate 99
Fenopron 148
fenoterol 136
fentanyl 64
Fentazin 44
Feospan 311
ferric ammonium citrate 312
Ferrograd/Ferrograd C/
    Ferrograd Folic 311
ferrous fumarate 311
ferrous gluconate 311
ferrous glycine sulphate 311
ferrous sulphate 311
Fersaday 311
Fersamal 311
Fertiral 193
Fesovit Z 311
fexofenadine 287
fibrates 99–100
fibroids 191
finasteride 189–90
fish oils 101
Flagyl/Flagyl Compak/
    Flagyl S 257–8
flavoxate 199
flecainide 107
Fleet Micro-enema 130
Fleet Ready-to-use Enema 129
Fletcher's Enemette 128
Fletcher's Phosphate Enema 129
Flixonase 238
Flixotide 141
Flomax MR 197
Florinef 173
Floxapen 248
flucloxacillin 248
fluconazole 188, 265
flucytosine 265
Fludara 297
fludarabine 297
fludrocortisone 173
flumethasone 236
flunisolide 238
flunitrazepam 28
fluocinolone 206
fluocinonide 206
fluocortolone 206
Fluor-a-day 315
fluoride preparations 314–15
Fluorigard 315
fluorometholone 227
fluorouracil 297
fluoxetine 37
flupenthixol 32, 42
fluphenazine 35, 43
flurandrenolone 207
flurazepam 28
flurbiprofen 148
flutamide 306
fluticasone 141, 207, 238
fluvastatin 98
fluvoxamine 37
FML/FML-Neo 227
Folex-350 311
folic acid 310, 312
follicle-stimulating hormone
    (FSH) 177, 191, 192

follitropin 192
Foradil 136
Forceval/Forceval junior 318
formaldehyde 214
formestane 306
Fortagesic 61
Fortespan 311
Fortipine LA 40 96
Fortral 65
foscarnet sodium 270
Foscavir 270
Fosfamax 159
fosfesterol 303–4
fosinopril 88
framycetin 216, 225
Friar's Balsam 143
Frisium 48
Froben/Froben SR 148
frusemide 80, 82
Frusene 82
FSH see follicle-stimulating
    hormone
Fucibet 206
Fucidin 217
    Fucidin H 207
Fucithalmic 226
Full Marks Liquid/Lotion 222
fungal skin infections 201,
    see also antifungal drugs
Fungilin 241, 264–5
Fungizone 264–5
Furadantin 258
Furamide 279
fusidic acid 217, 226, 257
Fusidin 257
Fybogel 127
    Fybogel Mebeverine 116
Fybozest Orange 101

G
GABA see gamma-
    aminobutyric acid
gabapentin 49
Galfer/Galfer FA 311
gall bladder conditions 113,
    130–1
Gamanil 34
gamma-aminobutyric acid
    (GABA) 26, 156
gamolenic acid 210
ganciclovir 270
Ganda 231
Garamycin 226, 235
gastro-oesophageal reflux
    112, 113, 118, 119
Gastrobid 73–4
Gastrocote 114
gastrointestinal infections
    246, 254
Gastromax 73–4
Gaviscon/Gaviscon Advance/
    Gaviscon Infant 114
Gelcosal 209
Gelcotar 209
GelTears 232
gemcitabine 298
gemfibrozil 100
Gemzar 298
genital infections 188, 214,
    215, 219, 246, 264, 268, 279
Genotropin 176
gentamicin 226
Gentisone HC 236
German measles see rubella
Gestone 187
gestrinone 193

gestronol 304
giardiasis 279, 280
gingivitis 242
Glandosane 241
glands 162-4
glaucoma 82, 224, 228-32
glibenclamide 168
gliclazide 168
gliquidone 168
glucagon 162, 169
Glucobay 167-8
glucocorticoid hormones 162, 164, 171
Glucophage 168-9
Glurenorm 168
glutaraldehyde 214
Glutarol 214
glycerol 128
glyceryl trinitrate 4, 6, 8-9, 93
Glypressin 176
Glytrin Spray 93
gold 151, 152
gonadorelin 177, 191, 193
gonadotrophin-releasing hormone 177
Gopten 89
goserelin 193
gout 145, 146, 147, 153-5
Graneodin 218
granisetron 72-3
Gregoderm 207
grepafloxacin 255
griseofulvin 266
Grisovin 266
growth hormone 176
guanethidine 231
guar gum 168
Guarem 168
Gyno-Daktarin 188

H
Haelan 207
haemophilia 176
Haemophilus influenzae vaccinations 321, 323-4
haemorrhoids 113, 130
Halciderm Topical 207
halcinonide 207
Haldol 43
Halfan 277
halofantrine 276-7
haloperidol 43
Harmogen 184
hayfever 234, 237-9, 284-8
hazards 10-11
heart, the 77
heartburn 72, 73
  see also antacids
heart problems 77-8, 82-6, 102-5, 109-10
  see also angina
HeliClear 120
Helicobacter pylori 112, 118, 120, 250
Heminevrin 30
heparin 102
heparinoid 222
hepatitis A vaccination 320, 324-5
hepatitis B 290
  vaccination 325-7
herbal remedies 12
heroin 20
herpes viruses 215, 217, 219, 224, 240, 268, 269, 270, 271, 274
Herpid 217
Hewletts Cream 203

hexachlorophane 217
Hexalen 293
hexamine 257
hexetidine 242
HFAs *see* hydrofluoralkanes
hiatus hernia 73, 112, 113
Hibiscrub 216
Hibisol 216
Hibitane 5% Concentrate/ Hibitane Obstetric 216
high blood pressure *see* hypertension
Hioxyl 217
Hiprex 257
hirsutism 189
Hirudoid 222
Hismanal 285
histamine 41, 285
  histamine H2 antagonists 117, 118-19
Hivid 274-5
Hodgkin's disease 295, 296, 299, 300, 301
Honvan 303-4
hormonal disorders 54, 55
hormone replacement therapy (HRT) 6, 10, 145, 158-9, 178, 183-6
hormones 162, 163
  antagonists 305-7
  anti-diuretic 175-6
  growth 176
  reproductive 177
Hormonin 184
HRT *see* hormone replacement therapy
Human Actrapid 167
human menopausal gonadotrophins 193
Humatrope 176
Humegon 193
Humiderm 203
Humulin S 167
Hycamtin 302
hydralazine 90, 91
Hydrea 298
hydrochlorothiazide 81, 82, 84, 85, 86, 87, 88, 89
hydrocortisone 151, 173, 207, 227, 236
  hydrocortisone butyrate 207
Hydrocortistab 151
Hydrocortisyl 207
Hydrocortone 173
hydrofluoralkanes (HFAs) 135
hydrogen peroxide 217, 242
Hydromol 203
hydromorphone 64
HydroSaluric 81
hydrous ointment 202
hydroxocobalamin 313
hydroxychloroquine 152
hydroxyethylcellulose 232
hydroxyprogesterone 187
hydroxyurea 298
hydroxyzine 287
Hygroton 81
hyoscine 73, 116
hypertension (*high blood pressure*) 7, 78, 82-6
  ACE inhibitors 86-9
  calcium channel blockers 94-6
hyperthyroidism 164, 171
hypoglycaemia 169-70
Hypolar Retard 20 96
Hypotears 233

hypothalamus 162, 177
hypothyroidism 164, 170
Hypovase 92, 197, 206
hypromellose 233
Hypurin Bovine Neutral 167
Hypurin Porcine Neutral 167
Hytrin/Hytrin BPH 92, 197

I
IBD *see* inflammatory bowel disease
Ibugel 148, 150
Ibumousse 148, 150
ibuprofen 3, 112, 148, 150
Ibuspray 148, 150
idarubicin 298
idoxuridine 217
ifosfamide 298
Ikorel 97
Ilosone 252
Ilube 232
Imdur 94
Imigran 68
imipramine 3, 32, 34
immunisation *see* vaccinations
immunoglobulins 319, 320, 322-3
Immunovir 271
Imodium 123
impetigo 201
impotence 194-5
Improvera 185
Imuran 308
incontinence, urinary 196, 198-9
  see also bedwetting
indapamide 81
Inderal/Inderal LA 86
indigestion 111-12
  see also antacids; anti-spasmodics
indinavir 271
indomethacin 148-9, 153
indoramin 90, 91, 197
Infacol 114
infections *see* antibiotics
  skin *see* anti-infective skin preparations
infertility 177, 178, 190, 192, 193, 194
inflammatory bowel disease (IBD) 112, 123-6, 139
influenza vaccination 320, 321, 327
inhalations 143
inhalers 16-17, 134-5
injections 9
Innovace 88
Innozide 88
inosine pranobex 271
inotropic drugs 109-10
insomnia 25, 26, 28, 29
insulin 7, 8, 162, 164-7
Intal 141
interactions, drug 12, 25, 23
interferon alpha 298
Intralgin 150
Intron A 298
Invirase 273
iodine 217
Ionamin 76
Ionax Scrub 213
Ionil T 209
ipratropium 138, 239
irbesartan 88
irinotecan 299

iron 20
iron-deficiency anaemia 310, 311-12
iron sorbitol 312
Irriclens 219
irritable bowel syndrome 73, 112, 113
  see also antispasmodics
Isib 60XL 94
Ismo/Ismo Retard 94
isocarboxazid 39
Isocard 94
Isogel 127
Isoket Retard 94
isomethepene 66-7
isoniazid 262, 316
Isopto Alkaline 233
Isopto Carbachol 230
Isopto Carpine 232
Isopto Frin 233
Isopto Plain 233
Isordil 94
  Isordil Tembids 94
isosorbide dinitrate 94
isosorbide mononitrate 94
Isotrate 94
isotretinoin 213
Isotrex 213
Isotrexin 213
ispaghula 101, 116, 126, 127
isradipine 95
Istin 95
itching skin 204-8
  see also eczema
itraconazole 266

J
Jectofer 312
joints 144
  disorders 144-6

K
Kalspare 82
Kalten 84
Kamillosan 203
kaolin and morphine 123
Kapake 61
Kaposi's sarcoma 296
Keflex 250
Kelfizine W 253
Kemadrin 53
Kemicetine 256
Kenalog 151, 173
Keri 203
Kerlone 84
ketacids 164
ketoconazole 218, 267
ketoprofen 149, 150, 153
ketotifen 287
Ketovite 318
kidneys, the 10
  diseases 15, 78, 293, 310, 313, 314, 317
Kinidin Durules 109
Klaricid/Klaricid XL 252
Kliofem 185
Kliovance 185
Kolanticon 116
Konakion 318
Konsyl 127
Kytril 72-3

L
labetalol 85
lacidipine 95
Lacri-Lube 233

LactiCare 203
lactitol 129
lactulose 128, 129
Lamictal 49
Lamisil 220, 267–8
lamivudine 271–2, 275
lamotrigine 49
Lanoxin/ Lanoxin PG 109–10
lansoprazole 120
Lanvis 301
Largactil 42
Lariam 277
Lasikal 80
Lasilactone 82
Lasix 80
Lasma 139
Lasonil 222
latanoprost 231
laxatives 4, 126–30
Ledermycin 251
Lederspan 151
Legionnaire's disease 252
leishmaniasis 279, 280
Lenium 210
Lentaron 306
lercanidipine 96
Lescol 98
letrozole 307
leukaemias 290, 293–8, 301, 302, 303
Leukeran 295
leukotriene receptor antagonists 142
leuprorelin 193
Leustat 295
levobunolol 231
levocabastine 228, 239
levodopa 55, 56
levofloxacin 255
levonorgestrel 178, 180, 181, 183
Lexotan 27
Lexpec 312
LH *see* luteinising hormone
Librium 27
lice 201, 221–2
Li-Liquid 46
linctuses 9
Lingraine 66
Lioresal 157
liothyronine sodium 171
Lipantil 99
lipid-lowering drugs 97–102
Lipobase 203
Lipobay 98
Lipostat 98
Lipton 98
liquid medicines 9, 16
liquid paraffin 126, 233
Liquifilm Tears 233
lisinopril 88
Liskonum 46
Litarex 46
lithium 46
lithium succinate 210
liver, the 10, 14
Livial 185
Livostin 228, 239
Locabiotal nasal spray 240
Loceryl 215
Locoid/ Locoid C/ Locoid Crelo 207
Locorten Vioform 236
Lodine/ Lodine SR 148
lodoxamide 228
Loestrin 180
lofepramine 32, 34

Logynon/ Logynon ED 180
Lomexin 188
Lomotil 123
lomustine 299
Loniten 92
loop diuretics 79, 80
loperamide 123
Lopid 100
loprazolam 28
Lopressor/ Lopressor SR 85
loratadine 284, 287
lorazepam 28
lormetazepam 28–9
Loron 161
losartan 88
Losec 120
Lotriderm 206
Loxapac 43
loxapine 43
Luborant 241
Lubri-Tears 233
Ludiomil 34
lung cancer 290, 294, 298, 302, 303
Lustral 37
luteinising hormone (LH) 177, 191
Lyclear 221
lymecycline 251
lymphomas 294, 295, 297, 298, 302, 303
lypressin 175, 176
lysuride 56–7

M

Maalox/ Maalox Plus/ Maalox TC 114
Macaroon 277–8
Macrobid 258
Macrodantin 258
macrolides 252
Madopar/ Madopar CR 55
Magnapen 248
magnesium carbonate 114
magnesium salts 128, 129
magnesium trisilicate 114–15
malabsorption 310, 317
malaria 275, 279
see also antimalarial drugs
malathion 221
male sex hormones 188–9
antagonists of 189–90
deficiences 178, 191, 192
Maloprim 278
Manerix 39
Manevac 128
mania 25, 40–5
see also antimanic drugs
Manusept 220
MAOIs *see* monoamine oxidase inhibitors
maprotiline 32, 34
Marvelon 180
Masnoderm 188, 216
Maxalt 67
Maxepa 101
Maxidex 227
Maxitrol 227
Maxolon/ Maxolon SR 73–4
MCR-50 94
measles vaccination 327–8, *see also* MMR
mebendazole 282
mebeverine 116
meclozine 73
Medihaler-Ergotamine 66
Medrone 173

medroxyprogesterone 187, 304
medroxyprogesterone acetate 183
mefenamic acid 149
mefloquine 277
mefruside 81
Megace 304
megesterol 304
Melleril 45
meloxicam 149
melphalan 299
menadiol 318
Ménière's disease 70, 71, 72, 74
meningitis 323, 331
vaccination 328–9
Menogon 193
menopause 178
Menophase 185
Menorest 184
menstrual disorders 178, 186–7, 190, 192
menstruation 177
Menthol and Eucalyptus inhalation 143
mepacrine 280
meprobamate 31
meptazinol 64
Meptid 64
mequitazine 287
Merbentyl 116
mercaptopurine 299
Mercilon 180
Merocet 242
mesalazine 125
mesterolone 188, 189
Mestinon 156
Metanium 204
Meted 210
Metenix 5 81
Meterfolic 311
metformin 168–9
methadone 64
methocarbamol 158
methotrexate 208, 299
methotrimeprazine 43
methylcellulose 127
methyldopa 90, 91
methylphenobarbitone 49–50
methylprednisolone 173
methysergide 69
metipranolol 231
metoclopramide 70, 73–4
metolazone 81
Metopirone 174
metoprolol 85
Metosyn 206
Metrodin High Purity 194
Metrogel 218
Metrolyl 257–8
metronidazole 16, 188, 218, 257–8, 279
Metrotop 218
metyrapone 174
mexiletine 107
Mexitil/ Mexitil PL 107
mianserin 32, 34
Micalcic 159–60
Micanol 209–10
Micolette Micro-enema 130
miconazole 188, 218, 242
Micralax Micro-enema 130
Microgynon 30/ Microgynon 30 ED 180
Micronor 182
Micronor HRT 187
Microval 182
Mictral 255

Midrid 66–7
migraine 26, 65–70, 82
Migraleve 66
Migranal 66
Migravess 66
Migril 66
Mildison 207
mineralocorticoid hormones 162, 164, 171
minerals 310, *see also* calcium; iron; magnesium; potassium; zinc
Minims Artificial Tears 232
Minims Chloramphenicol 225
Minims Dexamethasone 227
Minims Gentamicin 226
Minims Metipranolol 231
Minims Neomycin Sulphate 226
Minims Pilocarpine Nitrate 232
Minims Prednisolone 227
Minims Sodium Chloride 233
Minitran 93
Minocin MR 251
minocycline 251
minoxidil 92, 222
Mintec 117
Mintezol 283
Minulet 180
Mirena 182
mirtazapine 35
miscarriage, habitual 187
misoprostol 118, 121, 148, 149
mites 201
mitomycin 300
Mitomycin C Kyowa 300
Mitoxana 298
mitozantrone 300
mizolastine 287
Mizollen 287
MMR vaccination 320, 321, 331
Mobic 149
Mobiflex 150
moclobemide 39
Modalim 99
modified-release tablets 8
Modisal XL 94
Moditen 43
Modrasone 205
Modrenal 174
Moducren 86
moexipril 89
Moisture-eyes 233
moisturisers 202–4
Molcer 236
Molipaxin 35
mometasone 208, 239
Monit/ Monit SR 94
Mono-Cedocard 94
monoamine oxidase inhibitors (MAOIs) 33, 38–9
Monocor 84
Monomax SR 94
Monosorb XL-60 94
Monotrim 259
Monovent 137
Monozide 10 84
Monphytol 220
montelukast 142
moracizine 107–8
Morcap SR 64
Morhulin 203
morphine 20, 64
kaolin and morphine 123

Motens 95
Motifene 148
Motilium 72
Motipress 35
Motival 35
mouth conditions 240–4, 264
    ulcers 234, 235, 240, 241,
    243
mouthwashes 241–4
Movelat 150
moxonidine 92
MST 64
Mucaine 114
Mucogel 114
multiple sclerosis 25, 156
mumps vaccination 329, *see*
    MMR
mupirocin 218
muscle relaxants 156–8
muscle spasticity 146
MUSE 195
mustine 300
MXL 64
myasthenia gravis 26, 146,
    155–6
Mycardol 94
Mycobutin 262–3
mycophenolate 309
Mycota 220
Myleran 294
myocardial infarction 77
Myocrisin 152
Myotonine 198
Mysoline 50
myxoedema 164

N
nabumetone 149
nadolol 85
nafarelin 194
nalbuphine 64
nalidixic acid 255
nandrolone 175
nappy rash 204
Napratec 121, 149
Naprosyn/Naprosyn SR 149
naproxen 121, 149, 153
Naramig 67
naratriptan 67
narcotics 20
Nardil 39
NARIs *see* noradrenaline
    re-uptake inhibitors
Narphen 65
Nasacort 239
Naseptin cream 240
Nasonex 239
Natrilix/Natrilix SR 81
nausea 26, 70–5
Navelbine 303
Navidrex 81
Navispare 82
Navoban 75
nebulisers 134
nedocromil 141, 227, 228,
    239
nefazodone 37
nefopam 59, 61
Negram 255
Neisseria meningitidis 328–9
nelfinavir 272
Neo-Cortef 227, 236
Neogest 182
Neo-Mercazole 171
neomycin 218, 226
Neonaclex K 80
Neoral 308–9
NeoRecormon 313

Neosporin 226
neostigmine 156
Neotigason 208
Nephril 81
Nericur 212
Nerisone/Nerisone Forte 206
nervous system, the 24–5
Neulactil 44
neuroleptics *see* anti-
    psychotics
Neurontin 49
neurotransmitters 6, 8, 25,
    26, 40, 41
Neutrexin 281
*Neutrogena Dermatological
    Cream* 203
nevirapine 272
nicardipine 96
niclosamide 283
nicorandil 97
nicotinamide 213, 316
nicotinic acid 101–2
nicoumalone 103
nifedipine 84, 96
Nifedipress MR 96
Nifedotard 20 MR 96
Nifelease 96
Niferex/Niferex-150 312
nimodipine 96
Nimotop 96
Nipent 301
nisoldipine 96
nitrazepam 29
Nitro-Dur 93
nitrofurantoin 258
Nitrolingual Pump Spray 93
Nitromin 93
Nivaquine 276
Nivaten Retard 96
nizatidine 119
Nizoral 188, 218, 267
Nolvadex 307
non-steroidal anti-inflam
    matory drugs (NSAIDs)
    59, 121, 133, 146–50,
    153
noradrenaline 6, 7, 29, 32,
    41, 162
noradrenaline re-uptake
    inhibitors (NARIs) 39–40
Norditropin 176
norethisterone 178, 180, 182,
    183, 184, 185, 187, 304
norfloxacin 255
Norgalax Micro-enema 128
Norgeston 182
norgestrel 183
Noriday 182
Norinyl-1 180
Noristerat 182
Noritate 218
Normacol/Normacol Plus 127
Normasol 219
Normegon 193
Normin 180
nortriptyline 35
Norvir 273
nose, the 234–5
nose drops 18
notriptyline 32
Novantrone 300
NovoNorm 169
Nozinan 43
NSAIDs *see* non-steroidal
    anti-inflammatory drugs
Nubain 64
Nuelin/Nuelin SA 139
Nurofen 3
Nu-Seals Aspirin 104

Nutraplus 203
Nutrizym 131
Nuvelle/Nuvelle TS 185
Nycopren 149
Nystadermal 208
Nystaform 218
    Nystaform HC 207
Nystan 188, 218, 243, 267
nystatin 188, 218, 243, 267

O
obesity 75–6, 78
obsessional conditions 33,
    36, 37
occlusal 214
octreotide 300
Ocusert 232
Odrik 89
oesophageal cancer 290
oestradiol 184, 185
Oestradiol Implants 184
Oestrogel 184
oestrogens 163, 177, 184
ofloxacin 226, 255
Oilatum 203
    Oilatum Plus 203
olanzapine 43
Olbetam 100–1
olsalazine 125
omeprazole 120
Oncovin 302
ondansetron 74
One-Alpha 317
Optilast 228
Optimine 286
Orabase 241
Orahesive 241
oral hygiene 242–4
Oralbalance 241
Oraldene 242
Oramorph/Oramorph SR 64
Orap 44
orciprenaline 137
Orelox 249
Orgafol 194
Orimeten 305
orlistat 75–6
*Orovite Complement B6
    tablets* 316
orphenadrine 53
Ortho-Dienoestrol 186
Ortho-Gynest 186
Orudis 149
Oruvail 149, 150
Ossopan 314
osteoarthritis 144–5
osteomalacia 145, 146, 158
osteoporosis 145, 146, 158–
    60, 178, 183, 185, 313, 317
Ostram 314
Otex 236
Otomize 236
Otosporin 236
Otrivine-Antistin 228
ovarian cancer 294, 300, 302
ovaries 162, 163
    polycystic 189
overdosage, accidental 19
    first aid 20–1
Ovestin 184, 186
Ovran/Ovran 30 180
Ovranette 180
Ovysmen 180
oxazepam 29
Oxis 136
oxitropium 138
Oxivent 138
oxprenolol 85

oxybutinin 199
oxypertine 43
oxytetracycline 251

P
Pabrinex injection 316
paclitaxel 300
Paget's disease 146, 158,
    159, 160, 161
pain 25, 26
painkillers 20, *see also*
    analgesics
Palfium 63
Palladone/Palladone SR 64
Paludrine 277–8
Pamergan P100 65
pamidronate 160–1
pancreas 162
    diseases 113, 298
Pancrease/Pancrease HL 131
pancreatin 131
Pancrex/Pancrex V 131
panic attacks 36, 37
PanOxyl 212
pantoprazole 120
Papulex 213
paracetamol 12, 20, 59, 60–1
paraffin, yellow soft 233
Paramax 66
parasympathomimetics
    197–8
parathyroid glands 162
parenteral administration 9
Pariet 120
Parkinson's disease 25, 52–8,
    190
Parlodel 54–5, 190
Parnate 39
paroxetine 37
Parstelin 39
patches, skin 10
Pecram 139
Penbritin 248
penciclovir 218
Pendramine 153
penicillamine 151, 153, 318
penicillins 246, 247–8
Pentacarinat 280
pentaerythritol tetranitrate 94
pentamidine 280
Pentasa 125
pentazocine 61, 65
Pentostam 280
pentostatin 301
Pentrax 209
Pepcid 119
peppermint oil 116–17
peptic ulcers 112, 113,
    117–22
Percutol ointment 93
Perdix 89
pergolide 57
Pergonal 193
Periactin 286
pericyazine 44
Perinal spray 130
perindopril 89
permethrin 221
Permitabs 219
Peroxyl 242
perphenazine 33, 44, 70
Persantin/Persantin Retard
    104–5
pertussis *see* whooping cough
pethidine 65
Pevaryl 188, 216
    Pevaryl TC 208
Pharmorubicin 297

phenazocine 65
phenelzine 39
Phenergan 74
phenindamine 288
phenindione 103
phenobarbitone 49-50
phenothrin 222
phenoxymethylpenicillin 248
phentermine 76
phenylbutazone 149
phenytoin 50
pHiso-Med 216
phobias 25, 33, 37, 39
Pholcodine Linctus 143
Phosex 314
phosphates 129
  reducing levels 314
  supplements 314
Phyllocontin Continus 139
Physiotens 92
Phytex 219
phytomenadione 318
piles 113, 130
pill, the *see* contraception
pilocarpine 232, 243
Pilogel 232
pimozide 44
pindolol 85
piperazine 282-3
Piportil 44
pipothiazine 44
Piriton 286
piroxicam 150, 153
Pitressin 176
pituitary gland 162, 164, 177
pivampicillin 248
pizotifen 70
Plaquenil 152
Plavix 104
Plendil 95
Plesmet 311
pneumonia 331
  pneumocystitis pneu-
    monia 279, 280, 281
podophyllum 214
poisoning, accidental 19
polio vaccinations 320, 321,
  322, 332-3
polmyxins 219
polyestradiol 305
Polyfax 219, 226
polymixin B 226
polysaccharide-iron
  complex 312
Polytar Emollient 209
Polytar shampoos 209
polythiazide 81
Polytrim 226
polyvinyl alcohol 233
Pondocillin 248
Pork Velosulin 167
Posalfilm 214
potassium canrenoate 82
potassium channel activators
  97
potassium permanganate 219
potassium-sparing diuretics
  79, 82
povidone-iodine 188, 243
Powergel 149, 150
Pragmatar 209
pravastatin 98
prazosin 90, 92, 196, 197
Precortisyl Forte 173
Pred Forte 227
Predenema 124
Predfoam 124
Prednesol 173
prednisolone 124, 151, 173,
  227, 236

prednisone 173
Predsol 124, 227, 236
  Predsol N 227
Pregaday 311
pregnancy 14, 22, 78
  folic acid 312
  and vaccines 312-13
Pregnyl 191
Premarin 184, 186
Premique 185
Prempak-C 185
Prepulsid 117
Prescal 95
Preservex 147
pressure sores 204, 217
Prestim 86
Priadel 46
Primalan 287
primaquine 277
primidone 50
Primosten Depot 189
Primulot N 187, 304
Prioderm Lotion 221
Prioderm Shampoo 221
Pripsen 282-3
Probanthine 117
probenecid 153, 155
procainamide 108
procaine penicillin 248
procarbazine 301
prochlorperazine 44, 70
Proctocream HC 130
Proctofoam HC 130
Proctosedyl ointment/
  suppositories 130
procyclidine 53
Profasi 191
Proflex 148, 150
progesterone 163, 187
progestogen-only contra-
  ceptives 181-2
progestogens 177, 184,
  186-7
Progral 309
proguanil 277-8
Progynova/Progynova TS 184
Proleukin 293
Proluton Depot 187
promazine 44
promethazine 29, 74, 288
Pronestyl 108
Propaderm 205
propafenone 108-9
propamidine 226
propantheline 117
Propine 230
propiverine 199
propranolol 86
propylthiouracil 171
Proscar 189-90
prostaglandins 59, 194-5
Prostap 193
prostate gland:
  benign prostatic
    hyperplasia 196
  cancer 189, 191, 193, 297,
    303-6
  enlarged 196
Prothiaden 33
Protium 120
proton pump inhibitors
  117, 119-20
protozoa 279, *see also*
  antiprotozoal drugs
protriptyline 32, 35
Provera 187, 304
Pro-Viron 189
Prozac 37
pruritus *see* itching skin
pseudoephedrine 143

psoriasis 201, 202, 208-11,
  299, 308
Psoriderm 209
Psorigel 209
Psorin 209-10
puffers 134
Pulmicort 141
Pulmozyme 142
Puregon 192
Puri-Nethol 299
Pylorid 119
pyrazinamide 262
pyridostigmine 156
pyridoxine 316
pyrimethamine 278
Pyrogastrone 121

Q
Questran/Questran Light 100
quetiapine 45
quinagolide 194
quinapril 89
quinidine 109
quinine 278
Quinocort 207
Quinoderm 212
quinolones 254-5
Quinoped 216

R
rabeprazole 120
rabies vaccination 333-4
Rabthera 301
radiotherapy 321
  nausea from 72, 74, 75
raloxifene 185-6
raltitrexed 301
ramipril 89
ranitidine 119
ranitidine bismuth citrate 119
Rapitil 228
Rastinon 169
Raxar 255
razoxane 301
reboxetine 39-40
rectal administration 9
rectal cancer 297
Regaine 222
Regulan 127
Rehidrat 123
rehydration solutions, oral
  123
Relaxit Micro-enema 130
Relifex 149
repaglinide 169
reproductive system 177-8
  disorders 190-4
  impotence 194-5
reproterol 137
Requip 57
Respacal 138
respiratory problems 132-4,
  246, 252, 254
  see also asthma; bron-
    chiolitis; bronchitis;
    emphysema
Respontin 138
Restandol 189
restlessness, severe 43, 44
Retin-A 213
retinal detachment 224
Retrovir 275
Revanil 56-7
rheumatoid arthritis 125, 139,
  145, 147, 151-3, 308, 318
Rheumox 147
Rhinocort Aqua 237
Rhinolast 237

riboflavine 316
rickets 145, 146
Ridaura 152
rifabutin 262-3
Rifadin 263
rifampicin 263
Rifater 263
Rifinah 263
Rimactane 263
Rimactazid 263
Rinatec 239
ringworm 201, 213, 219, 264
risks 10-11, 13-15
  see also side effects
Risperdal 45
risperidone 45
ritonavir 273
rituximab 301
rivastigmine 59
Rivotril 48
rizatriptan 67
Roaccutane 213
Robaxin 158
Rocaltrol 317
Roferon A 298
Rohypnol 28
ropinirole 57
rotahaler 134
roundworm 281, 282
Rozex 218
rubella vaccination 330-1,
  see also MMR
Rynacrom 238
Rythmodan/Rythmodan SR
  106

S
Sabril 51
Saizen 176
Salactac 214
Salactol 214
Salagen 243
Salamol 137
Salazopyrin 125-6
salbutamol 137, 140, 141
salcatonin 159
salicylates 243
salicylic acid 210, 214, 219
Saliva Orthana 241
saliva, artificial 241
Salivace 241
Salivix 241
salmeterol 135, 137
Salofalk 125
Saluric 80
Salvese 241
Sandimmnun 308-9
Sandocal 314
Sandostatin/Sandostatin LAR
  300
Sandrena 184
Sanomigran 70
saquinavir 273
Savlon Dry Powder 218
scabies 201, 204, 220-2
Scheriproct ointment/
  suppositories 130
schizophrenia 25, 40-5
Scopoderm TTS 73
scurvy 316
Sea Legs 73
seborrhoeic dermatitis 201,
  210, 218
Secadrex 84
Sectral 84
Securon/Securon SR 96
selegeline 58
selenium sulphide 210
self-mutilating behaviour 46

Selsun 210
Semi-Daonil 168
Semprex 285
senna 127, 128
Senokot 128
Septrin 253
Serc 70-1
Serenace 43
Serophene 192
Seroquel 45
serotonin 8, 32, 41
  see also SSRIs
Seroxat 37
sertraline 37
Servent 137
Sevredol 64
sex hormones 162, 163, 164
  in cancer treatment 303-5
shingles 201, 268
side effects 6, 11-12, 13, 23
sildenafil 195
Simple Eye Ointment 233
Simple Linctus 143
Simplene 229
simvastatin 99
Sinemet/ Sinemet CR/
  Sinemet LS/ Sinemet-Plus
  55
Sinequan 34
Singulair 142
Sinthrome 103
Siopel 204
Skelid 161
skin, the 200
Skinoren 212
sleeping problems *see*
  insomnia
sleeping sickness 279
Slofedipine XL 96
Slo-Phylin 139
Slow Fe 311
  Slow-Fe Folic 311
Slozem 95
Sno Phenicol 225
Sno Pilo 232
Sno Tears 233
social anxiety 37
social phobia 39
sodium aurothiomalate 152
sodium bicarbonate 113, 115
sodium chloride 219, 233
sodium citrate 130
sodium clodronate 161
sodium cromoglycate 227,
  228
sodium ironedetate 312
sodium perborate 244
sodium stibogluconate 280
Sofradex 227
Soframycin 216, 225
Solian 42
Solpadol 61
Solu-Cortef 173
Solu-Medrone 173
Solvazinc 315
somatropin 176
Soneryl 29
Sorbichew 94
Sorbid SA 94
Sorbitrate 94
Sotacor 86
sotalol 86
Spasmonal 115
spasticity 156
spectinomycin 258
Spiroctan 82
Spiroctan-M 82
spironolactone 82
Sporanox 266

Sprilon 204
SSRIs (selective serotonin
  re-uptake inhibitors) 8,
  36-8
stanozolol 175
Staril 88
statins 98-9
stavudine 273-4
Stelazine 45
Stemetil 44
Sterac Sodium Chloride 219
sterculia 115
Sterexidine 216
Steripod Chlorhexidine/
  Cetrimide 216
Steripod Sodium Chloride 219
steroids 162
  anabolic 174-5
  see also corticosteroids
Ster-Zac 217
  Ster-Zac Bath Concentrate
  220
Stiedex 206
Stiemycin 212
stilboestrol 304-5
Still's disease 145
Stilnoct 31
storing medicines 19
Streptococcus pneumonia 331-2
streptokinase 102
streptomycin 263-4
strokes 102, 104, 105, 156
Stromba 175
Stugeron 71
sublingual tablets 8-9
sucralfate 117, 118, 122
Sudafed 143
Sudocrem 204
sulconazole 220
Suleo C 221
Suleo M 221
sulfadoxine 278
sulindac 150, 153
Sulparex 45
sulphadiazine 254
sulphadimidine 254
sulphametopyrazine 253
sulphasalazine 125-6, 151
sulphinpyrazone 153, 155
sulphonamides 253-4
sulpiride 45
Sulpitil 45
Sultrin 188
sumatriptan 68
suppositories 17
Suprax 249
Suprecur 191
Surgam/ Surgam SA 150
Suscard 93
suspensions 9
Sustac 93
Sustanon 189
sweating 222
Symmetrel 54
Synalar/ Synalar C/
  Synalar N 206
Synarel 194
Synflex 149
Synphase 180
Syntaris 238
Syntopressin 176
Syscor MR 96
systemic lupus erythmatosus
  308
Sytron 312

T
tablets 8-9, 16

tacalcitol 210
tacrolimus 309
Tagamet 119
Tambocur 107
tamoxifen 307
Tampovagan pessaries 186
tamsulosin 197
tapeworm 281, 283
Tarcortin 207
Targocid 259
Tarivid 255
Tarka 89, 96
Tavanic 255
Tavegil 286
Taxol 300
Taxotere 296
tazarotene 211
tear deficiency 232-3
tear production, excessive
  233
Tears Naturale 233
teething gels 241, 243
Tegretol 48
teicoplanin 259
Telfast 287
temazepam 29
Temgesic 62
Tenben 84
Tenif 84
Tenoret 50 84
Tenormin 3, 84
tenoxicam 150
Tensipine MR 96
Teoptic 230
terazosin 90, 92, 197
terbinafine 219, 267-8
terbutaline 137
terfenadine 288
terlipressin 176
Terra-Cortril 207
  Terra-Cortril Nystatin 207
Terramycin 251
Tertroxin 170
testes 162, 163, 177
  cancer 294, 297
testosterone 163, 164, 177,
  178, 188, 189
tetanus vaccination 321,
  322, 334-5
Tetrachel 251
tetracycline 212, 251
tetracyclines 250-1
Tetralysal 300 251
T/Gel 209
thalidomide 12
Theo-Dur 139
theophylline 139
Thephorin 288
thiabendazole 283
thiamine 316
thiazide diuretics 79, 80-1
thioguanine 301
thioridazine 45
thiotepa 301
threadworm 281, 282, 283
throat, the 234
  cancer 290
  infections 246
thrombophlebitis, superficial
  222
thrombosis 102
thrush 188, 264
  oral 242, 243
thymol 244
thymoxamine 195
thyroid gland 162, 164
  disorders 7, 82, 164, 170-1
thyroxine 162, 170
tiaprofenic acid 150

tibolone 185
Ticlid 105
ticlopidine 105
Tilade 141
Tilarin 239
Tildiem/ Tildiem LA/ Tildiem
  Retard 95
Tiloryth 252
tiludronic acid 161
Timodine 207
timolol 86, 230, 232
Timonil 48
Timoptol/ Timoptol LA 232
Tinaderm-H 219
tinea capitis/cruris/pedis/
  unguis 264
tinidazole 259, 279
tioconazole 220
Tisept 216
Titralac 314
tizanidine 158
Tofranil 34
Tolanase 169
tolazamide 169
tolbutamide 169
tolfenamic acid 68
tolterodine 199
Tomudex 301
Topal 114
Topamax 51
topical medicines 10
Topicycline 212
topiramate 51
topotecan 302
torasemide 80
Torem 80
toremifine 307
toxoplasmosis 279
tramadol 65
Tramake Insts 65
Trandate 85
trandolapril 89, 96
tranquillizers 20, 25, 26-31
  see also antidepressants;
  antipsychotics
transdermal administration
  10
Transiderm-Nitro 93
transplanted organs,
  rejection of 308, 309
Transvasin 150
Tranxene 27
tranylcypromine 39
Trasidrex 85
travel sickness 70-4, 284
Travogyn 188
Travsept 100 216
Traxam 150
trazodone 32, 35
treosulfan 301
tretinoin 213, 302
Tri-Adcortyl 208
  Tri-Adcortyl Otic 236
Triadene 181
triamcinolone 151, 173,
  208, 236, 239
triamterene 82
tribavirin 274
trichomonas vaginitis 188,
  279
trichomoniasis 279
triclofos 31
triclosan 220
tricyclics 32-5
Tridestra 185
trifluoperazine 39, 45, 70
Trifyba 127
tri-iodothyronine 162
trilostane 174

Triludan 288
trimeprazine 288
trimethoprim 259
trimetrexate 281
Tri-Minulet 181
trimipramine 32
Trimopan 259
Trimovate 206
Trinordiol 181
TriNovum 181
Triptafen/Triptafen M 33
triptorelin 194
Trisequens 185
Tritace 89
Trobicin 258
tropisetron 75
Trosyl 220
Trusopt 230
trypanasomiasis 279, 280
tryptophan 32
tuberculosis 260–4, 335–6
  vaccination 321, 336
tulobuterol 138
tumours *see* cancer
turbohaler 134
Tylex 61
typhoid vaccination 336–7

U
Ubretid 156, 198
Ucerax 287
ulcerative colitis 112, 113,
  123–6
ulcers, mouth 234, 235,
  240, 241, 243
ulcers, peptic 112, 113, 117–
  22
ulcers, skin 217
Ultrabase 204
Ultralanum Plain 207
*Ultraproct ointment/
  suppositories* 130
undecanoates 220
Unguentum Merck 204
Uniphyllin Continus 139
Unipine XL 96
Univer 96
Urdox 131
Uriben 255
urinary problems:
  incontinence 196, 198–9
  infections 196, 246, 254
  rash 204
  urine retention 196, 197–8
Urispas 199
urofollitrophin 194

ursodeoxycholic acid 131
Ursofalk 131
Ursogal 131
Utinor 255
Utovlan 187

V
vaccinations 319–23
Vagifem 186
vaginal infections 188, 264,
  279
valaciclovir 274
Valium 28
Vallergan 288
Valoid 71
valproate 51
valsartan 89
Valtrex 274
Vancocin 260
vancomycin 260
varicose veins 222
Vascace 88
Vaseline Dermacare 204
vasodilators 90–2
Vasogen 204
vasopressin 175, 176
Vectavir 219
Velbe 302
Velosef 250
venlafaxine 37
Ventide 140
Ventodiscs 137
Ventolin 137
Vepesid 297
Veracur 214
verapamil 89, 94, 96
Verapress MR 96
Vermox 282
verrucas 201
Verrugon 214
Vesanoid 302
Viagra 195
Viazem XL 95
Vibramycin/Vibramycin-D
  251
Videx 269
vigabatrin 51
Vigranon B syrup 316
viloxazine 32, 35
vinblastine 302
vincristine 302
vindesine 303
vinorelbine 303
Vioform Hydrocortisone 207
Viracept 272
Viraferon 298

Viramune 272
Virazid 274
Viridal 195
Virormone 189
viruses 268, *see* antiviral
  drugs
Viscotears 232
Viskaldix 85
Vista-Methasone 227, 235
  Vista-Methasone N 227,
  235, 240
Vistide 269
vitamins 12, 310
  vitamin A 315–16
  vitamin B group 316
  vitamin B12 deficiency
  310, 312, 313
  vitamin C 316
  vitamin D 316–17
  vitamin E 317
  vitamin K 317–18
Vivalan 35
Vividrin 238
*Voltarol/Voltarol Retard/
  Voltarol SR* 148
  Voltarol Emulgel 148, 150
vomiting 26, 70–5

W
warfarin 103
Warticon 214
warts 201, 214, 291
wax, ear *see* ear wax
Waxsol 236
Welldorm 30
Wellferon 298
Wellvone 279
whooping cough
  vaccination 321, 329–30
Wilson's disease 318
worms *see* ringworm;
  roundworm; tapeworm;
  threadworm
wounds 216, 217

X
Xalatan 231
xamoterol 110
Xanax 27
Xatral/Xatral SR 197
Xenical 75–6
xipamide 81
xylometazoline 240
*Xyloproct ointment/
  suppositories* 130

Y
yellow fever vaccination
  337–8
Yomesan 283

Z
Zaditen 287
zafirlukast 142
zalcitabine 274–5
Zamadol/Zamadol SR 65
Zanaflex 158
Zanidip 96
Zantac 119
Zarontin 48–9
Zavedos 298
Zelapar 58
Zemtard 300 XL 95
Zerit 273–4
Zestoretic 88
Zestril 88
Zidoval 188
zidovudine 275
Zimovane 31
Zinacef 250
Zinamide 262
zinc and caster oil ointment
  202
zinc cream/ointment 202
zinc sulphate 233
zinc supplements 315
Zineryt 212
Zinnat 250
Zirtek 286
Zispin 35
Zithromax 252
Zocor 99
Zofran 74
Zoladex 193
Zoleptil 45
zolmitriptan 68
zolpidem 31
Zomacton 176
Zomig 68
Zomorph 64
zopiclone 31
Zorac 211
zotepine 45
Zoton 120
Zovirax 215, 225, 240, 268
Z span 315
zuclopenthixol 45
Zumenon 184
Zydol/Zydol SR 65
Zyloric 154
Zyprexa 43